D1708844

PROTEIN FOLDS

A Distance-Based Approach

Edited by
Henrik Bohr and Søren Brunak

CRC Press

Boca Raton   New York   London   Tokyo

Library of Congress Cataloging-in-Publication Data

Protein folds : a distance based approach / edited by Henrik Bohr and Søren Brunak.
    p. cm.
Includes bibliographical references and index.
ISBN 0-8493-4009-8
1. Protein folding. 2. Protein binding. I. Bohr, Henrik. II. Brunak, Søren.
QP551.P695823   1995
574.19'.245--dc20

                            95-35601
                               CIP

THE EDITORS

Henrik Bohr, M.Sc., Ph.D., is associate professor at the Center for Biological Sequence Analysis at the Department of Physical Chemistry, the University of Denmark (Lyngby, Denmark). He has been visiting professor at the University of Arizona (1988), the University of Illinois at Urbana-Champaign (1990–1992), the Bechman Institute (1992–1993), and Heidelburg University (1993–1994).

Dr. Bohr received his M.Sc. degree in 1979 from the Niels Bohr Institute, Copenhagen University (Denmark). His thesis was evaluated as Ph.D. at London University (U.K.) in 1980. He has had postdoctoral appointments at Imperial College (London University) and ICTP/SISSA in Trieste (Italy).

Henrik Bohr has published approximately 140 scientific articles in international journals in the areas of theoretical physics, biophysics, and technology and has written 5 books in biophysics. He has presented over 80 invited talks at international meetings and has organized 2 international meetings and several workshops at the Center for Biological Sequence Analysis. Dr. Bohr has been permanent reviewer for *Reviews* since 1985. His current major research is focused on protein structure prediction and bio-molecular calculations.

Søren Brunak, M.Sc., Ph.D., is the director of the Center for Biological Sequence Analysis at the Department of Physical Chamistry, the Technical University of Denmark (Lyngby, Denmark).

Dr. Brunak received his M.Sc. degree in 1987 from the Niels Bohr Institute, Copenhagen University (Denmark) and his Ph.D. degree in 1991 from the Technical University of Denmark (Lyngby).

Søren Brunak is cofounder of the Danish Center for Neural Networks CONNECT (Copenhagen), a member of the board of the Center of Art, Science and Technology COAST(Denmark) and a memeber of the scientific board of NeuroTech A/S. He is also cofounder and Editor-in-Charge of the *International Journal of Neural Systems* which now enters its sixth year of existence. He functions as reviewer for the *Commission of the European Communities* (Brussels) and a number of scientific periodicals.

Dr. Brunak has presented more than 50 lectures at international meetings and seminars and has organized several international meetings besides the international meetings and workshops held at the Center for Biological Sequence Analysis. He has published over 40 scientific articles in international journals and has written and edited 5 books. His current research is focused on the analysis of the structure and function of biological sequences, mainly addressed by novel adaptive computational methods, such as data-driven artificial neural networks.

Contents

Overview

Protein-Ligand Complexes and Protein Biosynthesis

Profile Methods for Protein Structure and Fold Determination

Topological Aspects of Protein Folds

Protein Modelling and Docking

Introduction

Henrik Bohr and Søren Brunak

Center for Biological Sequence Analysis, The Technical University of Denmark,
DK-2800 Lyngby, Denmark

The present monograph contains contributions from molecular biology, biophysics and physical chemistry by a number of established scientists. The contributions provide aspects of protein structure, function and protein folding in a framework termed "the distance approach". The contributions arose from the symposium "Distance-Based Approaches to Protein Structure Determination II" held in Copenhagen in November 1994 being the succession of a similar symposium held in the previous year.

The subjects of protein structure determination and protein folding are topics of increasing importance and maintain a highly significant position in science. The importance is of course due to the relevance of protein folding for the fast growing biotechnological industry and of the importance to the genome projects. Here one should add that prediction of accurate 3-dimensional (3-D) structures of proteins from their sequence and an accurate theory of how they fold still is lacking. However, the amount of scientific literature concerned with these topics (with comprehensive reviews of protein folding [1]) is growing rapidly, making it necessary to be more specific and focussed when getting involved with the area. We have in this monograph focussed on the more limited distance geometry aspects of the field.

The distance geometry approach to protein structure determination is to be understood as protein structure analysis, experimentally as well as theoretically, carried out on the basis of exact distance measures. With respect to experimental techniques this implies that protein structures are described in time or space by means of detailed distance information within the molecule, rather than description in terms of a phenomenological study of *e.g.* bio-chemical reactions. The detailed experimental techniques can either be X-ray diffraction crystallography, nuclear magnetic resonance, NMR methods, circular dichroism methods, infrared spectroscopy or neutron scattering. The first technique being the most established, the second dealing with problems of solvents, the third, fourth and fifth being more straight forward to carry out and having advantages in particular structure studies but providing less accuracy. Almost half of the contributions in the book are devoted to the application of these techniques with which either protein-ligand complexes (S. Larsen, R. Bauer, J. Nyborg, J. Ulstrup) or membrane bound protein configurations (J. Findlay, D. Donnelly, T. W. Schwartz, R. Bywater) have been studied.

In theoretical studies the limitation of distance geometry approaches implies that protein dynamics and protein structure prediction are studied under the constraints of available experimental distance information or simply some distances being fixed within the protein in order to limit the degree of uncertainty in structure analysis or structure prediction.

Although the problem of protein structure prediction from sequence is greatly reduced, when knowledge is given about certain inter-molecular distances, one should still be aware of the complexity in generating a full and detailed 3-D protein structure from often sparse, and at best, incomplete distance information. In fact, many experiments can give distance inequalities only, rather than exact real valued distances and often in a 2-dimensional (2-D) form, *e.g.* in NMR, whereby the mathematical puzzle of generating the full 3-D structure is, in principle, rendered unsolvable. There are nevertheless various approximation techniques [2] that can circumvent these problems mostly with the use of computer simulation techniques. For a very detailed and thorough treatment of the mathematical problems in distance geometry analysis the reader is referred to the book by G. M. Crippen and T. F. Havel: "Distance Geometry and Molecular Conformations" [3, 4].

Apart from generation of 3-D structures of proteins from distance constraints the distance geometry approach to protein structure analysis has also been understood in a wider sense to encompass potential energy methods based on distances and angles in the molecules. In one approach [5] (P. G. Wolynes) the problem of protein structure prediction is transformed into the problem of minimizing an energy function for an analogous spin glass system [6], where the spin states correspond to protein configurations. This method is in line with distance geometry approaches in the sense that energy function optimization basically implies satisfying a great number of distance constraints and simultaneously comparing sequences corresponding to these protein configurations. Somewhat in the same spirit is comparative protein modelling, performed by satisfying a set of spatial restraints and aims at making exhaustive enumerations of protein conformations on a lattice, where the protein is highly idealized [7]. Such a study has the purpose of selecting the fittest conformations in an evolutionary sense.

A new-comer could be tempted to feel that in the past, theoretical studies of protein folding were quite abstract and the basic new knowledge of protein folding paths have been obtained by elaborate experiments. However, a new era has arrived with the use of lattice Monte Carlo techniques and spin glass models that can simulate folding processes and even evolution. A protein is schematically represented by links on a 3-D lattice, where the thermodynamics of the simulated protein folding processes can be measured (A. Šali, E. Shaknovich). Also various spin glass models can help understand the shape of the protein folding landscape (P. G. Wolynes, J. N. Onuchic, D. Thirumalai). One can also use distance methodology, or more precisely the distance matrix error, as a potential function to drive conformational searches (D. Eisenberg).

There has been a renewed interest in topological aspects of protein folding and in protein structure in general. In a chapter about topology of folds the origin of secondary structure formation has been related to the linking and twist of the backbone (J. Bohr, H. Bohr, S. Brunak) and many interesting structural features has been obtained by exploring the chirality of protein structures (T. Slidel). Furthermore, the dense packing of proteins side-chains that occur in the course of folding can be extracted from a study of internal cavities (P. Argos).

One of the modern themes recurrent throughout many of the contributions has been to discuss general classes of protein folds (M. Braxenthaler, W. Taylor, A. Aszodi, P. A. Lindgaard) rather than describing specific protein structures. It is believed that proteins appearing in organisms are based on a limited repertoire of different core structures or folding motifs. In the past it has been common to classify proteins with respect to sequence similarity for evolutionary purposes or, most commonly, to group proteins with respect to their function so that, for example, proteases go in one group, immunoglobulins in another, *etc.* The concept of protein folds [8] is, however, related to topological characteristics so that given folds belong to the same fold class if they share the same topological structure. A fold is a distinct geometrical domain [9] of a protein (*e.g.* a cluster of supersecondary structures), either of the whole protein or part of it. Often a necessary requirement, albeit not a sufficient, is that protein folds belong to the same class if they have more than 50% sequence identity. Proteases are for example divided into several fold-classes. A typical example of a fold class is the Tim Barrel class. One of the many questions concerning fold classes, addressed in this book, is the problem of being able to identify them from sequence studies and from distance geometry analysis (W. Taylor). Another problem is to find an appropriate choice of parameters to link the different classes, such as a parameter for packing of secondary structures. This question arises especially when an entirely new protein, with practically no sequence similarity to any known structure, has to fit into or establish a relationship to one of the known classes. A very relevant question is to ask how the most "extreme" classes could be characterized. An attempt to find the total number of possible fold classes in nature with the help of statistical mechanical arguments and polymer physics (P. A. Lindgaard, H. Bohr) is presented in a short contribution of this book.

Connected to these protein folds is the new idea of "threading" [10, 11, 12, 13, 14] (M. Braxenthaler, M. Sippl, D. Eisenberg, M. Gribskov, W. Taylor) meaning that protein sequences are being "threaded" through various different folding motifs in order to identify misfolded structures through an empirical evaluation function that can distinguish incorrect from correct folds. For reasons of simplicity folding motifs have been represented as linear profiles of local environmental properties independent of the type of fold being considered, *e.g.*, secondary structures, at each residue in a known protein structure. Specific sequences can be given evaluation scores depending on preferences of the aligned residues for their respective environmental categories. Instead of representing folding motifs as linear profiles they can be represented as 2-D contact matrices or as distance matrices [15, 16, 17, 18, 19] (W. Taylor). A special section has been devoted to the application of these profile methods for protein structure (M. Gribskov, M. Braxenthaler) and fold determination (W. Taylor, A. Aszodi).

Predicting which fold-class a given protein belongs to can further help the prediction of distance matrices and hence the construction of 3-D protein structures at higher accuracy than previously achieved. There are good reasons to believe that distance matrices can be correctly predicted by neural networks for proteins homologous to the ones the network has been trained on [5, 20]. The long term hope is to be able to develop prediction schemes for protein folds to understand which changes in their sequence are required for transforming a fold from one class into another (the inverse folding problem). In more direct words one could ask how many substitutions are needed to give, for example Lysozyme, the functionality of a Cytochrome.

The central subject of the book, distance-based protein structure prediction, was the target for a section where distance restrained methodologies (A. Aszodi), structure building from protein sequence families (G. Casari) and fitting of 1-dimensional predictions into 3-D structures (B. Rost) were presented.

A special section of the book is devoted to experimental and theoretical studies of membrane proteins. These studies have either been focussed on the role of G-binding proteins (J. Nyborg, D. Donnelly, J. Findlay), or on the role of more specific receptor proteins (T. W. Schwartz, R. Bywater) and of structural and functional aspects (*e.g.* electron transport) of metalloproteins (R. Bauer, J. Ulstrup).

A final section contained interesting contributions about protein modelling and docking analysis. New development has taken place in the area of drug design, where sophisticated techniques have been employed for designing drugs from models of protein structure. Studies have been concerned with modelling of specific proteins with the help of neural networks and molecular dynamics or specific homology modelling schemes (W. Taylor). One of the specific proteins was the photo-protein Obelin (T. Sandalova) and another was the HIV envelope protein complex of GP120 and GP 41 (J. L. Gabriel), where also a model for the interaction between GP120 and CD4 was presented.

The distance geometry approach to protein structure determination turns out to be an interesting and versatile forum for scientific discussions. All considered it seems that while the experimental efforts focus on still higher accuracy in protein structure determination, the theoretical counter part of prediction methodologies is occupied and content with the gross features of protein structure prediction at low resolution. Precise predictions of new protein structures from sequences has yet to come.

> *Nondum clivum exsuperavimus. (Seneca)*, ref. [21].

Acknowledgements

The Danish National Research Foundation and Novo Nordisk A/S are deeply acknowledged for their support. Neither the symposium nor this monograph would have been without them. We also wish to thank Mrs. Johanne Keiding, who has provided us with great and indispensable editorial work in connection with the book.

References

[1] T. E. Creighton (ed.), *Protein folding*, W.H. Freeman & co., 1992, and D. B. Wetlaufer, *The protein folding problem*, AAAS selected Symposium, Vol. 89, Westview Publisher, Boulder, USA 1984.

[2]   J. Bohr *et al.*, *J. Mol. Biol.*, 231, p. 861-869, 1993.

[3]   G. M. Crippen and T. F. Havel, *Distance Geometry and Molecular Conformation*, Wiley, New York 1988.

[4]   G. M. Crippen, *J. Mathematical Chemistry*, 6, p. 307-324, 1991.

[5]   R. A. Goldstein, Z. Luthey-Schulten and P. G. Wolynes, *PNAS*, 89, p. 4918-4922, 1992.

[6]   M. S. Friedrich and P. G. Wolynes, *Science*, 246, p. 371-377, 1989.

[7]   A. Ŝali, E. I. Shakhnovich and M. Karplus, *Nature*, 369, p. 248-251, 1994.

[8]   T. L. Blundell and M. S. Johnson, *Protein Science*, 2, p. 877-883, 1993.

[9]   S. Pascarella and P. Argos, *Prot. Eng.*, 5, p. 121-137, 1992.

[10] D. Jones and J. Thornton, *L. Comp. Aid. Mol. Design*, 7, p. 439-456 1993.

[11] J. Novotny, A. A. Rashin and R. E. Bruccoleri, *Proteins*, 4, p. 19-30, 1988.

[12] D. Eisenberg and A. D. McLachlan, *Nature*, 319, p. 199-203, 1986.

[13] J. S. Fetrow and S. H. Bryant, *Biotechnology*, 11, p. 479-484, 1993.

[14] L. M. Gregoret and F. E. Cohen, *J. Mol. Biol.*, 211, p. 959-974, 1990.

[15] W. Taylor, *Prot. Eng.*, 4, p. 853-870, 1991.

[16] J. T. Jones, W. R. Taylor and J. M. Thornton, *Nature*, 358, p. 86-89, 1992.

[17] G. M. Crippen, *Biochemistry*, 30, p. 4232-4237, 1991.

[18] M. J. Sippl, *J. Mol. Biol.*, 213, p. 859-883, 1990.

[19] L. Holm and C. Sander, *J. Mol. Biol.*, 233, p. 123-138, 1993.

[20] H. Bohr *et al.*, *FEBS*, 261, p. 43-46, 1990.

[21] Seneca, Epistolae Moralis: "Nobody has yet reached the summit", Nero court, Rome 0062.

Color Plates

Color Plates

Plate 1   In *Interplay between Metal Coordination Geometry and Protein Structure*, pages 31-42 (Rogert Bauer *et al*).

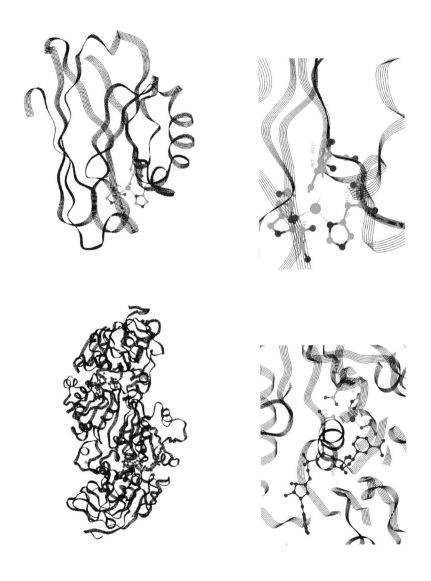

Left side top: the global structure of azurin, copper is green; left side bottom: the structure of the dimer of alcohol dehydrogenase from horse liver complexed with the coenzyme NADH and dimethylsulfoxide, note there are two structural zinc ions (green) and two catalytic zinc ions (violet), NADH is blue and dimethylsulfoxide red. Right side top: coordination geometry of copper in azurin showing the planar coordination geometry of two histidines and one cysteine (notice the sulfur from methionine 121 in yellow having no line connecting it to copper) and right side bottom: coordination geometry for one of the catalytic zinc ion in alcohol dehydrogenase including dimethylsulfoxide. Also shown is NADH which does not coordinate to zinc. The program InsightII from Biosym has been used to generate the graph. The coordinates were obtained from Brookhaven Protein data bank.

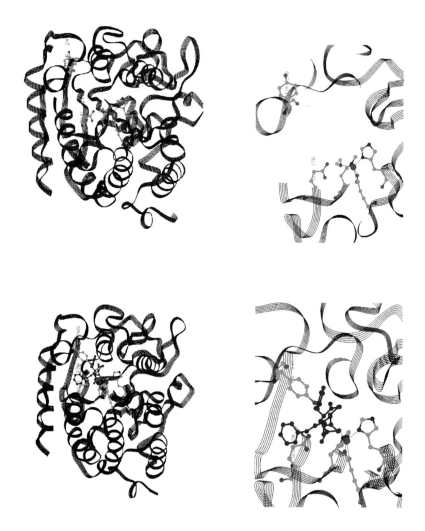

Left side top: the global structure of carboxypeptidase A; left side bottom: the global structure of carboxypeptidase A with a phophonate substrate analogue (blue). Right side top: coordination geometry of zinc (violet) for carboxypeptidase A having water as a solvent ligand to zinc (notice tyrosine 248 is far away from the metal), and right side bottom: coordination geometry of zinc for carboxypeptidase A with the phosphonate substrate analogue (notice tyrosine 248 is close to the substrate analogue and the metal). The program InsightII from Biosym has been used to generate the graph. The coordinates were obtained from Brookhaven Protein data bank.

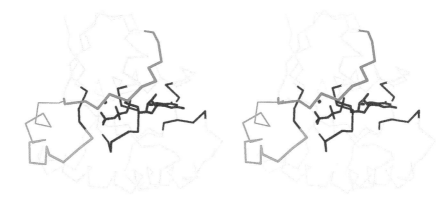

(a)

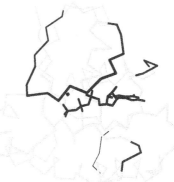

(b)

Stereo diagram of the generic structure of a G-domain. The protein backbone is shown in yellow and the GTP molecule in magenta. In (a) shown in red are the positions in the structure of the concensus sequences. In green is shown the position of the switch 1 (effector) region and in blue the switch 2 region. In (b) shown in red are the positions of major inserts.

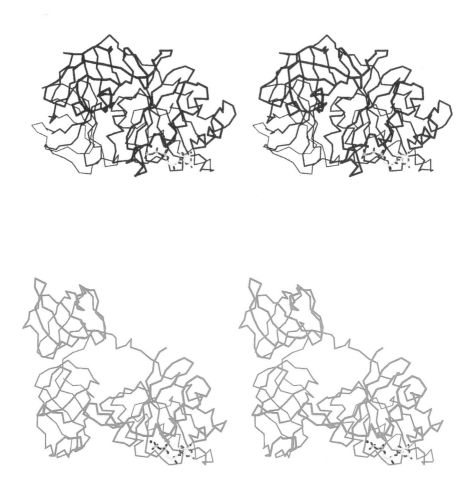

Stereo diagrams of the structures of EF-Tu:GDPNP and intact EF-Tu:GDP. At the top is shown the active EF-Tu:GDPNP with backbone in red. At the bottom is shown the inactive EF-Tu:GDP with backbone in blue. The direction of view of domains 1 in both molecules is the same and is approximately perpendicular to the plane of the base of the nucleotide. Notice the large relative shift of domains 2 and 3 and the strange hole in the structure of EF-Tu:GDP.

Plate 5 In *Elongation Factor Tu: A G-protein in Protein Biosynthesis*, pages **43-55** (**P. Nissen** *et al*).

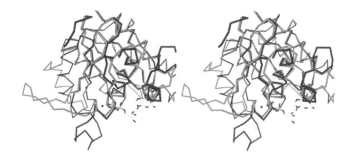

Stereo diagram of the G-domain of an inactive and active G-protein. In blue is shown the backbone of EF-Tu:GDP and in red the backbone of EF-Tu:GDPNP. The direction of view is as in color plate 4. The central β-sheet is very well aligned. At the bottom to the left is seen the switch 1 region, which in the EF-Tu:GDP is extended while in EF-Tu:GDPNP it is forming a short helix. Most helices are also wellaligned except helix B of switch region 2 shown to the left. The shift in the helix axis is easily seen.

Plate 6 In *Elongation Factor Tu: A G-protein in Protein Biosynthesis*, pages **43-55** (**P. Nissen** *et al*).

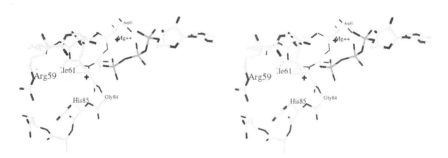

Stereo diagram of the detailed structure around the catalytic water in EF-Tu:GDPNP. The position of the water is shown as a red cross. Amino acid G84 is seen close to the γ-phosphate. The NH of its backbone is possibly hydrogen bonded to the phosphate.

Plate 7 In *Elongation Factor Tu: A G-protein in Protein Biosynthesis*, pages **43-55** (**P. Nissen** *et al*).

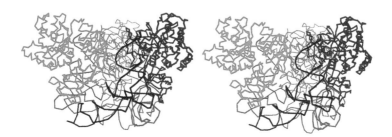

Stereo diagram of the structure of the trimer of ternary complexes. The three monomers are shown in red, blue and green.

Plate 8 In *Electron Transfer of the Di-Heme Protein*, pages 56-67 (Jens-Jakob Karlsson *et al*).

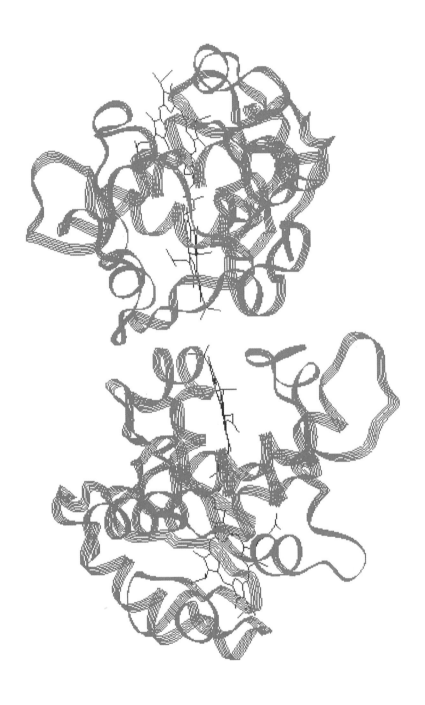

Plate 9 In *Protein Fold Determination Using a Small Number of Distance Restraints*, pages 85-97 (A. Aszódi, M.J. Gradwell and W.R. Taylor).

(a)

(b)

(c)

(d)

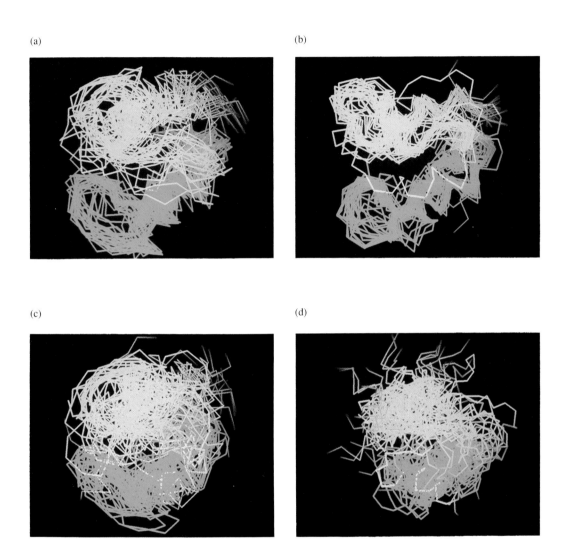

Model C_α backbones aligned to the native CABP structure 3ICB. Residue positions are color-coded from blue (N-terminus) to red (C-terminus) in a smooth range. A and B are models generated from 19 long-range restraints by DRAGON and X-PLOR, respectively. X-PLOR produced better structures in this case except one outlier which had a slightly incorrect topology. The DRAGON models were less accurate but all 25 models had correct topologies. C and D are models generated from 5 long-range restraints by DRAGON and X-PLOR. 20 out of 25 DRAGON models still had correct topologies, whereas 21 X-PLOR models were incorrect. Note that the X-PLOR model images were scaled down to fit in the screen.

Plate 10 In *Protein Fold Determination Using a Small Number of Distance Restraints*, pages 85-97 (A. Aszódi, M.J. Gradwell and W.R. Taylor).

(a)

(b)

(c)

(d)

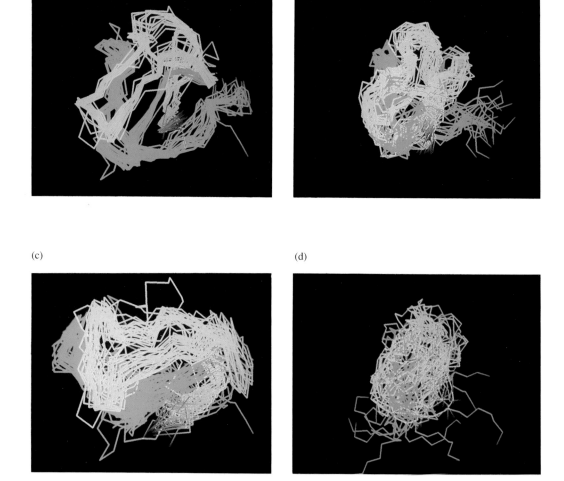

Model C_α backbones aligned to the native tendamistat structure 3AIT. Color codes as in color plate 8. A and B are models generated from 46 long-range restraints by DRAGON and X-PLOR, respectively. DRAGON produced markedly better results, whereas the X-PLOR models were more variable. C and D are models generated from 5 long-range restraints by DRAGON and X-PLOR. All DRAGON models still had correct topologies while the majority of the X-PLOR models became incorrect.

Plate 11 In *Protein Fold Determination Using a Small Number of Distance Restraints*, pages 85-97 (A. Aszódi, M.J. Gradwell and W.R. Taylor).

(a)

(b)

(c)

(d)

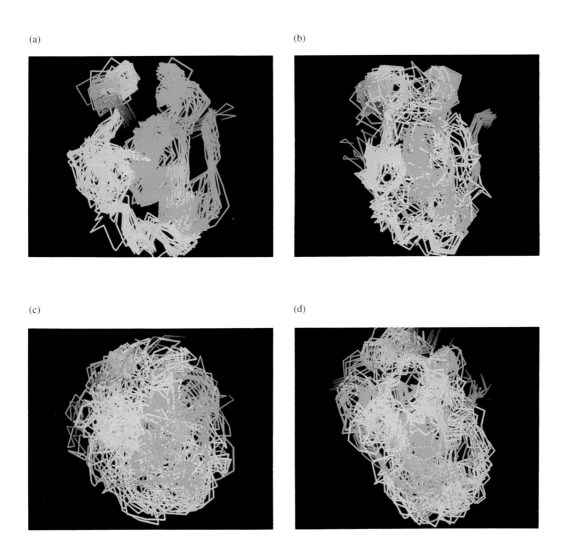

Model C_α backbones aligned to the native thioredoxin structure 2TRX (A-chain). Color codes as in color plate 8. A and B are models generated from 48 long-range restraints by DRAGON and X-PLOR, respectively. The DRAGON models were correct in all cases, while the X-PLOR produced a number of incorrect results. C and D are models generated from 20 long-range restraints by DRAGON and X-PLOR. Both methods located the correct topologies in about 10 cases out of 25 but the overall model quality was poor.

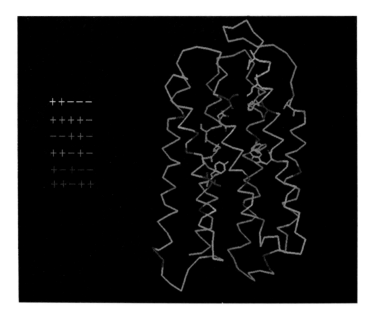

Side view of the D1 receptor backbone showing in color the sites at which correlated mutations (see text) are located. The color-coding is shown at the left, where the five columns represent the five dopamine receptor subtypes and the binding activities, shown as (+) or (-) for a panel of ligands sorted into six specificity categories. See reference [24], (page 185).

Plate 13 In *Chirality in Protein Structure*, page 251 (Timothy W.F. Slidel and Janet M. Thornton).

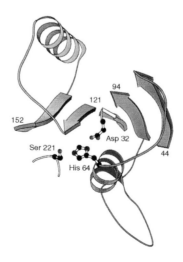

Right-handed (green) and left-handed (red) βαβ motifs from subtilisin (PDB code 1CSE). (See reference [29], page 262). This MOLSCRIPT (see reference [30], page 262) diagram shows how important the abnormal left-handed motif is in positioning histidine 64 in the catalytic triad. A right-handed motif would have placed the histidine on the opposite side of the β-sheet.

Plate 14 In *HIV GP120 Docking Interactions and Inhibitor Design Based on an Atomic Structure Derived by Molecular Modeling Using the DREIDING II Force Field*, pages 292-305 (Jerome L. Gabriel and William M. Mitchell).

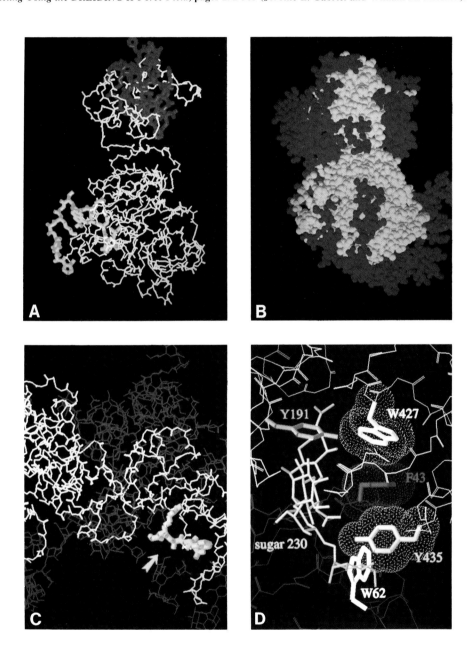

Structural features of the modeled gp120 moelcule. (a) Localization and solvent accessibility of CD4 domain (blue) and V3 loop (red). The remainder of the peptide backbone is depicted in yellow. (b) Topographical relationship of N-linked oligosaccharides (red) on the surface of folded gp120 protein (yellow). (c) Accessibility of conserved GPGR sequence as indicated by the arrow. Peptide backbone is depicted in yellow; oligosaccharide backbone in red. (d) van der Waals contacts in CD4-gp120 complex. F43 and W62 are CD4 residues; the remainder are gp120 residues. CD4 peptide backbone is in red; gp120 peptide backbone is in yellow. The N-linked oligosaccharide of N230 is illustrated in green.

Plate 15   In *HIV GP120 Docking Interactions and Inhibitor Design Based on an Atomic Structure Derived by Molecular Modeling Using the DREIDING II Force Field*, pages 292-305 (Jerome L. Gabriel and William M. Mitchell).

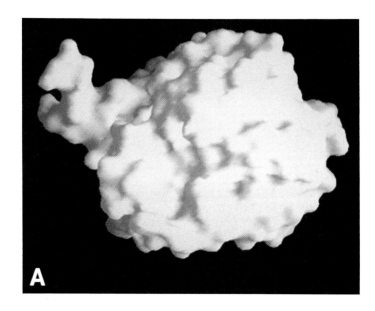

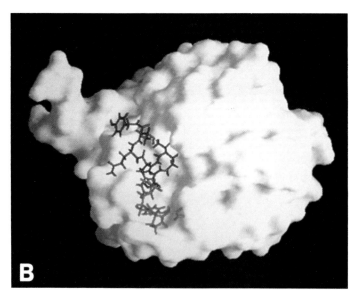

Molecular surface of CD4 binding domain on gp120. (a) No ligands. (b) CD4 mimetic bound to the upper site (red) and CPF bound to the lower site (blue).

Overview

Three Paradoxes of Protein Folding

Peter G. Wolynes

School of Chemical Science, University of Illinois, Urbana-Champaign,
505 S. Mathews Avenue, Urbana, IL 61801, U. S. A.

1   Introduction

It is most appropriate that a conference on protein folding like this one, should be held at the Royal Danish Academy of Sciences and Letters. Niels Bohr, whose spirit imbues this institution, had the hope that the physical study of biological problems would reveal new insights about the natural world. He also believed, as evidenced in his talk on "Light and Life", that as happened in the study of atoms, biological systems would present us with philosophical paradoxes which would force us to deepen our understanding [1]. Many early molecular biologists were drawn to the field from physics because of Bohr's views, but later on some have expressed the feeling that molecular biology progresses mainly without the need for revolutionary concepts and without the need for resolution of paradoxes, unlike the early days of quantum mechanics. I disagree with this latter view. At least, the field of protein folding has provided us with paradoxes and attempts at their resolution have required the introduction of new concepts and deepened our understanding. Many of these efforts are discussed in the other lectures at this conference.

In this lecture, I will describe three paradoxes of protein folding. Like all good paradoxes these paradoxes capture some basic worries about the basic biological and physical problems but require formulation and reformulation in order to have a precise form that can lead to intellectual progress. These three paradoxes are: (1) the Levinthal paradox which deals with the problem of how a biomolecule can find its low energy state in a time less than geological; (2) the Hoyle paradox which asks how foldable proteins could have evolved within the lifetime of a "big bang" universe; and (3) a third paradox which is only beginning to emerge that I will call the marginal stability or Honig paradox. — Why do proteins seem to have such a delicate compensation of entropy and energy during intermediate stages of the folding process? The first two paradoxes, at least, are clearly related to the fundamental ways in which information if transferred in biology.

All of the paradoxes of protein folding come from the more basic observation that spontaneous folding occurs and is largely a process of self-organization. This was shown by Anfinsen's groundbreaking experiments [2]. Without self-assembly life would be even more paradoxical. It is appropriate to quote an anecdote recounted by Gunther Stent concerning a conversation with Max Delbrück about folding [3]. He tells how Delbrück pointed out that one biological paradox was clear and had been described by Watson in his book. This is the so-called "enzyme cannot make enzyme paradox", which is resolved by the notion that DNA makes proteins which then fold spontaneously and become the enzymes. Delbrück writes:

> You might as well say that the resolution of this paradox by the reduction in dimensionality from three-dimensional continuous to one-dimensional discrete in the genesis of proteins is a new law of physics and one nobody could have pulled out of quantum mechanics without first having seen it in operation.

0-8493-4009-8/96/$0.00+$.50

The three paradoxes we speak about clearly proceed by further developing this paradox sensed by Delbrück. On the other hand, we should bear in mind that immediately upon making this remark about a "new law of physics" to Stent, Delbrück quotes Bohr as telling about a man who upon seeing a magician sawing a live woman in half, rises excitedly from his seat and shouts: "It's all a swindle!" Whether this is the reaction Bohr would have on listening to a protein folding conference is something we shall all meditate on.

2   The Levinthal paradox

The first paradox of protein folding is that protein molecules, in their functioning state, sample only a very small portion of the configuration space that such a large chain molecule has available to it. Indeed, at low resolution, one often thinks of a folded protein molecule as having a unique conformation, at least unique enough to give a well-defined X-ray structure. We actually know that even this well-defined x-ray structure allows the existence of functionally significant fluctuations [4], but it is clear that a dramatic reduction of the configuration space is involved in folding.

Levinthal, early on, made an estimate of this reduction in configuration space [5]. Roughly speaking, each amino acid in the protein chain has ten conformational states available to it. Thus a protein of length 100 possesses a complete configuration space spanning 10^{100} states. Even if the time to make a conformational transition is as short as a femtosecond, it is clear that not all conformational states can be searched if protein folding is to occur on physiological timescales of the order of a few seconds. Levinthal then introduced the notion of a pathway for a protein folding. Actually in reading his discussion of this, I find it not at all clear what he meant, but later workers often interpret this to mean a kinetic pathway with discrete states which could be studied by the classical methods of chemical kinetics [6]. Levinthal's paradox is then to understand how proteins organize themselves in extremely short times compared to this unguided conformational search time. Levinthal's paradox was ignored by physically-minded people for quite a long time. This is because the paradox seems so silly when it is applied to the usual systems studied by physicists and chemists. For example, a sample of water can crystallize and, thereby, find a very small part of its phase space. Indeed, since a water molecule hydrogen bonded to neighbors, might also have of the order of ten configurations, the time it would take to search all of the configurations of a bowl of water is of the order of $10^{10^{23}}$ which is an even more ridiculous time than that for a protein folding search.

Water crystallizes by first finding a critical nucleus which is followed by progressive growth. The resulting search time is considerably shorter than the cosmological time from the simple Levinthal estimate. It is interesting that the nucleation example which is even cited by Levinthal in his article, is an example where a traditional chemical kinetic pathway doesn't really exist. Experimentalists seem to have largely ignored this observation. What makes the Levinthal paradox interesting is that this *reductio ad absurdum* of the crystallization example is not a proof that complex information bearing molecule does not have a difficult conformational search problem facing it.

In 1987, Joe Bryngelson and I began to think about the role of the heterogeneity of the protein sequence in protein folding [7]. We tried to develop many models of heteropolymers which captured the essence of the idea that for most configurations of a heteropolymer, one would bring together segments of the protein which would have conflicting interactions. Examining each model convinced us that a random heteropolymer would have a good deal of "frustration", to use the term of Anderson and Toulouse [8, 9]. It had been known for quite a long time that random systems possess a more complicated configuration space and thermodynamics than do simple regular systems. This was most clear in the analysis of spin glasses — systems of two-state spins interacting by random interactions. The ferromagnet, having all the same sign spin spin interactions, possesses a very symmetrical ground state. This is because all of the interactions are harmonious and cooperative. If we assign interactions between the spins at random, one obtains a very different system which has extremely sluggish dynamics below a phase transition. This sluggish dynamics is connected with the search through a very rugged energy landscape resulting from the conflicts or frustration between the different random interactions.

Bryngelson and I came to the conclusion that almost all approximations for treating the randomness of the sequence in self-assembly lead to a very rough energy landscape and it seemed reasonable to us to make the most extreme ansatz as a starting point to understanding the consequences of this ruggedness. This extreme approximation is that the energy states of a heteropolymer can, in the main, be described by the most rugged energy landscape, the so-called random energy model of Derrida [10]. This model postulates that each conformation of a protein has an energy which can be taken as an independent random variable. Thus making a small change in conformation by changing one dihedral angle, for example, gives a wildly different energy. This, of course, is credible for polymers because a single dihedral angle change can bring together very distant parts of the sequence that had never been in contact before.

We were emboldened to make this hypothesis because of a good deal of work on the so-called "exotic" spin glasses known as Potts glasses. It had been shown by Gross and coworkers that the Ising spin glass is special and that most random systems of interacting objects which lacked the special symmetry of the Ising spins, possessed a phase transition that was similar to that of the random energy model [11]. Ted Kirkpatrick and I made this analogy more explicit by showing that the phase transition in Potts glasses corresponded to an entropy crisis like that in the random energy model(REM) [12]. One could define a coarse-grained energy landscape and show that within this energy landscape, the different states were uncorrelated and that, furthermore, the phase transition occurred via an entropy crisis in which whichever state happened to be the lowest free energy, becomes singled out below a transition temperature. This entropy crisis is very much like one believed to occur in liquids as they undergo their glass transition [13] and, indeed, has been used to understand the slow dynamics which occurs as the glass transition is approached [14, 15]. This universality of REM-like behavior lead to our expectation that a typical non-symmetrical polymer system with random interactions would have a configuration space that would be shattered into parts with large barriers between them and that the search between these parts would be essentially unguided. Thus the search through the coarse-grained energy landscape of a random heteropolymer to find its ground state should be a difficult and arduous process comparable to the situation envisioned by the Levinthal problem. Of course, this scenario allows the possibility that the number of states to be searched through reflects not the total entropy but still some sizeable fraction of it counting the number of distinct valleys. Nevertheless, it should scale to be cosmologically long in the limit of large protein structures. We made this argument more precise by examining the kinetics of the random energy model and showed that, indeed, the Levinthal paradox does emerge at a temperature low enough so that one could remain trapped in the low energy states [7]. The typical search time was of the order of the time to search through all configurations. How then did proteins evade the Levinthal paradox which should be a real one for most random hereropolymers?

We argued that the correct configurations of proteins were not highly frustrated but rather that kinetically foldable proteins resembled ordinary systems like the ferromagnet more than the spin glass, at least as they became more native-like. This idea seems certainly very plausible when one looks at the structures of completely folded proteins. They do not seem to be the result of simply satisfying a slight majority of some interactions but, instead, there seem to be at least locally, very nice themes of consistency and symmetry. Indeed, Go had talked about the consistency between a local structure and higher order structure before, specifically, worrying about how local interactions giving secondary structure and tertiary interactions combined [16]. But there are many ways to avoid frustration and in the model which we discussed, we argued that basically all the interactions of a protein are possible candidates for lowering the energy more than expected as the native structure is approached, giving a kind of ferromagnetic and consistent set of interactions. We argued then that the folding transition of proteins is distinct from the glass transition of heteropolymers, and we developed a kinetic theory of folding which showed if folding could go on at temperatures exceeding the glass transition, it could be relatively fast, occurring by either a downhill mechanism or one that involved forming a transition state which actually consists of a large set of configurations. Folding could be very facile if the folding temperature was much above the glass transition. Thus we showed that if a protein satisfied the "principle of minimal frustration", it could fold rapidly, at least within the approximations of our model.

Many simulations of minimalist models of proteins have shown great consistency with these ideas. Thirumalai and coworkers studied a model of a β-barrel whose sequences were designed thoughtfully[17]. They showed that the energy landscape of this model corresponded rather closely to that expected for the minimally frustrated random energy model; namely, first a low energy state which has some excitations which are closely related to it in structure and that are similar in energy to the ground state. Second when one went high enough in energy, one begins to encounter alternate structures that had no relationship to the ground state or each other but were, nevertheless, local minima that are competitive with each other in energy. If one, through the use of a Maxwell Demon, prevented a system from entering the region of phase space which was correlated with the ground state, one would see a very rough energy landscape. As the system cooled a glass transition would result.

The β-barrel structure is, however, highly symmetric and well designed. Is the behavior of more random sequences like that which the randomly frustrated energy landscape model predicts? A very clear hint of this comes from the study of Leopold, Montal and Onuchic [18] in which, again, they simulate the folding of a minimalist model; in this case, a 27 cube, a well designed, non-frustrated sequence here has an energy landscape similar to that of the minimally frustrated model with a very wide funnel leading to the ground state. Many states with similarity to the ground state are pulled down in energy so that Brownian diffusion more often takes you towards the ground state than away from it. On the other hand, Leopold, *et al.*, also deliberately frustrated their sequence and showed that in this case the configuration space fragments into many many funnels like those we would expect for the Potts spin glass and, in this case, folding was essentially unobservable on meaningful time scales.

The most definitive work on minimalist models addressing this point is contained in the recent series of studies by Shakhnovich and coworkers, some of which are reported on in this conference [19]. They have shown by simulating a large number of randomly selected sequence that for small lattice models only the sequences for which the folding temperature exceeds the glass transition temperature can be folded in sensible times.

The competition between the self-organization of folding and the kinetic trapping which occurs at the glass transition suggests a non-monotonic dependence of the folding rate on temperature for minimally frustrated systems. Detailed studies of folding vs. temperature have been undertaken by Socci and Onuchic [20] and by Chan, Dill and coworkers [21]. They are consistent with the energy landscape analysis.

How does minimal frustration overcome the Levinthal paradox? It does so by continuously

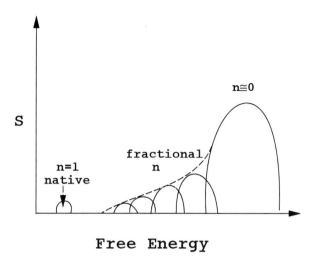

Figure 1: A schematic of the logarithmic density of states as a function of an order parameter for a minimally frustrated protein. Notice how the stratification of configuration space, representing a correlation in the landscape, leads to a low energy tail.

trading off entropy for energy. As the protein resembles the folded state more and more, entropy goes down. Because of the minimal frustration the energy goes down as well. If this process did not occur, there would be a huge entropy barrier which is effectively what Levinthal was talking about, but this entropy barrier is canceled by the energy term. Generally we would expect the cancellation of entropy and energy to be imperfect at the folding transition temperature itself. Because of the analogy to the ordinary first order phase transition, one expects a residual nucleation or activation barrier. If the overcoming of this activation barrier is limiting, there is no sign of the Levinthal paradox left. The process of folding is simple exponential. The only hint of glassy dynamics is in the strongly non Arrhenius temperature dependences of the rates which reflect both the cancellation of entropy and energy and the trapping processes. If the folded state is far more stable than the unfolded, however, the cancellation can be, in principle, more perfect. This leads to what we call downhill folding [18]. A bit of the Levinthal paradox now remains in this downhill folding scenario during the late stages of activated folding.

The density of states of minimally frustrated random heteropolymer is thought of in the Bryngelson and Wolynes analysis as a super position of densities of states at various levels in the protein folding funnel. This is pictured in figure 1. We can define a glass transition temperature for any value of the degree of nativeness. If the ruggedness of the landscape does not decrease with the approach to the folded state, the effective glass transition temperature becomes larger as the folded state is approached, since the configurational entropy surely decreases. Thus at a certain level in the funnel a glass transition can occur and search becomes rate limiting again. The search problem is, however, much smaller so the Levinthal paradox is partly solved. The Bryngelson/Wolynes analysis then would suggest that the folding rated is limited by that final search and is roughly approximated by the inverse Levinthal time corresponding to the number of states at the glass transition level.

In fact, the situation can be slightly worse than this in that it is possible that after the glass transition is encountered, the driving forces towards further native contacts are still very large but misguided, so one continues towards a more folded state but reaches some sort of topologically frustrated dead end. In this case one must backtrack from the dead end and there will be an additional factor in the rate corresponding to the activation from the dead end back to the place where many states emerge. Notice that this implies the increase of stability of a folded state can sometimes decrease the rate if there are topological dead ends. Some evidence for this has been seen in simulations by Camacho and Thirumalai [22].

It is also possible that the ΔE^2 does not remained fixed but decreases as one approaches the native, due to the increase of constraints. If this is the case, the glass transition may never be encountered. These seem to be non-universal properties of the various models. In simulations to be discussed later by Onuchic at this meeting the glass transition has been located in a realistic folded funnel. This does suggest that proteins indeed encounter the search problem at the very last stages of folding.

One might worry that the minimal frustration principle is only required to overcome the Levinthal paradox *in vitro*; other loopholes might apply *in vivo*. Of course there are many complications in the *in vivo* situation, such as the possibility of sequential folding and so on. Recently, one has seen the importance of chaperone molecules which catalyze folding [23]. A model of kinetic proofreading for folding with chaperones has been examined using energy landscape ideas by Gulukota and Wolynes and, at least, within these models also it seems to be impossible to avoid the invocation of a minimal frustration principle [24].

We see then that foldability is a non-trivial property of heteropolymers. Finding foldable heteropolymers is a problem that leads to our next paradox.

3   The Hoyle paradox

At first sight, the minimal frustration principle might merely trade one paradox for another. How difficult is it for a protein to have evolved whose sequence satisfies the principle of minimal frustration? This is a variant of what might be called Hoyle's Paradox, concerning the origin of life in a finite short amount of time [25, 26]. First, it is clear that not all proteins could have been made. The number of possible proteins of length 100 is 20^{100}. This exceeds by far the number of protons in the universe times the turnover time of a typical protein. Thus, it is hard to argue that any particular protein is the most perfect one for its task, despite the strong temptation to do so because of their remarkable properties. There are, of course, many beautiful examples of convergent evolution at the molecular level. These do suggest that many individual amino acids are highly adapted to their purpose in protein structure. One example of this is the existence of two distinct classes of serine proteases [27]. These two families have entirely different three-dimensional structure but have the same residues in the active site. Other examples occur in the evolution of hemoglobin [28, 29]. Two bird species of different families both fly to extraordinarily high altitudes. It is very desirable for these high fliers to have a high affinity oxygen binding form of hemoglobin. In both of these two species, the same amino acid, which is crucial for the adaptation is found at the same site. Similarly, there are examples of convergent molecular evolution for humans. In the various thalessemias, again, the same mutation has independently occurred in different lines of descent, both giving a hemoglobin which can dimerize in the low oxygen environment of a parasite-infected red blood cell which is infected by the malaria parasite.

The worry is then that achieving a minimally frustrated protein requires also this sort of fine tuning where each amino acid must be perfect. This would require a difficult search through a large sequence space. As it happens, achieving minimal frustration is not a terribly demanding computational task, at least if the random heteropolymer is well described by currently existing mean field theories. This realization was utilized in the efforts by my research group to decode protein sequence by finding energy functions that will give rapid folding for known proteins with known structures and sequence. Our strategy which was discussed at the first of these conferences by my coworker, Richard Goldstein [30, 31, 32], involved optimizing the ratio of the folding temperature of the protein to the glass transition temperature of the protein where each of these temperatures were estimated, using the simplest mean field theories. In this event, the folding temperature is directly related to the difference in energy between the correct folded structure and the ensemble of misfolded compact structures. Similarly, the glass transition temperature can be estimated using the simplest mean field theory as being proportional to the root mean square fluctuation of the energies of the misfolded structures. One can then ask what parameters in a given form of an energy function optimize the ratio of T_f[1] to T_g[2], indeed, a closed form unique solution is easily obtained. We showed that for two forms of Hamiltonians, one based on neural network ideas [31], and another more conventional Hamiltonian based on contact energies [32], that this procedure gives rise to energy functions that were extremely good at recognizing correct folded structures from a large family of alternatives in the case of associative memory Hamiltonians, the optimized energy functions generally gave good results even when used with molecular dynamic simulations. This showed that the energy landscape really was minimally frustrated and leads to a good folding funnel.

The same quantitative principle has been used by Shakhnovich in a somewhat different algorithmic form to design proteins which are minimally frustrated, assuming a given form for simple pair interactions[33]. This is an exercise of protein engineering, whereas our study was an effort in so to speak "reverse engineering". He formulates the algorithm in terms mathematically very closely related to the T_f/T_g criterion. Shakhnovich's protein design problem is precisely the one that would have been encountered in the Hoyle paradox, so we can say that within current understanding of heteropolymer theory, the core of the Hoyle paradox has been resolved.

A bit of a worry has emerged, however. Are the current ways of estimating T_f to T_g really good enough? Recently, we have tried to improve the statistical mechanical description of the random heteropolymer states in our efforts towards deducing energy functions that will reliably fold to the correct structure [34]. We did this because in surveying protein recognition problems, it was apparent that there are occasionally a few clinkers in the recognition process. A related but different tertiary structure is sometimes lower in energy than the native one, in the case of the reverse engineering or decoding problem. In the case of forward design, the desired structure for two letter code problems designed by the simple algorithm was found by Yue, *et al.*, to not always correspond to the actual lowest energy [35]. In our view the main problem here is that the density of states near the low energy end of the molten globule spectrum differs from the crudest random energy model expectations. One reason for this effect can be correlations in the energy landscape so a generalized REM should be used. Also the presence of new order parameters, such as degree of helicity, etc., makes a difference. As in figure 1, there should be a tail in the low energy density of states reflecting these partial orderings. In fact, we do find that usually the clinkers in recognition problems are configurations that have a similar amount of secondary structure to the correct one. Suppose such an additional order parameter as secondary structure plays a role. Then we expect the density of states of incorrect structures to be quite skewed. In fact, such a result is obtained when one uses optimal local Hamiltonians for alignment-based minimization.

A density of aligned minima is shown for the simple optimized Hamiltonian in figure 2.

---

[1]Folding temperature.
[2]Glass transition temperature.

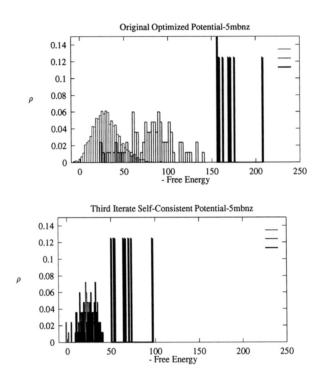

Figure 2: A comparison of the density of states and of local minima based on alignment for REM optimized and self-consistently optimized potential based on calculations of Koretke, Luthey-Schulten and Wolynes. The thick lines denote the homologous proteins, the medium line denote local minima obtained by alignment and the thin line denotes density of states for the "molten globule" configurations used to generate the REM optimized values.

The correct estimate for T_f/T_g then requires distinguishing the thermally occupied states in this ensemble from the folded one. To implement finding a completely minimally frustrated energy function then requires an iteration to self-consistency. First an energy function is deduced with the simple REM form of the minimal frustration principle. New energy minima are constructed on the basis of this energy function. This is then used to estimate the low energy density of states of incorrect structures and one goes through the loop. The reoptimized density of aligned minima is also shown in figure 2. In figure 3, we show some recognition results that Koretke, Luthey-Schulten and I have obtained with such a self-consistent iterated method compared with the recognition results with the simple REM optimized energy function one [34].

The self-consistency calculation for reverse engineering and decoding is analogous to the problem that laboratory protein designers have begun to worry about of explicit negative design. Not only must the folded structure be more stable than what we statistically expect to be the lowest energy state of the random heteropolymer, it must actually be confirmed that there are no intruder states from the molten globule for this particular energy function or sequence. Usually such intruders have a lot of structural similarity to the design goal.

Swissprot	Target Name		Predicted Homolog	EF	PC-GCG
	Name	PDB	Name		
B2MG_BOVIN	Bovin β-2 μ-globuline	3hfmh	IG∗G1 Fab Fragment	11.6	20.8
B2MG_MELGA	Turkey β-2 μ-globuline	2rhez	Bence-∗Jones Protein	11.5	21.4
B2MG_PONPY	Orangutan β-2 μ-globline	2rhez	Bence-∗Jones Protein	3.8	15.4
B2MG_RAT	Rat β-2 μ-globuline	2rhez	Bence-∗Jones Protein	14.3	13.2
HA2B_MOUSE	Mouse H-2 Histocomp. Antigen	3adkz	Adenylate Kinase	12.5	18.1
HA2P_HUMAN	Human H-2 Histocomp. Antigen	4fd1z	Ferredoxin	5.7	16.0
HA2Q_MOUSE	Mouse H-2 Histocomp. Antigen	2snsz	Staphylococcal Nuclease	6.4	12.1
HA2S_MOUSE	Mouse H-2 Histocomp. Antigen	4fd1z	Ferredoxin	4.7	12.3
HA2Z_HUMAN	Human HLA Histocomp. Antigen	2azaa	Azurin (Oxidized)	7.5	14.7
HB25_HUMAN	Human HLA Histocomp. Antigen	3hlaa	Human Class I Histocompatibility	15.8	22.9
HB2B_HUMAN	Human HLA Histocomp. Antigen	2rhez	Bence-∗Jones Protein	12.5	17.5
HB2G_HUMAN	Human HLA Histocomp. Antigen	3hfmh	IG∗G1 Fab Fragment	15.0	18.7
HB2S_HUMAN	Human HLA Histocomp. Antigen	2rhez	Bence-∗Jones Protein	11.4	17.5
KAC6_RABIT	Rabbit IG κ Chain	2pazz	Pseudoazurin (Cupredoxin)	9.0	16.8
KACA_RAT	Rat IG κ Chain	3hlaa	Human Class I Histocompatibility	20.4	21.6
KACB_RAT	Rat IG κ Chain	3hlaa	Human Class I Histocompatibility	17.3	23.7
KAC_MOUSE	Mouse IG λ Chain	2ssiz	Streptomyces Subtilisin Inhibi	13.0	19.4
LAC1_MOUSE	Mouse IG λ Chain	2rhez	Bence-∗Jones Protein	15.8	12.1
LAC2_MOUSE	Mouse IG λ Chain	1rela	Bence-∗Jones Immunoglobulin	10.0	15.0
LAC3_MOUSE	Mouse IG λ Chain	2pazz	Pseudoazurin (Cupredoxin)	5.1	13.7
LAC5_MUSSP	Mouse IG λ Chain	2rhez	Bence-∗Jones Protein	10.8	13.7
LAC_HUMAN	Human IG λ Chain	3hlaa	Human Class I Histocompatibility	22.2	22.2
LAC_RABIT	Rabbit IG λ Chain	3hlaa	Human Class I Histocompatibility	22.9	25.3

Figure 3: Recognition of various immunoglobin sequences using local Hamiltonians based on the simple REM and the self-consistent optimization. Notice the greater consistency of the self-consistent results.

At the moment, I do not know any rigorous proof that this self-consistency problem is not computationally difficult, but it certainly seems that the starting estimates of the amino acid interactions based on the simplest mean field theories are so good that, at least for ordinary proteins, only a local search is involved so the convergence problem should not really be exponentially difficult.

4 The marginal stability paradox

The two paradoxes which are just discussed are clearly inherent to the problem of how any information-bearing macromolecule can have evolved to spontaneously self-assemble into a complex form. Another conundrum of a more detailed nature arises when we try to account for experimental observations on the thermodynamics and kinetics of real protein folding. The route to the statement of the "paradox" is a bit circuitous. I was drawn to this problem through the effort of trying to understand the role of secondary structure formation in real protein folding [36]. Our attempt, undertaken in collaboration with José Onuchic, Zan Luthey-Schulten and Nicholas Socci [37], tries to bring together laboratory observations on folding kinetics with the theory of protein folding to quantify the statistical features of the energy landscape.

Onuchic's lecture will describe more of the details, so I will be brief. Our philosophy is based on the law of corresponding states in the theory of phase transitions [38]. Empirically, it is well known that phase transitions of very different systems at the microscopic level, often can be described by the same phase diagram and that the mechanism of kinetic structure formation depends largely on where one is in the phase diagram. The theory of magnetic domain formation and of condensation in a supercooled gas or bubble formation in the early universe are all very similar. Even more striking, as the critical point of a phase transition is approached, the microscopic details of the underlying energy function wash out and only truly universal global features of the energy landscape play a role in the critical phenomena. This is the basic idea of the renormalization group in which short range interactions are taken successively into account, leading eventually to a coarse grained description depending only on a few parameters measuring the proximity to the critical point [39].

Most of the work on the statistical mechanics of protein folding has been based on very simple models. These models are much simpler than real atomic level descriptions of proteins. At the lowest level, these models are characterized by two characteristic transition temperatures, the folding temperature, T_f and the glass transition temperature, T_g. Since a protein is a mesoscopic system and some of the motions involve, global topological changes, the size of the protein also matters and is most conveniently described as an effective configurational entropy. The characteristic temperatures, T_f and T_g, can be more picturesquely described as characterizing two aspects of the energy landscape [40]. T_g depends primarily on the mean square interaction energy fluctuations, ΔE^2, measuring the ruggedness of the landscape and in order to have a separate higher temperature folding transition, there must be also be an overall average gradient toward the folded state, ΔE_S. In visual terms, the energy landscape of a foldable protein is a funnel, at least for these simple models.

How can we characterize these various parameters and take into account the renormalizations of the underlying interactions that lead to these parameters emerging out of the complex micro physics of local structure formation? A formal renormalization treatment is complex so we carried this out using a combination of simple theory, simulation and some experimental results to estimate renormalized values of the funnel parameters. Secondary structure formation is a prominent feature of protein folding. First we ask, how much entropy is lost through this process? A direct measure of this is a bit difficult because it involves balancing fairly large energy terms and large entropy terms. Barry Honig has looked into such a microscopic approach and obtained the correct, but also initially surprising result, that the free energy scale for helix formation is effectively zero [41]. We know this is roughly correct because; in fact, helix-coil transitions do occur in isolated polymer chains around room temperature. Such transitions can be induced by only slight changes in the solvent environment. This is our first example of marginal stability! The entropy and energy of secondary structure formation almost cancel each other, even at this intermediate stage.

In long helix-forming polymers, the amount of entropy reduction can be quite dramatic from this mechanism since one forms in a helix-coil transition of a soluble homopolymer, helices of length 100 or so, and the small coil regions which are left, move up and down the polymer. The helix formation in protein folding, however, is not so simple since the protein must also collapse. Collapse works against the formation of such long helices since helices must come in contact with each in order to gain the hydrophobic energy interaction.

Bascle, Garel and Orland have discussed some rather simple models of this effect in a hydrophobic homopolymer [42]. A different approach was taken by my collaborators, Zan Luthey-Schulten, Ben Ramirez and me, in which we highlight the conflict between helix-coil transitions and collapse rather directly in heteropolymers [36]. An interesting feature of our analysis is that it is important to take into account that while helix formation is in some ways frustrated by collapse, the helices are also partly encouraged by the collapse transition, since aligned helices have less excluded volume than disordered random coils. There is, hence, a liquid crystal transition as well as a helix-coil transition in a collapsed polymer. In quantifying the protein folding funnels landscape, we assume the funneled search for correct topology occurs from such a collapsed liquid crystalline polymer state. The helical content of an equilibrium collapsed state depends on the effective hydrogen bond strength which, presumably, is the result of many conflicting terms as described by Honig. In this theory, the conformational entropy is also a function of that effective hydrogen bond strength, so measurements of helical content can tell us what the appropriate conformational entropy is. When we use measured values of molten globule helicity of around 65%, the theory gives an entropy of $.6k_B$ per monomer unit which is to be contrasted with the free chain value of 2.3 per monomer unit. Thus indiscriminate helix formation in collapse dramatically reduces the entropy through a phase transition possessing a latent heat of only $.15k_BT$ per monomer unit, or $9k_BT$ for an entire 60 amino acid helical protein. Again, there are the signs of marginal stability. This analysis shows that the renormalized entropy of the different topologies of 60 amino acid protein with fluctuating helices is very comparable to that of the 27-mer lattice models that have been studied so much. The barriers to this helical ordering transition must also be quite small, since they basically involve largely one-dimensional ordering effects.

We imagine then that after the indiscriminate helix formation, helices come and go at will within the collapse structure and the chain tries out various different topological configurations. The time scale of these sets the energy scale for the ruggedness. Since microscopic reconfiguration times are of the order of a nanosecond and fluctuations within the molten globule take a few milliseconds, the simplest estimate of the energy landscape ruggedness can be obtained using the theory based on the random energy model where a zeroth order estimate of the reconfiguration time is $\tau_{\text{reconfig}} = \tau_0 \exp(\Delta E^2/2T^2)$. This may be something of an overestimate since we might imagine smaller scale motions playing the most important role, but with this value, one obtains a ruggedness scale, $\Delta E^2/2T_{f^2}$ of the order of 11 to 18. When this is combined with the entropy estimate from the indiscriminate helical collapse, we would find that the molten globule entropy is still further reduced to a value of the order 21 k_B for a 60 amino acid chain. Since the protein folds at T_f, we know this overall entropy is balanced by the energy loss. Thus we obtain a value for the energy gradient of the funnel of the order $\Delta E_S/T_f = S_L + \Delta E^2/2T_{f^2}$. Here we have also taken into account the fact that the energy scale ruggedness means that the low energy states of the globule will be preferentially occupied.

The resulting value for the energy gradient tells us that it is roughly ten times larger than the root mean square energetic ruggedness. Together with the configurational entropy estimate then, the thermodynamic glass transition temperature is T_g of order $.6T_f$. This ratio is larger than that for the two-letter code models most studied and is very close to that for a three-letter code model. So we can say that the lower part of the protein folding funnel, after helical collapse, resembles that of the three-letter code 27 mer simulations. A sketch of the resulting "realistic" folding funnel is shown in figure 4.

We have now examined how entropy and energy are traded off for each other within this folding funnel. This can be done by monitoring the density of states as a function of various reaction coordinates like the fraction of correct contacts made in the protein (Q) or the fraction of angles which are correct (A). These scales are indicated on the plot of the folding funnel. In this representation, the thermodynamic barrier between the folded state and the molten globule occurs with a Q value between .57 to .64 and an A value between .84 and .92. This transition state region is a thermodynamic bottleneck to folding. What is interesting is how modest the thermodynamic barrier is. Even at Tf, the thermodynamic activation barrier is only of order 2.4 k_BT_f. Details of these results will be discussed in Onuchic's contribution to this volume. But, what is interesting here is how small the barrier is. This is a sign of marginal stability. Again, the energy and entropy have compensated each other as one goes through the folding funnel. The apparent large activation free energies for folding really are a result of trapping within states in this bottleneck region and don't reflect the compensation of energy and entropy directly very well.

The small barrier suggests again a kind of fine tuning of the folding process. Like the entropy energy compensation in helix formation, this may also seem paradoxical. Of course, the overall folding transition must have a compensation between energy and entropy that is the definition of the folding transition temperature. The interesting thing is that this compensation

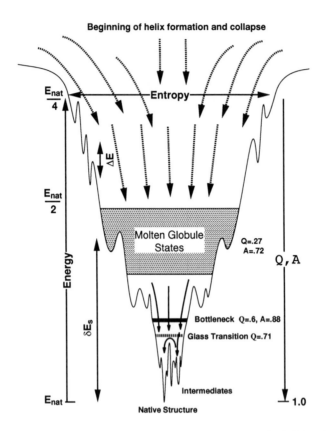

Figure 4: A schematic representation to scale of a realistic protein folding funnel based on calculations of Onuchic, *et al.* [37]. The molten globule, bottleneck region and the local glass transition are indicated Q and A are order parameters measuring the fraction of native contacts and correct angles, respectively.

occurs in such a way that no overall large barrier is encountered by it. We see a realistic folding funnel describes a marginally stable system. Even at intermediate degrees of order, energy and entropy compensate each other. This is like a system near its critical point and may be a clue for understanding the sensitivity of folding to external conditions.

The marginal stability is both a hindrance and a help for further work by theoreticians. If marginal stability applies for every order parameter, it will be difficult to distinguish rival theories of dominant ordering processes. At this point the resolution of the marginal stability paradox seems to be related to both the polymeric nature of proteins and evolutionary constraints. Polymers are notorious for having low surface tensions, i.e., they fluctuate a lot [43]! Also from the evolutionary viewpoint, the relative small size of thermodynamic barriers would be ideal. This is something like Albery and Knowles' description of a "perfect enzyme" which is diffusion limited because each of the microsteps has been optimized sufficiently to give a low barrier [44].

The marginal stability paradox was encountered by those who wish to use microscopic theories to understand folding *ab initio*. Honig, who estimated entropy and energy changes in the collapse to the molten globule from such microscopic theories, also ended up with very small, nearly cancelling contributions. Perhaps then we should call this marginal stability paradox the Honig paradox, since he was one of the first to popularize the puzzle in the microscopic context. Sadly then marginal stability makes *ab initio* theories difficult to use, but it becomes a license for describing the physics at a different energy scale and allows us to think about effective models just as in low temperature physics where again those transitions that do occur at low temperatures involve highly renormalized interactions between highly organized low entropy objects. If we want to characterize folding completely, the lesson of low temperature physics where many different phases come into play by virtue of the low entropy density gives us hope. From this perspective, the marginal stability paradox gives us insight into the role of subtle features in protein folding and biomolecular physics in general and holds open the prospect of considerably more interesting work with simple models.

5   The role of paradoxes in biomolecular theory

I hope my lecture has made clear how the physical study of protein folding has provided challenging paradoxes that have called upon us to develop new concepts for understanding biological systems. Probably none of these are nearly as profound as Niels Bohr imagined would be needed to understand life. But the intellectual adventure is just beginning! So far most of molecular biology has been concerned with identifying the players. So much progress is made so quickly by molecular biologists that there has been little time to contemplate the principles needed to understand the inner workings of biology. Folding is the first area where the quantitative understanding of biological self-organization has been faced. There are many more complex situations concerned with the structure of the biological cell and its organelles, regulatory networks and embryonic development where new problems of information transfer and self-organization must be solved. Like protein folding, once a quantitative basis for these is obtained experimentally at the molecular level, the resolution of mathematically posed paradoxes will likely play a role in achieving an understanding of these problems too.

Even within the confines of folding problems, I am sure new more refined paradoxes will continue to emerge and entertain us.

Acknowledgements

I thank the organizers, Søren Brunak, Henrik Bohr and Johanne Keiding for putting together an excellent symposium in an inspiring locale. I also thank my collaborators, Zan Luthey-Schulten, Ben Ramirez, Kris Koretke, José Onuchic, Nicholas Socci, Richard Goldstein, Kamalakar Gulukota and Joe Bryngelson whose work I discussed. Discussions with Henrik Bohr, Dev Thirumalai, E. Shakhnovich, Barry Honig, Jeff Saven, Jin Wang, Bill Eaton, Hans Frauenfelder and Ken Dill have also contributed to my understanding of the folding paradoxes. Our work at the University of Illinois is supported by NIH Grant, PHS R01 GM44557.

References

[1] N. Bohr, Light and life, *Nature*, 131, p. 421-23, 1933;
Light and life (revisited), Essays 1958-1960, Atomic Physics and Human Knowledge, Wiley, New York, 1965.).

[2] C. Anfinsen, E. Haber, M. Sela and F. H. White, The kinetics of formation of native ribonuclease during oxidation of the reduced polypeptide chain, *PNAS*, 47, p. 1309-14, 1961.

[3] G. Stent, That was the molecular biology that was, *Science*, 160, 390-95, 1968.

[4] H. Frauenfelder, F. Parak and R. D. Young, Conformational substates in proteins, *Ann. Rev. Biophys. Chem.*, 17, p. 451-79, 1988.

[5] C. Levinthal, How to fold graciously, *Mossbauer Spectroscopy in Biological Systems*, Proceedings of a meeting held at Allerton House, Monticello, Illinois, P. deBrunner, J. Tsibris and E. Munck (eds.), University of Illinois Press, Urbana, Illinois, 1969.

[6] P. S. Kim and R. L. Baldwin, Specific intermediates in the folding reactions of small proteins and the mechanism of protein folding, *Ann. Rev. Biochem.*, 51, p. 459-89, 1982.

[7] J. D. Bryngelson and P. G. Wolynes, Spin glasses and the statistical mechanics of protein folding, *PNAS*, 84, p. 7524-28, 1987;
     J. D. Bryngelson and P. G. Wolynes, Intermediates and barrier crossing in a random energy model (with applications to protein folding), *J. Phys. Chem.* (R. Zwanzig special issue), 93, p. 6902-15, 1989.

[8] P. W. Anderson, The concept of frustration in spin glasses, *J. Less-Common Metals*, 62, p. 291-94, 1978.

[9] G. Toulouse, Theory of the frustration effect in spin glasses I, *Comm. in Phys.*, 2, p. 115, 1977.

[10] B. Derrida, Random-energy model: An exactly solvable model of disordered systems, *Phys. Rev.*, B24, p. 2613-26, 1981.

[11] D. Gross, I. Kanter and H. Sompolinsky, Mean field theory of the Potts glass, *Phy. Rev. Lett.*, 55, p. 304, 1985.

[12] T. Kirkpatrick and P. G. Wolynes, Stable and metastable states of mean field potts and structural glasses, *Phys. Rev.*, B36, p. 8552-64, 1987.

[13] C. A. Angell, D. R. MacFarlane and N. Oguni, The Kauzmann Paradox, metastable liquids and ideal glasses: A summary, *Ann. N. Y. Acad. Sci.*, 484, p. 241, 1987.

[14] P. G. Wolynes, Aperiodic crystals: Biology, chemistry and physics in a fugue with stretto, *Proc. Intl. Symposium on Frontiers in Science* (H. Frauenfelder Festschrift), S. Chan and P. deBrunner (eds.), Am. Inst. Phys., 1989.

[15] T. Kirkpatrick, D. Thirumalai and P. G. Wolynes, Scaling concepts for the dynamics of viscous liquids near an ideal glassy state, *Phys. Rev. A*, 40, p. 1045-53, 1989.

[16] N. Gó and H. Takemoto, Reoperative roles of long and short range interactions in protein folding, *Biomol. Struct., Proceedings International Symposium*, Srinarasan (ed.), Pergamon, N.Y., 1981.

[17] J. D. Honeycutt and D. Thirumalai, Metastability of the folded states of globular proteins, *PNAS*, 87, 3526-29, 1990;
     Z. Guo, D. Thirumalai and J. D. Honeycutt, Folding kinetics of proteins, *J. Chem. Phys.*, 97, 525-35, 1992.

[18] P. E. Leopold, M. Montal and J. N. Onuchic, Protein folding funnels: A kinetic approach to the sequence-structure relationship, *PNAS*, 89, 8721-25, 1992.

[19] A. Sali, E. Shakhnovich and M. Karplus, How does a protein fold?, *Nature*, 369, 248-51, 1994.

[20] N. Socci and J. Onuchic, Folding kinetics of protein-like heteropolymers, *J. Chem. Phys.*, 101, 1519-28, 1994.

[21] H. S. Chan and K. Dill, Transition states and folding dynamics of proteins and heteropolymers, *J. Chem. Phys.*, 100, 9238-57, 1994.

[22] H. Bohr and P. G. Wolynes, *Phys. Rev. A.* , 46, 5242-5248, 1992.

[23] C. Camacho and D. Thirumalai, Modeling the role of disulfide bonds in protein folding entropic barriers and pathways, preprint, 1994.

[24] S. M. van der Vies, A. A. Gatenby, P. V. Viitanen and G. Lorimer, Molecular chaperones

and their role in protein assembly in protein folding *in vivo* and *in vitro*, *American Chemical Society*, Washington DC, 1993.

[25] K. Gulokota and P. G. Wolynes, Statistical mechanics of kinetic proof-reading in *in vivo* protein folding, *PNAS*, 91, 9292-96, 1994.

[26] F. Hoyle, *The Black Cloud*, Harper, New York, 1957.

[27] K. F. Lau and K. Dill, Theory for protein mutability and biogenesis, *PNAS*, 87, 638-42, 1990.

[28] C. Branden and J. Tooze, *An Introduction to Protein Structure*, Garland Publishing, New York, p. 62, 1991.

[29] J. Gillespie, *The Causes of Molecular Evolution*, Oxford, 1991.

[30] R. E. Dickerson and I. Geis, *Hemoglobin: Structure, Function, Evolution and Pathology*, Benjamin, Menlo Park, California, 1983.

[31] R. A. Goldstein, Z. A. Luthey-Schulten and P. G. Wolynes, Optimized energy functions for tertiary structure prediction and recognition, *Protein Structure by Distance Analysis*, H. Bohr and S. Brunak (eds.), IOS Press, Amsterdam, p. 135-44, 1994.

[32] R. A. Goldstein, Z. A. Luthey-Schulten and P. G. Wolynes, Optimal protein folding codes from spin glass theory, *PNAS*, 89, p. 4918-22, 1992.

[33] R. A. Goldstein, Z. A. Luthey-Schulten and P. G. Wolynes, Protein tertiary structure recognition using optimized Hamiltonians with local interactions, *PNAS*, 89, p. 9029-33, 1992.

[34] E. Shakhnovich, Proteins with selected sequences fold into unique native conformation, *Phys. Rev. Lett.*, 72, p. 3907, 1994.

[35] K. Koretke, Z. Luthey-Schulten and P. G. Wolynes, in preparation.

[36] K. Yue, K. Fiebig, P. D. Thomas, H. S. Chan, E. I. Shakhnovich and K. S. Dill, A test of lattice protein folding algorithms, *PNAS*, to appear 1995.

[37] Z. Luthey-Schulten, B. E. Ramirez and P. G. Wolynes, Helix-coil liquid crystal and spin glass transitions of a collapsed heteropolymer, *J. Phys. Chem.*, to appear 1995.

[38] J. Onuchic, P. G. Wolynes, Z. Luthey-Schulten and N. D. Socci, Towards an outline of the topography of a realistic protein folding funnel, *PNAS*, to appear 1995.

[39] L. D. Landau and E. M. Lifshitz, Statistical Physics, Part I, 3rd edition, *Course of Theoretical Physics, 5*, p. 531-37, J. B. Sykes and M. J. Kearsley (eds.), Pergamon Press, Oxford, 1980.

[40] N. Goldenfeld, *Lectures on phase transitions and the renormalization group*, Addison Wesley, Reading, Pennsylvania, 1992.

[41] J. Bryngelson, J. Onuchic, N. Socci and P. G. Wolynes, Funnels, pathways and the energy landscape of protein folding, *Proteins: Structure, Function and Genetics* (and references therein, to appear 1995.

[42] B. Honig, Macroscopic treatments of electrostatic and hydrophobic free energies: Applications to protein folding, *Book of Abstracts, 208th ACS National Meeting, Part II*, American Chemical Society, Washington DC, 1994.

[43] J. Bascle, T. Garel and H. Orland, Formation and stability of secondary structures in globular proteins, *J. Phys. II*, (France), 3, p. 245-53, 1993.

[44] P. G. deGennes, *Scaling Concepts in Polymer Physics*, Cornell Press, Ithaca, 1979.

[45] W. J. Albery and J. R. Knowles, Evolution of enzyme function and the development of catalytic efficiency, *Biochemistry*, 15, p. 5631, 1976.

Protein-Ligand Complexes and Protein Biosynthesis

Conserved Water Molecules and Protein Folding in Fungal Peroxidases

Sine Larsen and Jens F. W. Petersen

Centre for Crystallographic Studies, University of Copenhagen, Universitetsparken 5,
DK-2100 Copenhagen, Denmark

Abstract

The recently increased knowledge of peroxidase structures provides the basis for a detailed structural comparison of the crystal structures of the fungal peroxidases. A ligninase from *Phanerochaete chrysosporium* (LiP) and the peroxidases from *Coprinus cinereus* (CiP) and *Arthomyces ramosus* (ARP) are compared internally and with the structure of yeast cytochrome c peroxidase (CCP) with which they share less than 20% sequence identity. The peroxidases have the same overall folding, which is mainly helical but also outside the helical regions there are similarities between CCP and the fungal peroxidases. The presence of two independent molecules in the crystal structures of LiP and CiP has enabled us to identify the structurally bound water molecules in these proteins. The role of the surrounding media is elucidated by a comparison of the water molecules in ARP and CiP which are known to be identical from the amino-acid sequence, but their crystals were grown under different conditions. 30 water molecules are conserved in the structures of the fungal peroxidases. Several of these are found close to the active site and it is likely that they play a role in protein catalysis.

1 Introduction

Heme-containing peroxidases constitute an important group of enzymes that catalyze the oxidation of a variety of substrates by hydrogen peroxide. The peroxidases convert the two electron oxidation ability of hydrogen peroxide to two one electron oxidation processes. Based on the sequence alignment Welinder [1] was able to divide the heme containing peroxidases from bacteria, fungi and plants into three classes. There is less than 20% identity between the amino acid sequences of peroxidases belonging to the different classes.

Yeast cytochrome c peroxidase belonging to class I of the plant peroxidase superfamily was for many years the only peroxidase with known structure [2]. Recently, the knowledge of peroxidase structure has increased dramatically. In 1993 the structure of a lignin peroxidase isolated from *Phanerochaete chrysosporium* (LiP) was determined by two different groups [3, 4] and in 1994 the structures of two closely related fungal peroxidases from *Coprinus cinereus* (CiP) [5] and *Arthomyces ramosus* (ARP) [6] were established. It has been shown by Kjalke *et al.* [7] that the only difference between the last two enzymes appears to be in their degree of glycosylation and a possible extra amino acid of ARP at the N-terminus.

The different characteristics of the known peroxidase structures are given in Table 1. This increased insight in peroxidase structures made it possible to make a detailed analysis of the overall folding of peroxidases, e.g. the relations between class I (CCP) and class II peroxidases

Table 1: Characteristics of the "known" peroxidase structures.

Name	Acronym	Type	Number of amino-acids residues	Ca^{2+} ions present	Number of independent molecules in the crystal
Yeast Cytochrome c peroxidase	CCP	Class I	294	0	1
Ligninase from *Phanerochaete chrysosporium*	LiP fungal	Class II	343	2	2
Coprinus cinereus peroxidase	CiP	Class II fungal	343	2	2
Arthomyces ramosus peroxidase	ARP	Class II fungal	344	2	1

(LiP, CiP and ARP) and a study of the similarities and differences between the structures of the different fungal (class II) peroxidases.

Crystal structure determinations for proteins also includes a description of some of the solvent molecules found in the crystal. The position of some of the water molecules in a protein structure may depend on the crystallization conditions: pH, precipitant etc., whereas other water molecules constitute an integral part of the protein and can be regarded as "structural water". The structure of CiP to 2.0 Å resolution [8] was determined from crystals grown at pH=7.0 with PEG 6K as the precipitating agent, they contain two crystallographically independent molecules, whereas crystals grown at pH=5.0 with $(NH_4)_2SO_4$ as precipitant were used for the determination of the ARP structure to 1.9 Å resolution. These crystals contain only one independent molecule pr. asymmetric unit. This rare incidence of structures of two identical enzymes in different solvents determined to a rather high resolution has enabled us to identify structurally conserved water molecules in CiP/ARP and to compare them with water molecules in the other fungal peroxidases.

2   The folding of peroxidases

The overall folding of the peroxidases is mainly helical. The single polypeptide chain of 294 amino-acid residues of cytochrome c peroxidase (CCP) folds to form 10 helical segments of different length (labelled A to J). In addition CCP contains two antiparallel β pairs and small β-sheet. The fungal peroxidases LiP, CCP and CiP have longer polypeptide chains and share less than 20% sequence identity with CCP. Still the overall folding of peroxidases is very similar.

The LiP, CiP and ARP structures have only helices as their secondary structural elements, LiP has one, CiP and ARP two additional helices inserted between helices B and C of CCP. In order to be able to compare the folding in peroxidases an overall pairwise alignment of the polypeptide chains was made. The Cα atoms from two different structures were superimposed using the least squares algorithm in Turbo-Frodo [9] which minimizes the root mean square

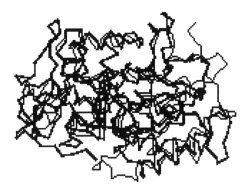

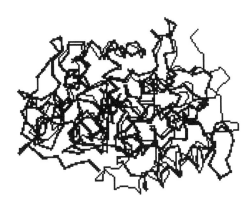

Figure 1: A stereo pair showing the overall alignment of the polypeptide chain of one of the independent molecules in the *Coprinus cinereus* peroxidase, CiPa, with the polypeptide chain of yeast cytochrome c peroxidase, CCP. The latter is shown as the thin lines and CiPa with a heavier line. The heme group almost in the center of the peroxidase structures. The N terminus starts in the top of the drawing.

deviation, RMSD, between Cα atoms within a chosen cut-off value. The number of Cα atoms used in the alignment with the associated RMSD are listed in Table 2 for different cut-off radii.

The overall agreement between the two independent CiP molecules is very good. The alignment based on all the Cα atoms in the model (it was impossible to locate the first 7 residues of the N-terminus) has a RMSD of 0.25 Å. Similar agreement is found between the two independent molecules in the LiP structure.

CiP and ARP have been shown to have identical structure and function [7] and this is also reflected in the agreement between their folding which is comparable to the internal agreement between the two CiP molecules.

CiP and LiP share ca. 45% sequence identity as indicated by the numbers in Table 2. The overall folding in these two structures is very alike. Compared to CCP the fungal

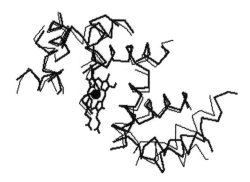

Figure 2: A pairwise alignment of the polypeptide chains of CCP and CiPa similar to the one shown in figure 1 but only showing the helical segments. CiPa is shown with the heavier lines.

Table 2: Pairwise alignments of peroxidase structures.

Cut-off (Å)	1.0 Å		2.0 Å	
	RMSD/Å	No. of Cα atoms	RMSD/Å	No. of Cα atoms
CiPa-CiPb	0.25	336	0.15	336
LiPa-LiPb	0.25	336	0.29	340
CiPa-ARP	0.25	332	0.28	334
CiPa-LiPa	0.60	223	0.90	303
CiPa-CCP	0.64	73	1.20	182

peroxidases have ca. 40 additional amino-acid residues, which are located to the C-terminus. Not unexpectedly do the CiP and CCP structures compare less well considering that they display less than 20% sequence identity. If one inspects the overlay of the two structures shown in figure 1 it is obvious that their overall structure is similar. However if one only looks at helical segments of CCP and CiP the overall similarity between the two structures is even more pronounced as shown in figure 2.

Two structurally bound Ca^{2+} ions have been found in the known fungal peroxidase structures. The topology of the peroxidases is described relative to the heme group which almost divides the structure into two domains. The bottom domain in figure 1 carries the coordinating (proximal) His 183 therefore the Ca^{2+} ion close to this group is referred to as the proximal Ca^{2+} ion. Another His is found in the upper domain adjacent to the heme group, but too far away to be coordinating. Therefore this upper domain which also contains a Ca^{2+} ion is referred to as the distal domain. The sequence alignments of the Ca^{2+} binding regions are shown in Table 3.

There is very little sequence homology between CCP and the two fungal peroxidases which contain Ca^{2+} ions. The Ca^{2+} ion in the distal domain is seven coordinated, the protein provides five of the ligands the remaining two are water molecules. The overall alignment of the CCP is shown in figure 3. We find it remarkable that the two proteins which differs so much in their sequence are so similar in their folding.

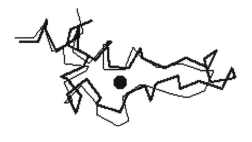

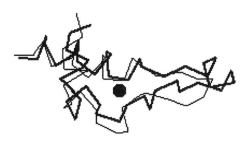

Figure 3: A stereo pair showing the folding of the polypeptide chains of CiPa and CCP in the region of the distal Ca^{2+} site in CiP. CiP and CCP are drawn as in figure 1 and 2.

Table 3: Regions in amino acid sequences in peroxidases[1].

Around the distal Ca^{2+} site

```
CCP         50A  W  H  T    S  G  T  W  D  K  -  -  -  -  -  -  H  D  N  T  G    G  S    Y    G  G    T  Y
(-Ca2+)
CIP         53V  F  H  D    A  I  G  F  S  P  A  L  T  A  A  G  Q  F  G  G  G    G  A    D    G  S    I  I
LIP         45V  F  H  D    S  I  A  I  S  P  A  M  E  A  K  G  K  F  G  G  G    G  A    D    G  S    I  M
Ca2+ Ligands     OD                                                          O     OD   OG
+2H2O            O
```

Around the proximal Ca^{2+} site

```
CCP         175  H  A  L    G  K  T  H  L  K  N  S  G  Y  E  G  -  -  P  W  G  A  A  N    N  V    F  T    N  E
(-Ca2+)
CIP         183  H  S  K    A  S  Q  E  G  L  -  N  S  A  I  F  R  S  P  L  D  S  T  P    Q  V    F  D    T  Q
LIP         176  H  S  V    A  A  V  N  D  V  -  D  P  T  V  Q  G  L  P  F  D  S  T  P    G  I    F  D    S  Q
Ca2+ Ligands     OD                                                     OD  OG          O    OD
                 O                                                      OD  O
```

Two of the eight ligands of the proximal Ca^{2+} site come from a Ser residue close to the His 55 which is a ligand to Fe in the heme group. The overall folding of CCP and

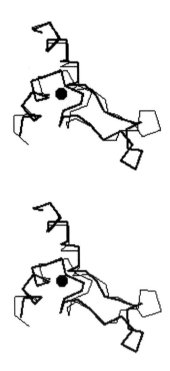

Figure 4: A stereo pair showing the protein folding of CCP and CiP close to the proximal Ca^{2+} site in CiP. CiP and CCP are drawn as in figure 1 and 2.

CiP in the region of the proximal Ca^{2+} ions binding site is shown in figure 4. Considering the differences between the amino-acid sequences of CCP and CiP we find that the overall similarity between the folding of CiP and CCP is striking. We have examined the structure of CCP for possible interatomic interactions that could account for the folding of CCP in these regions. It appears that the folding in CCP is stabilized by hydrogen bonds between the protein and water molecules in the pockets that is occupied by Ca^{2+} in the fungal peroxidases. This significance of water molecules in the protein structures leads us to the next part of this paper.

3 Conserved water molecules

Water molecules are normally introduced in the final stages of the refinement of the protein structure. They model peaks in the residual electron density in order to get a decrease in the crystallographic R-value. One should be aware that the introduction of water molecules into a protein structure is a subjective process and that the peaks in the residual electron density could also reflect different experimental errors. Therefore great care should be taken when water molecules are modelled into a protein structure.

The final model of CiP structure contains 470 water molecules [8], distributed on and between the two independent molecules. The following criteria were employed in the introduction of water molecules: They should represent density in the residual $(F_o\text{-}F_c)$ electron density map above 4σ and have density in the $(2F_o\text{-}F_c)$ map above 1σ. More importantly they should have chemically reasonable distances to potential hydrogen bond donors/acceptors, and

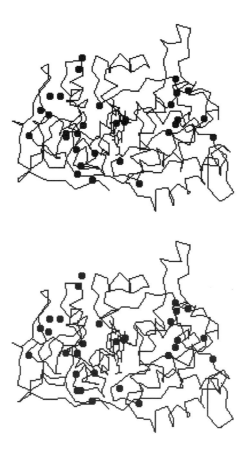

Figure 5: A stereo pair of CiP showing the distribution of the 30 water molecules that are conserved in all fungal peroxidases.

finally their refined thermal parameters should be less than 50 Å^2. The improvement of the model was monitored by both the conventional R and the free R value [10].

After a pairwise alignment of the Cα atoms had been performed as described above using a cut-off radius of 1 Å, the structurally homologous water molecules were identified as those being closer than a given cut-off radius. The results from this alignment of water molecules using cut-off radii of 0.5 Å and 1.0 Å are listed in Table 4. In the subsequent comparison of water molecules in the different peroxidase structures, we will use cut-off radii, that reflect the agreement between structures listed in Table 2.

It is noteworthy that of the 470 water molecules, which were introduced in the CiP structure, 286 (cut-off radius of 0.5 Å) represent water found at almost the same location in the two independent CiP molecules. Similar agreement can be observed for the water molecules in the LiP structure. The effect of the surrounding media is reflected in the difference in conserved water molecules (CiPa-CiPb) versus CiPab~ARP, only 85 of the 143 structural water molecules in CiP are found in ARP, which is crystallized at a different pH 5.0 instead of 7.0 and with $(NH_4)_2SO_4$ as precipitant instead of PEG 6K.

Comparing the positions of the water molecules in the fungal peroxidases we find that with a cut-off radius of 1.0 Å, 30 water molecules are found in the same place. The stereo pair

Table 4: Conserved H_2O molecules in peroxidase structures.

	0.5 Å cut-off	1.0 Å cut-off
CiPa-CiPb	143	163
LiPa-LiPb	86	124
CiPab-ARP	85	107
(CiPab-ARP)-LiPab	15	30
CiPab-ARP-LiPab-CCP	2	4

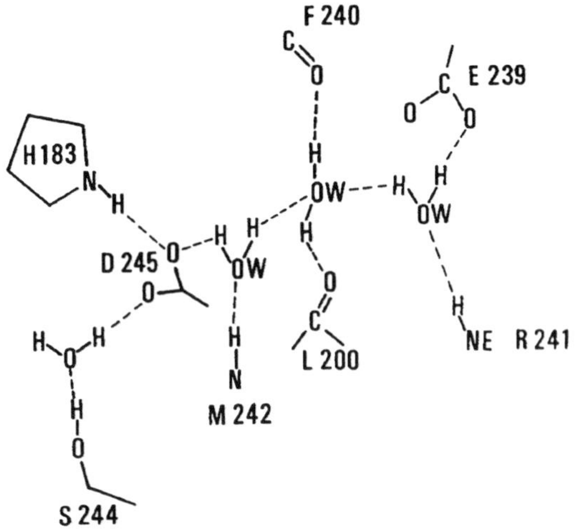

Figure 6: A schematic drawing of the hydrogen bonding system involving the four water molecules found on the proximal side of the heme group. These four water molecules are conserved in the structures of all the fungal peroxidases.

in figure 5 shows how they are distributed over the CiP structure. Six of the water molecules are close to the Ca^{2+} ions either directly as ligands or indirectly through hydrogen bonds to the ligands. It is characteristic that many of the conserved water molecules are involved in hydrogen bonding to salt bridges that are structurally conserved in the fungal peroxidase structures. In addition a fairly large fraction of the conserved water molecules are found close to the heme group. Four of these are part of an extensive system of hydrogen bonds that involve the catalytically important residues, the proximal His 183 and Asp 245.

In figure 6 a schematic drawing is shown of this system of hydrogen bonds. It is not possible to locate hydrogen atoms in a protein structure determined from X-ray diffraction data, however if one makes use of the general chemical knowledge of chemical bonding and hydrogen bond formation, it is obvious that the hydrogen atom can only be arranged in the way indicated on the schematic drawing.

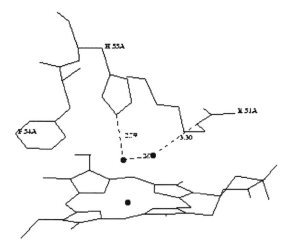

Figure 7: A drawing showing the hydrogen bonding of the two water molecules that are conserved in all peroxidase structures.

CCP differs from the fungal peroxidases by having a Trp residue at close to the heme group which carries the free radical in the catalytic cycle. Therefore this could explain why the system of hydrogen bonds shown in figure 6 is not preserved in the structure of CCP. Of the 4 water molecules that are conserved in CCP and the fungal peroxidases, two are found very close to the heme group. A common feature of all peroxidase structures is the presence of a water molecule close to the iron atom in the heme group. The refined Fe-O distances are all in the range 2.4 – 2.7 Å and are obviously dependent of the model used in the refinement. This water molecule is hydrogen bonded to another water molecule which also is preserved in all peroxidase structures. The water molecule closest to Fe is hydrogen bonded to the distal His 55 residue and the second water molecule is involved in a hydrogen bond to Arg 51 which is known also to play a role in the enzyme catalysis. These interactions are shown in Fig. 7. The first step of the catalytic cycle is the reaction with H_2O_2, and it cannot be excluded that the two conserved water molecules play a role in this process.

4   Conclusion

Despite the differences in the sequences of the polypeptide chains of peroxidases belonging to different classes they show great similarities in their overall folding.The conserved water molecules in peroxidase structures have been identified. The analysis showed that a large fraction of the water molecules introduced during the refinement of a protein structure can be regarded as structural, in the sense that they are important for the folding and the function of the protein.

Acknowledgements

This research is supported by the Danish National Research Foundation.

References

[1] K. G. Welinder, Superfamily of plant, fungal and bacterial peroxidases, *Curr. Opinion in Struc. Biol.*, 2, p. 388-393, 1992.

[2] B. C. Finzel, T. L. Poulos and J. Kraut, Crystal Structure of Yeast Cytochrome c Peroxidase Refined at 1.7 Å resolution, *J. Biol. Chem.*, 259, p. 13027-13033, 1984.

[3] T. L. Poulos, S. L. Edwards, H. Wariiski and M. H. Gold, Crystallographic Refinement of Lignin Peroxidase at 2 Å, *J. Biol. Chem.*, 268, p. 4429-4440, 1993.

[4] K. Piontek, T. Glumoff and K. Winterhalter, Low pH crystal structure of glycosylated lignin peroxidase from Phanerocheate crysosporium at 2.5 Å resolution, *FEBS Lett.*, 315, p. 119-124, 1993.

[5] J. F. W. Petersen, A. Kadziola and S. Larsen, Three dimensional structure of a recombinant peroxidase from Coprinus cinereus at 2.6 Å resolution, *FEBS Lett.*, 339, p. 291-296, 1994.

[6] N. Kunishima, K. Fukuyama, H. Matsubara, H. Hatanaka, Y. Shibano and T. Amachi, Crystal Structure of the Fungal Peroxidase from Arthromyces ramosus at 1.9 Å resolution, *J. Mol. Biol.*, 235, p. 331-334, 1994 .

[7] M. Kjalke, M. B. Andersen, P. Schneider, B. Christensen, M. SchΛlein and K. G. Welinder, Comparison of structure and activities of peroxidases from *Coprinus cinereus, Coprinus macrorhizus* and *Arthromyces ramosus*, *Biochim et Biophys. Acta*, 1120, p. 248-256, 1992.

[8] J. F. W. Petersen and S. Larsen in preparation.

[9] A. Roussel and C. Cambillau, Turbo-Frodo, Biographics, LCC MB-CNRS, Bvd. Pierre Dramard, F-13916 Marseille Cedex 20, France 1989.

[10] A. T. Brünger, The Free R value: A Novel Statistical Quantity for Assessing the Accuracy of Crystal Structures, *Nature*, 355, p. 472-474, 1992.

Interplay between Metal Coordination Geometry and Protein Structure

Rogert Bauer, Morten Bjerrum, Eva Danielsen, Esben Friis*, Jan M. Hammerstad*, Lars Hemmingsen, Marianne V. Pedersen* and Jens Ulstrup*

Department of Mathematics and Physics, Royal Veterinary and Agricultural University, Thorvaldsensvej 40, DK-1871 Frederiksberg C, Denmark
* Department of Chemistry A, Building 207, The Technical University of Denmark, DK-2800 Lyngby

Abstract

Metal containing proteins are important in numerous biological processes. The structure of the metal coordination geometry for many metal containing proteins has been determined by X-ray diffraction. A prominent feature of calcium proteins, also seen in some zinc proteins, is a flexible structure manifested in large stretches of α-helices. This is in contrast to small electron transporting copper proteins, which are very rigid in structure brought about by the presence of β-sheets. However, not much knowledge exists about the interplay between protein rigidity/flexibility and metal coordination geometry for metalloproteins. In solutions where most of these proteins function even less is known about the coordination geometry. By the nuclear technique Perturbed Angular correlation of γ rays (PAC) important information about this aspect has been derived both in the solution and crystalline state for a number of different metalloproteins. The results from this technique show that the designed rigid structure for the small blue copper proteins also is reflected in a rigid metal coordination geometry. Furthermore, the results show that the metal coordination geometry for a zinc enzyme is flexible in solution, but rigid in the crystalline state. Nevertheless, the active substrate/enzyme complex in solution is rigid probably to ensure the optimal geometry for catalysis.

1　Life, metal ions and proteins

1.1　Importance of metal ions for living species

Metal ions are important for life via many different functions [1] although metal ions themselves essentially can be characterised by rather few important properties. First of all a metal ion has a positive charge. Another important property is the ability to change oxidation state, a characteristic of the transition metals.

The concentration of copper and zinc ions is about a factor 10^5 higher in human blood than in sea water [1] whereas Al^{3+} ions have about the same abundance in blood and in sea

Metal	Flexible	Strong protein affinity	Redox properties
Calcium	Yes	No	No
Zinc	Yes	Yes	No
Copper	No	Yes	Yes

Table 1: Selected properties of the three metal ions calcium, zinc and copper including their affinity to proteins.

water indicating the biological importance of copper and zinc and the lack of importance of aluminum. However, also the concentration of Ca^{2+} ions is the same in blood and sea water in spite of the paramount importance of this element. The explanation is simple, there is plenty of Ca^{2+} ions in sea water to accommodate the biological need of man. Why, however, do biological species make use of metal ions such as Zn^{2+}, Cu^+ or Cu^{2+} when so little of them is present in nature. That mammals really need Zn^{2+} is demonstrated by the lack of growth for a diet without zinc. Similarly the use of energy stored in molecular dioxygen is impossible without copper proteins. In the next section we shall offer some explanation of why calcium, zinc and copper are used by biological species.

1.2   Interplay between protein structure and metal ion properties

The question arises whether the function of a metal ion in a protein is primarily related to the metal ions own properties, or if it an interplay between the protein structure and coordination geometry of the metal ion. To investigate this we can look at properties of importance for their interaction with proteins for the three metal ions calcium, zinc and copper. A schematic view of this is shown in table 1.

Calcium

Calcium ions have low stability constants when associated with proteins [1] whereas both zinc and copper in general have high stability constants. Calcium can therefore be used to regulate physiological processes by association and dissociation to and from a specific protein, performing its action only when calcium ions is bound to the protein. The divalent ions of calcium and zinc lack any preference for a specific coordination geometry because of their closed shells of electrons. For calcium ions this means that it can easily adapt to an environment where it is protein-bound as well as in an environment where it is not protein-bound. An important example of this is illustrated by the calcium binding protein troponin C which changes conformation upon binding of calcium ions. This is possible because of a very flexible protein structure originating from a high degree of α-helix (figure 1), and in contrast to the structure of azurin of which a large part of the structure is β-sheets (Color plate 1, page xvii).

Zinc

The flexibility in coordination geometry for zinc ions is of importance for the extremely fast catalysis for example by the zinc enzyme carbonic anhydrase, converting at a tremendous rate the massive amount of carbon dioxide produced by metabolism to bicarbonate, and then back to carbon dioxide in the lung. Such a catalysed reaction requires that the coordination sphere

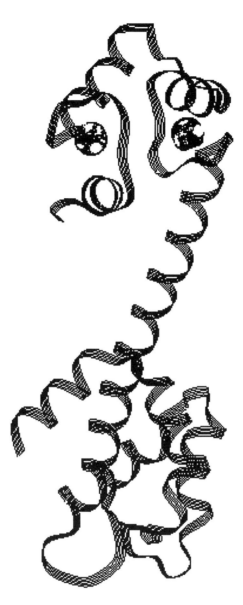

Figure 1: The structure of troponin C shown as the backbone conformation. Two out of the four calcium sites are occupied with calcium shown as solid circular objects. The program InsightII from Biosym has been used to generate the graph. The coordinates were obtained from Brookhaven Protein data bank.

of zinc in the enzyme can change with maximum speed from a geometry without substrate bound to one with substrate, and then to one with product bound. With steric restrictions a large energy barrier would be present between these states, lowering the rate of catalysis.

Copper

The only metal among these three which can change oxidation state is copper and a role as redox reagent is prominent for copper. A natural preference for specific coordination geometries only applies to copper in its oxidised form because of its unclosed d shell. The preference for a planar geometry would be accommodated when copper is incorporated for example in a heme group. It is to be expected that the protein constitutes a firm matrix for delivering a well defined coordination geometry for copper, optimal for electron transfer.

1.3 Spectroscopic techniques relevant for protein structure and metal coordination geometry

X-ray crystallography is the technique of choice if possible in order to derive detailed structural information about protein structure. Solving the three-dimensional structure of a metalloprotein does of course also give the coordination geometry of the metal. There are, however, a couple of features which X-ray diffraction does not solve. One of the most important of these concerns the structure of the protein in solution in contrast to that in the crystalline state derived from X-ray diffraction. Another feature not covered by protein crystallography is the electronic configuration of the metal ion in the protein. Particularly for metalloenzymes this is of importance because properties such as the degree of positive charge on the metal ion is decisive for the catalytic efficiency of the enzymes. For details about protein structure in solution NMR has already solved the structure for a few small proteins [2].

The local structure of a specific metal site in a metalloprotein has been studied by a number of different spectroscopic techniques. These include visual absorption spectroscopy, electron paramagnetic resonance, NMR applied to specific metals such as cadmium, magnetic circular dichroism, extended X-ray absorption spectroscopy, perturbed angular correlation of γ rays, and resonance raman spectroscopy [3].

2 Perturbed Angular Correlation of γ rays (PAC) applied to the study of metalloproteins

2.1 Simplified description of the principle of PAC spectroscopy

The technique Perturbed Angular Correlation of γ rays (PAC) can supply information about the metal coordination geometry and its possible interplay with the protein structure. The PAC method gives information about types and positions of ligands, and is very sensitive to changes in the first coordination sphere, where movement of a ligand of just a few degrees is detectable. A brief introduction to PAC-theory is given here, while a more detailed discussion can be found in Frauenfelder and Steffen [4]. The application of PAC to studies of metalloproteins is described in Bauer [5].

PAC measures the electric hyperfine interaction between a nucleus and its surroundings and requires a radioactive isotope decaying with two γ rays in succession. The following applies to the the decay of the 49 minutes ($T_{\frac{1}{2}}$) state in ^{111m}Cd.

An anisotropic distribution of angular momentum is created for the nucleus in the intermediate state reached after emission of the first γ ray in a specific direction. The electric hyperfine interaction affects this anisotropy by rotating the angular momentum of the nucleus. For a given value of the angular momentum of the intermediate state this affects the probability of emitting the second γ ray at an angle θ at time t after emission of the first γ ray. This can be expressed as

$$P(\theta, t) \propto e^{-t/\tau}(1 + A(\theta)G(t)) \tag{1}$$

where θ is the angle between the two γ rays, τ the lifetime of the intermediate state, $A(\theta)$ the anisotropy of the angular correlation resulting from the anisotropic distributions of angular momentum, and $G(t)$ describes the influence from the electric hyperfine interaction. $A(\theta)$ has a maximum in 180° and a minimum in 90°. In the absence of hyperfine interaction $G(t)$ is 1.

$G(t)$ can be written as a sum of cosines

$$G(t) = \sum_{i=1, j=1}^{2I+1} a_{ij} cos(\omega_{ij} t) \tag{2}$$

where ω_{ij} is related to the energy states E_i and E_j by $\omega_{ij} = (E_i - E_j)2\pi/h$ and h is Planck's constant. The different energies i, j come from the $2I + 1$ orientations of the angular momentum I for the intermediate state.

For ^{111m}Cd in the absence of an external magnetic field only the electric hyperfine interaction must be considered. In contrast to magnetic hyperfine interaction the electric hyperfine interaction is not a dipole interaction. This is because nuclei (in general) have no electric dipole moment. The first contribution which can affect the orientation of an angular momentum is the second derivative of the electrostatic potential equivalent to the derivative of the electric field. It is therefore called the electric field gradient. The electric hyperfine interaction is inversion symmetric, the center of the nucleus being the inversion center, with the consequence that orientations of the angular momentum opposite to one another affect $G(t)$ identically. The consequence of this is that with the angular momentum equal to $\frac{5}{2}$ for the intermediate state in ^{111m}Cd only three cosine oscillation plus a constant term (i = j) remain in $G(t)$.

The electric field is a vector with three components (x,y,z). The electric field gradient is therefore a tensor with nine components (α, β) with α and β = x,y or z. Only two parameters are needed to describe the electric field gradient for a randomly oriented ensemble of identical molecules in solution, namely the numerically largest element in the diagonalized EFG-tensor, V_{zz} and the asymmetry parameter $\eta = |V_{yy} - V_{xx}|/|V_{zz}|$. η thus ranges from 0 to 1 the value 0 representing axial symmetry, and 1 is sometimes denoted rhombic symmetry. Instead of V_{zz} we determine a parameter denoted ω_0 which is proportional to V_{zz}. The Fourier transform of $G(t)$ determined from a PAC spectrum on a ^{111m}Cd substituted metalloprotein consists of three peaks for each metal site. Situated in several different metal sites the number of lines in a Fourier transform of a PAC spectrum consists of three times the number of cadmium sites (figure 2).

In the data analysis of PAC spectra it is necessary to include rotational diffusion and frequency distributions in $G(t)$. The Brownian motion of the molecules infers that the electric field gradient at the ^{111m}Cd nucleus reorients. The reorientation is characterized by τ_r, the rotational diffusion time and its effect on $G(t)$ has been calculated [6]. Small structural variations in the coordination geometry for ^{111m}Cd in the ensemble of molecules lead to a distribution of EFG values. This can be described by a Gaussian distribution of EFG's with a relative width of δ. This frequency distribution is a measure of the rigidity of the metal site. The effect of δ representing a Gaussian distribution can be seen in figure 2.

Given the crystal structure of a cadmium complex, ω_0 and η can be calculated using the Angular Overlap Model [7].

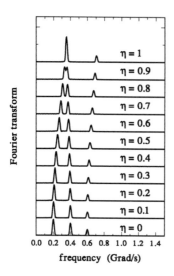 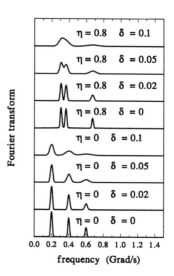

Figure 2: Fourier transform of theoretical PAC spectra. Left part: For $\omega_0 = 200$ Mrad/s the three lines are shown for $\eta = 0$ - 1. Right part: For $\omega_0 = 200$ Mrad/s and two different values of η (0 and 0.8) the three lines are shown for four different values of δ (0,0.02,0.05,0.1). δ is a relative Gaussian width of distributions of electric hyperfine interactions.

2.2   Experimental details in PAC spectroscopy

2.2.1 ^{111m}Cd production

^{111m}Cd is produced by irradiating ^{108}Pd deposited on graphite (to avoid foreign metals) with 21 MeV α particles [8]. ^{108}Pd can be separated from ^{111m}Cd on a column containing an anion exchange gel. The metals are first dissolved in *aqua regia*, whereafter the metal ions are dissolved in dilute hydrochloric acid. Under these circumstances palladium primarily exists in the form of $[PdCl_4]^{2-}$, due to its strong affinity to Cl^-, while cadmium primarily exists as the neutral $[CdCl_2]$ complex. This means that $^{111m}CdCl_2$ passes freely through the anion exchange gel column whereas $[^{108}PdCl_4]^{2-}$ is firmly attached to the column. In this manner the total amount of metal ions including the $^{111m}Cd^{2+}$ ions can be kept below 50 pmol which make PAC spectroscopy with ^{111m}Cd a very sensitive technique. After separation of palladium and cadmium adjustment of pH and buffer can be made.

2.2.2   Loading a metalloprotein with ^{111m}Cd

For details in isolating the used metalloproteins and the preparation of ^{111m}Cd substituted metalloproteins we refer to the literature [8, 9]. Adding ^{111m}Cd in the form of a convenient salt such as $^{111m}CdCl_2$ to a metalloprotein such as a copper or zinc protein does not always result in substitution of its native metal with cadmium, at least not within a few hours. This is a consequence of the tight binding of the metal ion in zinc and copper metalloproteins. Thus it is necessary first to remove the native metal ion first by prolonged dialysis against a strong metal chelator. Surprisingly the apoprotein (metalloprotein without its metal ion) does not normally collapse. This makes it possible to reconstitute an apoprotein to its native form by simply adding a salt of the native metal ion. This in itself gives important information about the interplay between protein structure and metal coordination geometry. The protein has a pre-formed configuration of the amino acids involved for metal coordination. In this way an efficient geometry for a specific catalytic function can be made.

2.2.3 PAC setup

The PAC spectrometer consists of 6 detectors arranged such that each detector is directed towards one plane of an imaginary cube, in the center of which the sample is positioned [10]. Only detector combinations in 90° and 180° are used. 6 combinations of 180° coincidence-spectra and 24 combinations of 90° coincidence spectra are collected.

3 Metal coordination geometry and protein structure for selected metalloproteins: A PAC study

3.1 Azurin

Azurin belongs to the group called blue copper protein. Azurin is a small electron transport protein with a mass of 14 kDa. Cu^{2+} accepts an electron and become Cu^+. Such a process is fast and there is no rearrangement in the protein structure during electron transfer. This is reflected in the rigid three dimensional structure of azurin from Pseudomonas aeruginosa (Color plate 1, page xvii) [11]. However, it is also characteristic that the Fourier transform of a PAC spectrum shows sharp lines for this protein with cadmium substituted for copper. This strongly indicates that not only is the overall protein structure of this protein rigid but so is also the metal coordination geometry. Interpretation of ω_0 and η derived from the three frequencies observed in the PAC spectrum from azurin from Pseudomonas aeruginosa (figure 3) leads to the conclusion that the metal geometry is triply coordinated with two histidines and one cysteine as ligands [9].

This protein has been the subject of numerous work on site directed mutants. In particular work has been performed with the amino acid methionine at position 121 in the sequence substituted with almost all known amino acids [12]. The interest in this resides in the fact that it is close to the copper ion (0.3 nm) and that there are speculations about its importance in electron transport. PAC spectra with mutants of azurin where methionine 121 is substituted with other amino acids can be found in Danielsen et al. [9]. As an example we show here a spectrum from Met121− Asp (figure 3). It is noteworthy that the lines are much broader than for wild type azurin. The rigidity in the structure of azurin [11] and its metal site [9] can thus be relaxed for the metal geometry to exhibit a larger degree of flexibility by substituting methionine with a smaller amino acid such as aspartic acid.

3.2 Carboxypeptidase A

Carboxypeptidase A is an enzyme which catalyses the cleavage of the carboxy terminal amino acid in peptides. Peptides with an aromatic amino acid at the carboxy are preferentially cleaved. It has a molar mass of 35 kDa and contains one zinc ion essential for catalysis. The three-dimensional structure is known [13] and it can be seen (Color plate 2, page xviii) that in contrast to azurin α helix is prominent. This suggest a more flexible structure than for azurin. Indeed, X-ray diffraction experiments have revealed that when substrate-like molecules bind a tyrosine residue swings in position to lock the substrate (Color plate 2, page xviii).

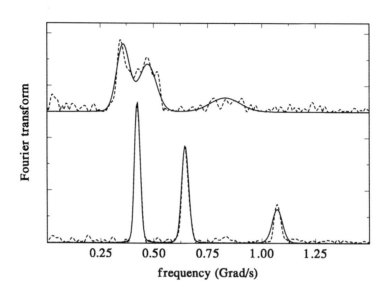

Figure 3: Fourier transform of PAC spectra from azurin (bottom) and azurin where methionine 121 is substituted with an aspartic acid residue (top). The dotted lines represent Fourier transforms of the PAC spectra and the solid lines Fourier transforms of fits to the spectra.

Whether this globally results in a more rigid structure or whether it has any consequences for the metal coordination geometry cannot be decided from the three dimensional structures available from x-ray diffraction. There exists PAC measurements both for carboxypeptidase dissolved and in the crystalline state (figure 4) [14]. The three frequencies in the PAC spectra are almost identical for the solution and crystalline states.

However, the crystalline state exhibits sharp lines whereas in solution the lines are much broader (figure 4). This could indicate that crystal packing forces a protein into a structure which has very little flexibility, whereas the protein in its native state exhibits flexibility. A particularly interesting feature using PAC is that it is possible to derive a spectrum *during* catalysis at least under steady state conditions [15]. The results of such experiments with carboxypeptidase A during peptide hydrolysis is shown in figure 4. There are two important features to note for this substrate experiment. First the frequencies are very different from the case without substrate present and secondly the lines are sharp even though the spectrum comes from carboxypeptidase A in solution. We can thus observe that the flexible coordination geometry observed for carboxypeptidase in solution becomes fixed for the substrate complex, probably because this is the most favourable geometry for catalysis.

3.3   Alcohol dehydrogenase

Alcohol dehydrogenase from the liver of a horse is like carboxypeptidase an enzyme. However, in contrast to carboxypeptidase A it is a redox enzyme. It catalyses the conversion of alcohols to aldehydes and vice versa in the presence of the coenzyme nicotinamide-adeninedinucleotide (NAD). The enzyme is a dimer with a total molar mass of 80 kD. Each monomer contains two zinc ion, one coordinated to four cysteines important for the integrity of the protein structure and one coordinated to two cysteines, one histidine and a solvent water molecule important for

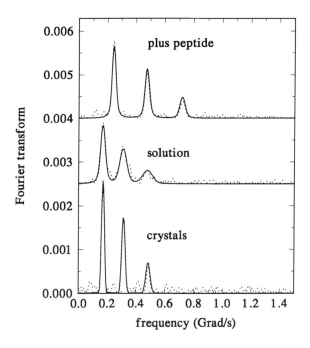

Figure 4: Fourier transform of PAC spectra from carboxypeptidase A crystallized (bottom), in solution (middle) and in solution while converting a peptide (top). The dotted lines represent Fourier transforms of the PAC spectra and the solid lines Fourier transforms of fits to the spectra.

catalysis [16]. The three-dimensional structure of alcohol dehydrogenase has been obtained not only for the native enzyme but also for its binary complexes with the coenzyme and ternary complex with coenzyme and various inhibitors and slowly converting substrates [17]. One very interesting fact relevant to this work is that the native enzyme exists in the crystalline state in a so-called open conformation and in the ternary complexes in a so-called closed conformation [17]. It appears as if the enzyme tightens its structure to fit exactly to coenzyme and inhibitor/substrate (see Color plate 1, page xvii). The spectral parameters ω_0 and η found for ^{111m}Cd in the catalytic site of alcohol dehydrogenase at low pH, in the presence of coenzyme (reduced form) and for the ternary complex between alcohol dehydrogenase, reduced coenzyme and dimethylsulfoxide agree well with the crystal structure of the ternary complex between the native zinc enzyme, reduced coenzyme and dimethylsulfoxide inhibitor [18]. The difference in ω_0 values between the three cases can be explained by movements of the coordinating groups of the order of $5°$. However, there is an important difference which can be seen in figure 5. For the free enzyme at low pH we find only one coordination geometry for cadmium in the catalytic site, although with a large frequency distribution corresponding to a flexible ligand sphere. This means that from one molecule to the next the coordination sphere is slightly different in the ligand-Cd-ligand angles. The PAC spectrum for the binary complex with NADH contains six lines all being relatively sharp corresponding to two well defined coordination geometries, i.e. the ligands are strongly fixed at their respective positions.

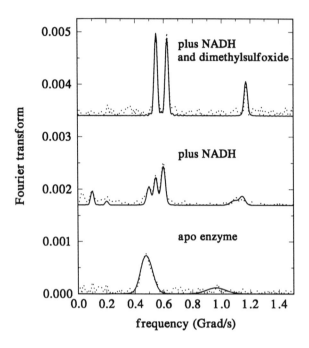

Figure 5: Fourier transform of PAC spectra from alcohol dehydrogenase (bottom), plus reduced coenzyme and with the molecule dimethylsulfoxide and reduced coenzyme. The dotted lines represent Fourier transforms of the PAC spectra and the solid lines Fourier transforms of fits to the spectra.

It can therefore be concluded that coenzyme binding to the enzyme produces a more rigid metal site. It is possible to crystallize the enzyme/reduced-coenzyme complex in both the open and the closed conformation, depending on the conditions for the crystallization [17]. The presence of two conformations for the binary complex between the enzyme and reduced coenzyme, observed via PAC spectroscopy, could be related to this. The near 50 % presence of each coordination geometry could also arise from minor differences between the two subunits not observable by X-ray diffraction. It is further striking that upon addition of both reduced coenzyme and dimethylsulfoxide three and only three sharp frequencies are observed (figure 5). We take this as representing one unique geometry optimised for catalysis as we did for carboxypeptidase A in the presence of a peptide.

4   Conclusion

To conclude we have demonstrated via combined information from X-ray diffraction data and PAC measurements that rigidity in the metal coordination sphere is imposed from the protein in azurin. We have further demonstrated that for the two zinc enzymes carboxypeptidase A and alcohol dehydrogenase they exist in solution as flexible structures with reference to the local active site near the metal. For the productive substrate complex we have shown for carboxypeptidase A that the metal geometry is rigid, as opposed to the situation without substrate. Rigidity is also obtained for the catalytic metal site in alcohol dehydrogenase when ternary complexes are formed including aldehyde substrates [15].

Acknowledgements

This work has been supported by the Danish Natural Science Council via the programme for Bioinorganic Chemistry.

References

[1] J. J. R. Frausto da Silva and R. J. P. Williams, *The Biological chemistry of the elements*, Clarendon Press, Oxford, 1991.

[2] K. Wütrich, Protein structure determination in solution by NMR spectroscopy, *J. Biol. Chem.*, 265, p./ 22059-22062, 1990.

[3] I. Bertini, C. Luchinat, W. Maret and M. Zeppezauer, *Zinc Enzymes*, Birkhauser Boston Inc., 1986.

[4] H. Frauenfelder and R. M. Steffen, Angular Distribution of Nuclear Radiation, in *Alpha-Beta and Gamma-ray Spectroscopy*. K. Siegbahn (ed.), vol. 2, North-Holland, Amsterdam, p. 97-1198, 1965.

[5] R. Bauer, Perturbed angular correlation spectroscopy and its application to metal sites in proteins: possibilities and limitations, *Quart. Rev. of Biophysics*, 18, p. 1-64, 1985.

[6] E. Danielsen and R. Bauer, Analysis of perturbed angular correlation spectra of metal ions bound to proteins with rotational correlation times in the intermediate region, *Hyp. Int.*, 62, p. 311-324, 1992.

[7] R. Bauer, S. J. Jensen and B. Schmidt-Nielsen, The angular overlap model applied to the calculation of nuclear quadrupole interactions, *Hyp. Int.*, 39, p. 203-234, 1988.

[8] R. Bauer, M. J. Bjerrum, E. Danielsen and P. Kofod, Coordination geometry of cadmium at the zinc and copper sites of superoxide dismutases: A study using perturbed angular correlations of x-rays from excited 111Cd, *Acta Chem. Scand.*, 45, p. 593-603, 1991 B.

[9] E. Danielsen, R. Bauer, L. Hemmningsen, M. Andersen, M. J. Bjerrum, T. Butz, W. Tröger, G. W. Canters, C. W. G. Hoitink, G. Karlsson, Ö. Hansson and A. Messerschmidt, Structure of metal site in azurin, Met121 mutants of azurin, and stellacyanin investigated by 111mCd Perturbed angular correlation, *PAC*, 270, p. 573-580, 1995.

[10] T. Butz, S. Saibene, T. Fraenzke and M. Weber, A "TDPAC-camera", *Nuclear Instruments and Methods in Physics Research*, A284, p. 417-421, 1989.

[11] H. Nar, A. Messerschmidt, R. Hubert, M. van de Kamp and G. W. Canters, Crystal structure analysis of oxidized Pseudomonas aeruginosa azurin at pH 5.5 and pH 9.0, A pH induced conformational transition involves a peptide bond flip, *J. Mol. Biol.*, 221, p. 765-772, 1991.

[12] B. G. Karlsson, M. Nordling, T. Pascher, L. Tsai, L. Sjölin and L. G. Lundberg, Cassette mutagenesis of met121 in azurin from Pseudomonas aeruginosa, *Prot. Eng.*, 4, p. 343-349, 1991.

[13] D. W. Christianson and W. N. Lipscomb, Carboxypeptidase A, *Acc. Chem. Res.*, 2, p. 62-69, 1989.

[14] R. Bauer, C. Christensen, J. T. Johansen, J. L. Bethune and B. L. Vallee, Perturbed angular correlation γ ray PAC spectroscopy of 111Cd carboxypeptidase A α, *R. Biochem. Biophys. Res. Comm.*, 90, p. 679-68x, 1979.

[15] R. Bauer, H. W. Adolph, I. Andersson, E. Danielsen, G. Formicka and M. Zeppezauer, Coordination geometry for cadmium in the catalytic zinc site of horse liver alcohol dehydrogenase, p. studies by PAC spectroscopy, *Eur. Biophys. J.*, 20, p. 215-221, 1991.

[16] H. Eklund, A. Jones and G. Schneider, Active site in alcohol dehydrogenase, in *Zinc Enzymes*, I. Bertini, C. Luchinat, W. Maret and M. Zeppezauer (eds.), Birkhauser Boston Inc, p. 377-392, 1986.

[17] E. Cedergren-Zeppezauer, Coenzyme binding to three conformational states of horse liver alcohol dehydrogenase, in *Zinc Enzymes*, I. Bertini, C. Luchinat, W. Maret and M. Zeppezauer (eds.), Birkhauser Boston Inc, p. 393-416, 1986.

[18] S. Al-Karadaghi, E. S. Cedergreen-Zeppezauer, K. Petratos, S. Hovmoeller, H. Terry and K. S. Wilson, Refined crystal structure of liver alcohol dehydrogenase NADH complex at 1.8 A resolution, *Acta Cryst.*, D50, p. 793-807, 1994.

Elongation Factor Tu:
A G-protein in Protein Biosynthesis

P. Nissen, M. Kjeldgaard, S. Thirup, L. Reshetnikova*, G. Polekhina, B. F. C. Clark and J. Nyborg

Institute of Chemistry, Aarhus University, Langelandsgade 140, DK-8000 Aarhus C, Denmark and
* Engelhardt Institute of Molecular Biology, Russian Academy of Sciences, 15 Vavilov Str., Moscow, Russia

Abstract

Elongation factor Tu (EF-Tu) binds guanosine phosphates as co-factors. It was the first structurally known member of the now large super-family of G-proteins. All G-proteins are found in an active state with GTP as co-factor while the proteins with GDP as co-factor are inactive. All G-proteins have a special domain (the G-domain) binding the co-factors. This domain has well conserved sequences mainly involved in co-factor binding. All G-proteins have intrinsic GTP-ase activities which eventually will shut off the active state. The GTP-ase activity can be stimulated by GTP-ase activating proteins. The members of the super-family have very diverse biological functions. The major families are:

1. The small G-proteins, which have only one domain, the G-domain. They are involved in transduction of cell signals. The best known of these is the *ras* oncogene product p21, which is involved in cell proliferation. Single point mutants of p21 are found in large amounts in cancer transformed cells.
2. The heterotrimeric G-proteins, which are composed of three different subunits. They are involved in the transduction of extracellular signals such as hormones, neuro transmitter molecules, light, taste and smell.
3. The elongation factors, which have several domains. They take part in the protein biosynthesis of every living cell.

EF-Tu:GTP binds aminoacylated tRNA (aa-tRNA), protects it from deaminoacylation and transports aa-tRNA to the ribosome where EF-Tu catalysts the recognition of specific codons on mRNA. Hereby a protein with a sequence coded for in a given gene can be synthesized on the ribosome. The structures of the inactive EF-Tu:GDP, the active EF-Tu:GTP and of aa-tRNA:EF-Tu:GTP are presented and discussed. There is a surprisingly large conformational change associated with the activation of EF-Tu. The active form provides binding clefts for aa-tRNA. The crystal structure of aa-tRNA:EF-Tu:GTP is very elongated and has a surprising similarity to the structure of EF-G:GDP.

1   Introduction

The field of G-protein function and structure is expanding rapidly in this period of time. Significant new information on the function of the ras-oncogene product p21 is found in almost every issue of every journal of biochemistry. During the last few years structures of many important G-proteins have appeared in the literature. It is therefore strange to witness this revolution in knowledge and interest in G-proteins for a group of researchers who have worked for the last 25 years on protein biosynthesis and especially on ribosomal protein factors. For about 15 years it was thought that proteins using GDP/GTP as co-factors to switch between an inactive and active form of the protein was an oddity for some strange evolutionary reasons only restricted to protein biosynthesis. The discovery in 1985 by Karen Halliday [1] that there were common sequence homologies between Elongation Factor Tu (EF-Tu) and p21 opened up the work of defining G-protein consensus sequences [2, 3]. The consensus sequences were almost immediately realized from the structure of the G-domain of EF-Tu to be determined for the main part by the binding of the co-factor GDP [4].

Now G-proteins are found in many important areas of biology and medicine. They generally work as molecular switches where they when bound to GTP record that an important biological event has happened thus transducing and amplifying a signal to places where the effect of the event has to result in specific biological actions. Normally after some time the switch is turned off either by intrinsic hydrolysis of GTP to GDP or stimulated by the resulting action of other biological events. The molecular switch is turned off in its GDP form until it is re-activated by a new biological event. In the ras oncogene studies it is now known that point mutations interfering with the hydrolysis of GTP will transform normal cells into cancer cells [3].

The present paper describes crystal structures as determined in our laboratory of some of the complexes of EF-Tu. However, some of the conclusions which can be drawn from our work seem to be general enough to be applicable to the other G-proteins. As a general background we will give the present biochemical knowledge on protein biosynthesis. Thereafter we will discuss the general features of all G-proteins. And finally we will try to demonstrate that structural knowledge about one member can shed some light on other members of this large family of biologically important proteins.

1.1   Protein biosynthesis

The genetic information found on DNA in all living cells contains instructions on how to produce proteins. The information for a given protein (or small groups of proteins) is transcribed into shorter pieces of messenger RNA (mRNA). The transcription process is controlled by transcription factors, which again are controlled by a cascade of enzymes (usually kinases) derived from internal or external biological events. In higher organisms the mRNA is further processed as the genetic information normally is spread out over a longer stretch of DNA with intervening nonsense DNA (introns). Part of the information on the mRNA is translated into a specific sequence of amino acids in the given protein using triplets of RNA bases according to the genetic code. The mRNA contains specific start and stop codons (triplet of bases). Furthermore the mRNA contains stretches of bases outside the coding area which is used by protein initiation factors and ribosomal RNA (rRNA) to recognize and initiate the start of protein biosynthesis.

The actual translation takes place on a very large complex of proteins and rRNAs called the ribosome. The purpose of the ribosome is to promote the peptide bond formation between amino acids in the correct sequence as coded for on mRNA. Single amino acids are brought to the ribosome by amino acid specific transfer RNA (tRNA) which at one end contains the

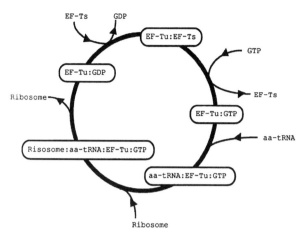

Figure 1: EF-Tu cycle. Around the circle are shown in boxes the complexes in which EF-Tu participate in one complete round of peptide elongation.

anticodon (a triplet of bases that can hydrogen bond to a codon) and at the other end the amino acid coded for by the codon. The ribosome particle has two subunits, which in bacterial systems are called the 50S and the 30S particle according to their sedimentation constants.

The translation process is divided into three different steps: initiation, elongation and termination. The initiation is catalyzed by initiation factors, the purpose of which is to recognize the initiation signals on the the mRNA and to assemble the two ribosomal particles and a special initiator tRNA (always attached to the amino acid fMet) in a so-called initiation complex. The termination is catalyzed by specific termination factors which will release the final product, a newly synthesized protein, from the ribosome particle. Elongation is a cyclic process involving two elongation factors. One called elongation factor G (EF-G) catalyzes the translocation of the ribosome particle on the mRNA, so that the next codon is exposed. During this process there are always two tRNAs on the ribosomal particle each attached to two consecutive codons. The purpose of the other, EF-Tu, is to protect the ester bond between an amino acid and its tRNA against hydrolysis. Furthermore it catalyzes the recognition between the anticodon on tRNA and the codon on mRNA. It also catalyzes the transformation of the ribosome into a form where the incoming amino acid can be coupled via peptide bond formation to the growing polypeptide.

1.2   EF-Tu cycle

During one round of peptide formation on the ribosome EF-Tu goes through its own specific cycle [5] as seen in figure 1.

The biochemically stable and inactive form of EF-Tu is the complex with the co-factor GDP, EF-Tu:GDP. The elongation factor Ts (EF-Ts) is a nucleotide exchange factor which catalyzes the exchange of the co-factor GDP for the co-factor GTP thus transforming EF-Tu into its active state. As far as known at the present the action of EF-Ts is not controlled, a fact which is significantly different from other G-proteins. In its active state EF-Tu:GTP can recognize aminoacylated tRNA (aa-tRNA) and form the socalled ternary complex, aa-tRNA:EF-Tu:GTP. This ternary complex enters the recognition process on the ribosome. A complex with a tRNA which can form hydrogen bonds to the exposed codon (a cognate tRNA) will enter into the elongation step. When a ternary complex is bound to the ribosome a GTP-ase activating center on the ribosome stimulates the GTP hydrolysis and EF-Tu leaves the ribosomal particle as inactive EF-Tu:GDP. The tRNA is now left in the A (aminoacyl-tRNA) site of the ribosome while the growing peptide is attached to a tRNA in the P (peptidyl-tRNA) site. A transpeptidylation reaction is catalyzed by the ribosome. This reaction leaves the elongated peptidyl-tRNA in the A-site and the now free tRNA in the P-site. EF-G catalyzes the translocation along mRNA and of peptidyl-tRNA into the P-site and free tRNA into the E (Exit) site. The ribosome particle is now ready for the next round of elongation.

2 G-proteins

The cyclic reactions of EF-Tu as shown in figure 1 are quite general for all G-Proteins. The transformation between the inactive and the active state is catalyzed by a G nucleotide exchange factor (GEF), which in most cases (but not in protein biosynthesis) is controlled by other proteins. The transformation between the active and the inactive state is controlled by an intrinsic GTP-ase activity the speed of which can vary. This transformation can also be catalyzed by GTP-ase activating proteins (GAPs) which rapidly shuts down the active state of the G-protein. In its GTP form the G-protein is interacting with its effector molecule which is perhaps the first one in a longer cascade of enzymes responsible for the biological response to the G-protein signal.

The amino acid sequences of G-proteins all have the same set (or subset) of five consensus elements as seen in figure 2.

All of the elements have amino acids involved in GDP/GTP binding while some are responsible for a molecular switch mechanism. This mechanism signals to other proteins the presence or absence of GTP in its binding pocket. The first element (G/A)XXXXGK(T/S) is a phosphoryl binding loop. The two small amino acids are there to introduce flexibility into the loop. Mainchain NHs are involved in binding of the β-phosphate. The sidechain of K is making a saltbridge to β- and γ-phosphates while T/S provides a sidechain oxygen as ligand to Mg^{++}. In the second element T the sidechain of T has an oxygen as ligand to Mg^{++} in the GTP form while it is not part of the coordination sphere in the GDP form. This element was for obvious reasons not easily recognized as important in the first attempts at defining consensus elements, but was defined after the structures of p21:GDP and p21:GTP were known [6, 7]. It is often found at the C-terminal end of a loop between two helices. This loop varies both in length and in sequence. It is supposed to interact with a specific effector molecule. It is termed the effector loop and the variation is likely due to the variation in structure and function of effector molecules. It is also sometimes termed the switch 1 loop as it is one of two (or three) loops which undergoes larger structural changes in response to the type of the co-factor. In the third element DXXG the D sidechain makes one hydrogen bond to T/S in the first element and probably stabilizes a water in the coordination sphere of Mg^{++}. The G residue is very important in transmitting the type of bound nucleotide to the switch 2 region which follows in sequence and which comprises a loop, a helix and a loop. The fourth element NKXD provides part of the specific recognition of the Guanine base as D makes hydrogen bonds to N1 and N2. The side chain of K makes a hydrogen bond with the endocyclic O of the ribose while N most likely provides a structural link between element one and element five. The fifth element SA (which is not found in all G-proteins) provides further recognition of the G base by a mainchain NH and S sidechain OH hydrogen bond to O6.

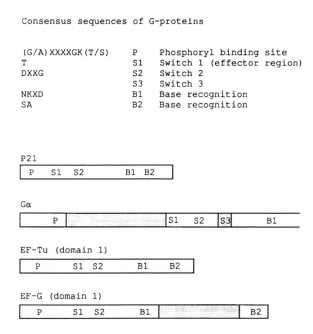

Figure 2: G-protein consensus sequences. At the top is shown in the first column the consensus sequences, in the second column a notation for a function of the sequence and in the third column the function in text. In the panels below are shown schematically the length in amino acids of G-domains from different proteins. The positions of consensus sequences are indicated. Shadowed areas give parts that represent major inserts.

2.1 The major families

The super-family of G-proteins comprises a very diverse set of biological functions some of which will not be mentioned here. However, there are three major families with comparable functions and overall structure.

The first of these is the family of small G-proteins. They are all of the approximate size of 21 kDa the main part of which is the G-domain responsible for GDP/GTP binding. The *ras* oncogene product p21 (deriving its name from its size) is one representative. There are however sub-families of this family. It is now known that p21 is transducing an extracellular control signal determining cell proliferation. This is why single point mutations of p21 are found as a major form of oncogenic protein in many forms of cancer. The structures of p21:GDP and of p21:GTP are known [6, 7]. This pair of structures were the first to indicate the important structural differences between the active and inactive state of a G-protein. It is characteristic for this family that they all have a relatively short effector loop.

The next one is the family of heterotrimeric G-proteins. They are composed of three different subunits Gα, Gβ and Gγ. They all are associated with the cytosolic part of a transmembrane receptor, which when activated by an external signal works as a nucleotide exchange factor. In its inactive state this G-protein binds GDP to its Gα subunit which is associated with the G$\beta\gamma$ subunits. When activated Gα:GTP dissociates from G$\beta\gamma$. A classical function of this type of G-proteins is transduction of hormonal signal where the direct intracellular effect is activation of adenylate cyclase and elevated concentrations of cAMP. Another well described function is that of transducin which interacts with rhodopsin in the eye and activates cGMP phosphodiesterase which decreases the concentration of cGMP. Such G-proteins are also involved in the transduction of taste and smell. Some G-proteins called Gi transduce inhibition signals. During the last few years the crystal structures of transducin Gtα:GTP [8] and transducin Gtα:GDP [9] have been determined. Very recently also the structure of Giα:GTP has been published [10]. These structures show a G-domain with essentially the same structure as p21. However there is a large inserted extra domain at the place of the effector loop (Fig. 2). This domain covers the nucleotide binding site. The structures indicate that this family of G-proteins have a third switch region as seen in figure 2.

The last major family comprises the elongation factors. It is not large but is distinctly different from the others and is probably the oldest family. Its nucleotide exchange factors are either not controlled (EF-Tu) or non existent (EF-G). They are all multidomain proteins with varying sizes. Their effector molecules are very different: aa-tRNA for EF-Tu and the ribosome for EF-G. The crystal structures of EF-Tu:GDP [11] and EF-Tu:GTP [12, 13] are known. Recently the structures of nucleotide-free EF-G [14] and EF-G:GDP [15] have been determined after many years of very difficult work on fragments of EF-G [16]. The N-terminal domain of both factors is a G-domain. EF-G has a rather large insert into this domain. The second domain of both is very similar. The third N-terminal domain of EF-Tu is similar to its second domain. EF-G has three N-terminal domains all similar to different known ribosomal proteins. This family comprises furthermore the initiation factor IF-2 and release factor RF-3.

2.2   The general G-Domain

The structure of the G-domain is that of a typical nucleotide binding protein. It has a central six stranded β-sheet where all strands except one are parallel. This sheet is surrounded by five or six α-helices. Comparing structures of the known G-proteins reveals the common structurally stable scaffold but also areas of some structural variability. A generic G-domain is seen in color plate 3 (See page xix). This should be compared to the sequence overview of the three major families in figure 2. It is obvious that all β-strands of the central β-sheet are well preserved in all known structures. Helix A with its dipole towards the phosphates of the nucleotide is also preserved although it has varying length, 9 residues in p21, 12 residues in heterotrimeric G-proteins and 16 residues in elongation factors. The effector (switch 1) loops have greatly varying sizes. In Heterotrimeric G-proteins this is a complete domain of about 120 residues. The loop-helix B-loop motif of the switch 2 region also displays some very interesting small differences. In most G-proteins the C-terminal loop is rather short, while in EF-Tu it is longer. This could account for the larger movement of helix B in the switch mechanism of EF-Tu. There is a large insert of about 90 residues between helix D and strand 6 in EF-G making the G-domain somewhat larger for this protein. Finally there is some variability in structure between strand 6 and helix E. EF-Tu has an extra helix here, which in thermophilic bacteria are longer than in *E. coli*. In p21 this helix is not present. All of these differences most likely point to areas responsible for the divergent functions of the different G-proteins.

2.2.1   GTPase activity

The G-proteins have greatly varying intrinsic GTP-ase activities. The lowest one is that of EF-Tu while that of p21 is slightly higher. The intrinsic GTP-ase activity of heterotrimeric G-proteins is relatively high. It is tempting to see this difference as expressing two types of switches. The switch of the heterotrimeric G-proteins could be described as timer switches which will turn off on its own after some time. The slow activity switches could then be described as time-delayed switches waiting for specific events to happen that will trigger the turn off.

The actual mechanism of the intrinsic GTP-ase activity has been a matter of some dispute. An early observation showed the surprising fact that none of the conserved residues pointed to a common mechanism. However, it was shown that His84 of EF-Tu when mutated to Gly showed a 20-fold reduction in activity. A similar 15-fold reduction was found in p21 of the structurally equivalent mutant Gln61 to Leu. However, it has been disputed that Gln61 can act as a general base in the catalysis. A recent paper points to the possibility that the γ-phosphate could act as the base in its own hydrolysis [17].

2.2.2 Switch regions

Switch regions in the G-proteins are defined as areas of the protein which will adopt different structures depending on the type of co-factor. Such switch regions are most likely recognized by molecules that are influenced by the inactive or active state of the G-protein. The switch 1 region is between helix A and strand b. In the p21 structure this is termed the effector loop because point mutations in this region affect the interaction with the effector molecule. The switch 2 region is loop-helixB-loop. In the EF-Tu structure this is the interface of the G-domain with the rest of the molecule. It is responsible for a very large conformational change of EF-Tu during switching as can be seen in color plate 4 (See page xx). Similar but not identical changes in this region can be seen in other G-proteins. However, nothing is known about the effect of possible partners binding to this region. The switch 3 region unique to the heterotrimeric G-proteins lies between strand 4 and helix C. The function of this region is at present unclear [18].

3 Structures of inactive and active forms of EF-Tu

The obvious goals of the structural work performed in our group on EF-Tu has been to investigate as many as possible of the complexes around the EF-Tu cycle as seen in figure 1. From the outset it was quite natural to choose to work on the binary complex EF-Tu:GDP, as this is the biochemically most stable of all complexes, apart from the complex EF-Tu:EF-Ts, which at the time was thought to be too big for an easy structural investigation. The reasons for the relative biochemical instability of the other complexes are that the co-factor GTP is rather easily hydrolyzed in water, that EF-Tu has an intrinsic GTPase activity and that the ester bond between an amino acid and the 3'-terminal ribose in aa-tRNA is hydrolyzed in water although this bond is protected to some degree against hydrolysis in the ternary complex aa-tRNA:EF-Tu:GTP.

The choice of EF-Tu:GDP as the first subject for crystal structure determination was in retrospect very unfortunate. The structure is not very stable, as can be seen from elevated temperature factors of one structural domain [11]. Furthermore the complex is very easily modified by proteases, which introduce hydrolysis at Arg44 and Arg58 (*E. coli* numbering) within the first minute of treatment with trypsin and further hydrolysis at Arg263 after prolonged trypsin treatment. Finally for many years only protein with the 14 amino acid peptide (44 to 58) removed gave crystals suitable for X-ray diffraction. The many years of frustrating work in our group and in others are described in the paper by Kjeldgaard and Nyborg [11]. Intact EF-Tu:GDP does give mainly smaller rod-like crystals. However, at present the use of synchrotron radiation and cryo-techniques can give data of a quality that allows structural determination on problems, which only a few years ago were intractable. The structural determination of the ternary complex also benefited from this development in data collection techniques as well as developments in methods for Molecular Replacement and Computer Graphics.

3.1 Structure of EF-Tu:GDP

Here we describe for the first time the crystal structure of the intact form of EF-Tu:GDP. The structural determination of this complex has recently been made more important by several comments by our colleagues about the possibility that the structure of the modified EF-Tu:GDP [11] could be an artefact of the crystal packing or not presenting the physiologically important structure. This was mainly spurred by the discovery of a very large conformational change between the structure of modified EF-Tu:GDP and intact EF-Tu:GTP [12, 13], which is described in more details later. The viewpoint received extra support from the structure determinations of nucleotide-free EF-G [14] and EF-G:GDP [15]. These structures showed two structural domains, domains 1 and 2, very similar to domains 1 and 2 of EF-Tu:GTP also in their relative orientation.

The present structure of intact EF-Tu:GDP from *E. coli* is based on data to 3.8 Å resolution. This of course does not allow us to give a very detailed account of the structure. However it does allow us to answer the question of whether the large conformational change is an artefact. First the structures of modified EF-Tu:GDP and of intact EF-Tu:GDP are indeed very similar. The structure consists of three structural domains. Domain 1 (residues 1 to 200), which has a central six-stranded β-sheet surrounded by six α-helices in a fold characteristic of nucleotide binding proteins, does contain the binding site for the co-factors GDP or GTP. Most of the conserved residues in the general G-protein consensus sequence are explained by the nucleotide binding as seen in color plate 3 (See page xix). The two other domains, domain 2 (residues 209 to 292) and domain 3 (residues 300 to 393), are both antiparallel β-barrels. Domains 1 and 2 are linked together by a short 8 residue long peptide of irregular structure, thus creating a strange hole in the structure (see Color plate 4, page xx).

3.2 Structure of EF-Tu:GTP

The structure of the active form of EF-Tu has been determined in a complex with the non-hydrolyzable analogue GDPNP, where the bridging oxygen between the β- and γ-phosphate has been replaced by NH. This structure is determined for proteins from *Thermus thermophilus* and from *Thermus aquaticus* [12, 13]. The structure shows the same three domains as found in the the inactive EF-Tu:GDP. Domains 2 and 3 essentially have the same structure. Their relative relationship is well maintained, but moving as a rigid body they have a completely new spatial relationship to domain 1 (the G-domain). The structure of domain 1 is also for a major part the same as found in EF-Tu:GDP. However the important switch regions display major local structural changes as seen in color plate 5 (See page xxi). As one of these regions, switch 2, in both structures form part of the interface between domain 1 and domains 2+3 the large conformational change is due to the local structural change of switch 2. The nucleotide binding site is surprisingly little affected by the introduction of GDPNP instead of GDP. The GDPNP co-factor binds for most part exactly as the GDP co-factor. The extra phosphate group is held by Lys24 (*E. coli* number) which forms a contact with one oxygen. However, this residue is already in the GDP structure involved in contacts with the β-phosphate. Another oxygen of the γ-phosphate is replacing one water as ligand to the Mg^{++} ion. The last oxygen is apparently involved in a hydrogen-bond contact with backbone NH of Gly83. Relative to the EF-Tu:GDP structure the peptide bond before the conserved consensus Gly83 is flipped by approximately 150°. This minor distortion of the co-factor binding pocket results in the major overall structural change of the protein upon binding of the GDPNP co-factor. Finally a rather noticeable feature of the structure is the entrapped catalytic water as seen in color plate 6 (See page xxi). Details about the shift in ligands around the Mg^{++} ion cannot be given here due to the low resolution of the GDP structure. However, it is reasonable to assume that Thr61, which is a ligand in the GDPNP structure, is forced out of the coordination sphere and replaced by water in the GDP structure in analogy with what is seen in the structure of p21 [6, 7].

The overall structure of EF-Tu:GTP displays a narrow cleft between domains 1 and 2, thus closing the strange hole in the GDP structure. It also forms a much wider cleft between domains 1 and 3. Both clefts were thought to be part of the binding site for aminoacylated tRNA [13].

3.3 Structural delineation of the switch mechanism

As can be seen from color plate 4 (See page xx) the effect of exchanging the co-factor from GDP to GTP has a major effect on the overall structure of EF-Tu. If domains 2 and 3 of the two structures are superimposed the relative shift of the position of domain 1 corresponds to a rotation of about 90°[13]. This is not just a sliding rotation of the two parts of the molecule relative to each other. It does imply a temporary dissociation followed by a re-association of the two parts. This is reminiscent of the function of the heterotrimeric G-proteins, where the $G\alpha$ subunit corresponds to the G-domain of EF-Tu [13]. Here it is known that upon activation of the receptor the $G\alpha$ subunit exchanges its GDP co-factor for GTP. In its GDP form $G\alpha$ forms a tight complex with $G\beta\gamma$. However, after nucleotide exchange $G\alpha$ dissociates.

At least part of what is happening in the switch between the two structural forms can be postulated from the structural comparison of EF-Tu:GDP and EF-Tu:GDPNP. As mentioned above the only immediate result of the change of the co-factor from GDP to GTP seems to be a flip of the peptide before Gly83 (and possibly a displacement of Thr61 from the coordination-sphere of Mg^{++}). However, the conformation of the main-chain at this glycine is apparently critical for the structure of the following helix B. In the GDP structure this helix starts at the next residue His84. The structure thus has a rather short loop from β-strand b to helix B. On the other hand the loop from helix B to β-strand c is rather long (residues 94-100). This longer N-terminal loop is in strange contrast to the structure of p21 [6]. In the GTP structure the C-terminal loop now becomes longer while the N-terminal loop is shorter. This amounts to a sliding of the helix structure by about 4 residues along the sequence. This simultaneous change in length of the two loops forces the helix to rotate about 45° around an axis perpendicular to the helix axis as seen in color plate 5 (See page xxi). As helix B together with helix C forms the interface to domain 3 the GDP structure collapses, the domains dissociate and re-associates to form the GTP structure and thereby exposing the binding sites for aminoacylated tRNA.

4   Structure of a G-Protein effector complex

One of the central questions in the field of structural studies of G-proteins is how a G-protein interacts with its nucleotide exchange factor. At present no answer can be given to this. However, it is quite obvious from comparisons of amino acid sequences that there most likely is no unifying scheme. Another central question is how G-proteins interact with their effectors. Again the nature and structure of effector molecules are seen to be very divergent and dependent on the nature of the biological process controlled by the G-protein. In protein biosynthesis the immediate effector molecule is even an RNA molecule, aminoacylated tRNA.

EF-Tu:GTP enters into the ternary complex aa-tRNA:EF:Tu:GTP in order to protect the ester bond between the amino acid and the 3'-terminal ribose of tRNA. Furthermore it catalyzes the recognition between the anticodon on tRNA and the codon on mRNA. Finally it assists in placing the aa-tRNA molecule in the A-site of the ribosome. Now for the first time we can report on the structure of a G-protein effector complex.

4.1   Structure of the ternary complex of aa-tRNA:EF-Tu:GTP

The preliminary crystal structure of the ternary complex of *Thermus aquaticus* EF-Tu:GDPNP with yeast Phe-tRNA ^{Phe} is seen in figure 3. It is seen that the complex is rather elongated with a very small contact area in the complex. This is very much in contrast with previous speculations and models based on biochemical data. The main reason for this discrepancy seems to be that an elongated molecule was thought to have unfavourable hydrodynamic properties. However, in the crystal the asymmetric unit packing shows a trimer of ternary complexes as seen in figure 3. In this trimer the tRNA crystal contacts are similar to those of the crystal structure of free tRNA[19,20].

The contact areas between the RNA and protein molecules are found in clefts of EF-Tu. One narrow cleft is accommodating the single-stranded CCA-end. At this end the amino acid is attached and protected by the protein in this cleft. This binding cleft is easily seen in the crystal structure of EF-Tu:GTP [12,13] and has earlier been the basis of several models of the ternary complex. None of these earlier models are in agreement with the preliminary crystal structure. The binding mode is also as expected very different from the ones now known from several structures of tRNA synthetases, however, much detail remains to be determined. The T- and D-loops of tRNA are not in contact with the protein. The binding area on the protein was proposed earlier [13].

4.2   Is a Trimer found in solution?

It is very tempting to speculate that the trimer of ternary complexes is also found in solution. Such an assumption is in contrast with some observations, of which we will mention low angle scattering studies [21]. However, biochemical foot-printing experiments on tRNA indicate correctly the contact area with EF-Tu. Furthermore they show further protections of tRNA, which are in good agreement with such a proposed trimer [22]. Some of the contrasting experiments and especially the low angle scattering experiments should be redone with the view of testing such an hypothesis.

We can immediately see some advantages of such a trimer. It would have improved hydrodynamic properties over the monomer. And assuming a random content of tRNAs in the trimers they could deliver at the same time three aa-tRNAs for testing in the recognition process on the ribosome. At the relative high concentrations of ternary complexes in the cell packing these into trimers where they could be stored until needed in protein biosynthesis could be a further advantage.

4.3   Structural similarity EF-Tu:GTP and EF-G:GDP

A very unexpected feature of the structure of EF-Tu:GTP came to light when someone asked the question why the relative orientations of domains 1 and 2 are so similar in EF-Tu:GTP [13] and in EF-G:GDP [15]. It was not at all obvious that the inactive form of EF-G should have a structure similar to that of the active form of EF-Tu.

By overlaying the two domains from the two structures it is found that the structures of the two N-terminal domains of EF-G are indeed similar to the ones of EF-Tu as can be seen from

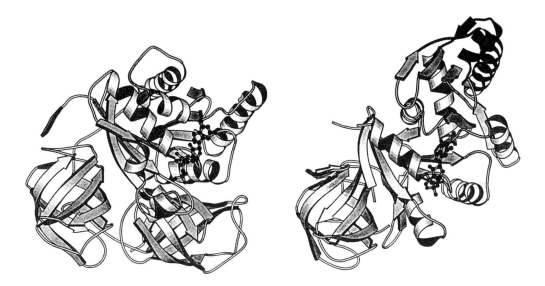

Figure 3: Structures of EF-Tu:GDPNP (left, domains 1, 2 and 3) and EF-G:GDP (right, domains 1 and 2) in the same relative orientation. The nucleotides are shown in ball-and-stick representation. EF-G contains a small insert, approximately 50 residues long, seen in a darker shade at the top right hand corner. Notice the similarity in the folding of domain 2 in the two structures (lower left). Although domain 1 in the two structures appear somewhat different, the details of the nucleotide binding are extremely similar.

figure 3. The domains 3 and 5 of EF-G are seen to be very similar to a number of known ribosomal proteins for reasons that are still unclear. Domain 4 has a very unusual structure in that one helix cross-over between two β-strands is left-handed [14,15]. This is found in only very few proteins all of which are involved in RNA or DNA interactions [23]. However, the structures of these three C-terminal domains are presumably such that they are ideally suited for interaction with other ribosomal proteins and with ribosomal RNA. This is to our knowledge the first time that it has been demonstrated that the long known structural similarity of G-domains can now be extended to include another domain.

4.4   Immediate conclusions

Why this striking similarity? The similarity of the relative orientations of domains 1 and 2 of EF-Tu and EF-G in retrospect could have been much more expected. The two factors are catalyzing two oppositely directed transformations of the ribosome. And quite obviously EF-G after it has done its job is followed by the step on the ribosome which is the decoding and the binding of the ternary complex. Moreover, we can now conclude that the folding and structure of domain 2 is common to EF-Tu and EF-G and most likely also for all other G-proteins in protein biosynthesis.

5   Concluding remarks

We are eagerly waiting to see the structure of EF-G:GTP. This perhaps will give us the first glimpse of the conformational state of the other main form of the ribosome. We are also eagerly waiting to see whether the structural similarity of domains 1 and 2 of EF-Tu and EF-G will be shown to exist also in other G-proteins of protein biosynthesis. We are thus planning to determine the structure of IF2 and RF3.

We hope to see very soon the first experimental indications of whether the trimer of the ternary complex is found in solution. We ourselves will work on the structures of ternary complexes of other aa-tRNAs in order to see whether the trimer will be found also in other crystal structures. At the same time we want to structurally investigate the nature of the observed differences in stabilities of different ternary complexes.

The structural determination of the ternary complex of EF-Tu, the dream goal of so many crystallographers over the past 25 years, as usual for crystallographic results answered many questions in an unexpected way. It certainly also immediately raises a number of new challenging questions to be answered in the coming years.

Acknowledgements

We would like to thank for the excellent technical help provided by G. Siboska and L. Bich Van. We have received invaluable help with data collection from P. F. Lindley and his staff at SRS, Daresbury. The work has been supported by the Danish Natural Science Research Council through its Programme for Biotechnology in the Protein Engineering Research Center and by networks for Protein Crystallography and for Elongation Factor Tu supported through the Human Capital and Mobility Programme at EU.

References

[1] K. R. Halliday, Regional homology in GTP-binding proto-oncogene products and elongation factors, *J. Cyc. Nucl. Prot. Res.*, 9, p. 435–448, 1984.

[2] T. E. Dever, M. J. Glynias and W. C. Merrick, The GTP-binding Domain: Three Consensus sequence Elements with Distinct Spacing, *Proc. Natl. Acad. Sci. USA*, 84, p. 1814–1818, 1987.

[3] H. R. Bourne, D. A. Sanders and F. McCormick, The GTPase superfamily: Conserved structure and molecular mechanism, *Nature*, 349, 117–127, 1991.

[4] F. McCormick, B. F. C. Clark, T. F. M. la Cour, M. Kjeldgaard, L. Nørskov-Lauritsen and J. Nyborg, A model for the tertiary structure of p21, the product of the *ras* oncogene, *Science*, 230, p. 78–82, 1985.

[5] Y. Kaziro, The role of guanosine 5-triphosphate in polypeptide elongation, *Biochem. Biophys. Acta*, 505, p. 95–127, 1978.

[6] E. Pai, U. Krengel, G. A. Petsko, R. S. Goody, W. Kabsch and A. Wittinghofer, Refined crystal structure of the triphosphate conformation of H-*ras* p21 at 1.35 Å resolution: Implications for the mechanism of GTP hydrolysis, *EMBO J.*, 9, p. 2351–2359, 1990.

[7] L. Tong, A. M. d. Vos, M. V. Milburn and S. -H. Kim, Crystal structures at 2.2 Å resolution of the catalytic domains of normal *ras* protein and oncogenic mutants complexed with GDP, *J. Mol. Biol.*, 217, p. 503–516, 1991.

[8] J. P. Noel, H. E. Hamm and P. B. Sigler, The 2.2 Å crystal structure of transducin-α complexed with GTPγS, *Nature*, 366, p. 654–663, 1993.

[9] D. G. Lambright, J. P. Noel, H. E. Hamm and P. B. Sigler, Structural determinants for activation of the α-subunit of a heterotrimeric G protein, *Nature*, 369, p. 621–628, 1994.

[10] D. E. Coleman, A. M. Berghuis, E. Lee, M. E. Linder, A. G. Gilman and S. R. Sprang, Structures of Active Conformations of Giα1 and the Mechanism of GTP Hydrolysis. *Science*, 265, p. 1405–1412, 1994.

[11] M. Kjeldgaard and J. Nyborg, Refined structure of elongation factor EF-Tu from *Echerichia coli*, *J. Mol. Biol.*, 223, p. 721–742, 1992.

[12] H. Berchtold, L. Reshetnikova, C. O. A. Reiser, N. K. Schirmer, M. Sprinzl and R. Hilgenfeld, Crystal structure of active elongation factor Tu reveals major domain rearrangements, *Nature*, 365, p. 126–132, 1993.

[13] M. Kjeldgaard, P. Nissen, S. Thirup and J. Nyborg, The crystal structure of elongation factor EF-Tu from *Thermus aquaticus* in the GTP conformation, *Structure*, 1, p. 35–50, 1993.

[14] A. Ævarsson, E. Brazhnikov, M. Garber, J. Zheltonosova, Y. Chirgadze, S. Al-Karadaghi, L. A. Svensson and A. Liljas, Three-dimensional structure of the ribosomal translocase: elongation factor G from *Thermus thermophilus*, *EMBO J.*, 13, p. 3669–3677, 1994.

[15] J. Czworkowski, J. Wang, T. A. Steitz and P. B. Moore, The crystal structure of elongation factor G complexed with GDP, at 2.7 Å resolution, *EMBO J.*, 13, p. 3661–3668, 1994.

[16] L. S. Reshetnikova, M. B. Garber, N. P. Fomenkova, S. V. Nikonov and Y. N. Chirgadze, Crystallographic Study of the Large Tryptic Fragments of Elongation Factor G from *Escherichia coli*, *J. Mol. Biol.*, 160, p. 127–132, 1982.

[17] T. Schweins, M. Geyer, K. Scheffzek, A. Warshel, H. R. Kalbitzer and A. Wittinghofer, Substrate-assisted catalysis as a mechanism for GTP hydrolysis of *ras* p21 and other GTP-binding proteins, *Nature Struct. Biol.*, 2, p. 36–44, 1995.

[18] N. Spickofsky, A. Robichon, W. Danho, D. Fry, D. Greeley, B. Graves, V. Madison and R. F. Margolskee, Biochemical analysis of the transducin-phosphodiesterase interaction, *Nature Struct. Biol.*, 1, p. 771–781, 1994.

[19] J. D. Robertus, J. E. Ladner, J. T. Finch, D. Rhodes, R. S. Brown, B. F. C. Clark and A. Klug, Structure of yeast phenylalanine tRNA at 3 Å resolution, *Nature*, 250, p. 546–551, 1974.

[20] S. -H. Kim, F. L. Suddath, G. J. Quigley, A. McPherson, J. L. Sussman, A. Wang, N. C. Seeman and A. Rich, Three-Dimensional Tertiary Structure of Yeast Phenylalanine Transfer RNA, *Science*, 185, p. 435–440, 1974.

[21] R. Österberg, B. Sjöberg, R. Ligaarden and P. Elias, A Small-Angle X-ray Scattering Study of the Complex Formation between Elongation Factor Tu·GTP and Valyl-tRNA^{Val} from *Escherichia coli*, *Eur. J. Biochem.*, 117, p. 155–159, 1981.

[22] F. P. Wikman, G. E. Siboska, H. U. Petersen and B. F. Clark, The site of interaction of aminoacyl-tRNA with elongation factor Tu, *EMBO J.*, 1, p. 1095–1100, 1982.

[23] A. G. Murzin, A ribosomal protein module in EF-G and DNA gyrase, *Nature Struct. Biol.*, 2, p. 25–26, 1995.

Electron Transfer of the Di-Heme Protein: *Pseudomonas stutzeri* cytochrome c_4

Jens-Jakob Karlsson, Anders Kadziola*, Allan Rasmussen[†], Thomas E. Rostrup and Jens Ulstrup

Chemistry Department A, The Technical University of Denmark, Lyngby,
* Institute of Biotechnology, The Technical University of Denmark, Lyngby and
[†] Department of Chemistry, Chemistry Lab. IV, University of Copenhagen, Denmark

Abstract

Individual multi-center metalloproteins and metalloprotein complexes are of vital importance for respiratory electron transfer (ET). We report a study of the di-heme protein cytochrome c_4. This protein presumably participates in respiratory electron transfer. Cytochrome c_4 was isolated from the bacterium *Pseudomonas stutzeri* for which the growth procedure has been optimised. The crystal structure of cytochrome c_4 with a resolution of 2.2 Å is obtained. The X-ray structure shows that cytochrome c_4 is a dipolar protein, and that the propionates from the heme groups are facing each other and are within hydrogen-bonding distance.

The reaction kinetics of cytochrome c_4 with $[Co(terpy)_2]^{2+/3+}$ and with $[Co(bipy)_2]^{2+/3+}$ have been studied. The data are in line with either bi- or tri-exponential kinetics. The former correspond to weak interaction between the heme groups, the latter to notable interaction effects. Arguments in favour of the latter mechanism and a co-operative two-electron transfer pattern are given. All phases are approximately proportional to the Cobalt-complex concentration, implying that intramolecular electron transfer is unlikely in this time range. The reduction potentials have been calculated from the forward and reverse rate constant ratios. The values are 241±5 and 328±2 mV *vs.* SHE if bi-exponential kinetics is used and interaction between the heme groups ignored. The tri-exponential, co-operative model gives intrinsic microscopic reduction potentials closer in value. This model transfers 30-40 mV to electrostatically dominated interaction potentials.

1 Introduction

Metalloproteins play a very important role in electron transport in so diverse organisms as bacteria, plants and animals. These metalloproteins contain iron, nickel, molybdenum, copper and other metals which are of crucial importance for its function. Individual multi-center metalloproteins and metalloprotein complexes dominate respiratory electron transfer [1, 2, 3, 4]. This is necessary to ensure facile long-range directional electron transfer by favourable electronic coupling between close and mutually oriented individual metalloproteins [3]. Other crucial features of this organisation are the co-operativity and electronic communication between the centres. Electric field changes associated with a given ET step may thus generate electrostatic

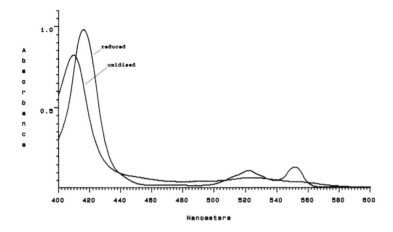

Figure 1: UV/VIS absorption spectrum of oxidised and reduced cytochrome c_4.

or conformational changes in other centres, poising the latter for favourable subsequent ET in a co-operative multi-center ET pattern [5, 6, 7, 8, 9].

Bacterial di-heme proteins are encountered in aerobic [10, 11, 12], nitrate [13], nitrite [14], ammonia [15], and methylothrophic respiration [16], in the enzymes cytochrome c peroxidase [17, 18] and fumarate reductase [19] and in the cytochrome cl and cytochrome b/cytochrome c peroxidase complexes [20].

The bacterial metalloprotein cytochrome c_4 has a polypeptide chain of 190 amino acids with a molecular mass of $\sim$ 20 kDa. It is a di-heme protein with two similar domains and the axial ligands for both hemes are histidine and methionine (*vide infra*). Cytochrome c_4 is characterised by the fact that it is a membrane-bound protein [21, 22]. Nearly 85% is strongly attached to the cell membrane facing the periplasm and approximately 15% is in the periplasm itself (this is almost unaffected by the growth conditions) [23].

Figure 1 shows the absorption spectrum of oxidised and reduced cytochrome c_4. Cytochrome c_4 has a low and a high absorption coefficient of the α- and Soret-band, respectively, compared with cytochrome c [24]. It is also distinctive of cytochrome c_4 that it has a low α/β-ratio of approximately 1.18 and that the absorption maxima of the α-, β-, and Soret-bands are at 551, 552 and 415 nm, respectively.

Cytochrome c_4 was first isolated from the bacterium *Azotobacter vinelandii* in 1956 by Tissiéres and Burris [24, 25]. Cytochrome c_4 has since been isolated from *Pseudomonas stutzeri* [11, 26, 27] (strains A.T.C.C. 11607 and 17591), *Pseudomonas aeruginosa* [28] (strain N.C.T.C. 10332), and *Alcaligenes sp.* [29] (formerly *Pseudomonas denitrificans*) (N.C.I.B. 11015). Cytochrome c_4 may also be present in *Pseudomonas perfectomarinus*, *Paracoccus denitrificans* [23], *Pseudomonas mendocina* [28], *Alcaligenes faecalis* [13], and *Thiobacillus denitrificans* [13].

Cytochrome c_4 is believed to participate in respiratory electron transfer but the exact function (or position in the ET chain) is still unknown. It is somewhat strange that cytochrome c_4 is isolated from both the strict aerobe *Azotobacter vinelandii* and from denitrifying bacteria grown under anaerobic conditions. One possibility is that cytochrome c_4 might establish an important link in both aerobic and anaerobic respiration. In cases where the bacteria have

Ps. stutzeri	A	G	D	A	E	A	G	Q	G	K	V	A	V	C	G	A	C	H	G	V	D	G	N	S	P	25
A. vinelandii	A	G	D	A	A	A	G	Q	G	K	A	A	V	C	G	A	C	H	G	P	D	G	N	S	A	
Ps. stutzeri	A	P	N	F	P	K	L	A	G	Q	G	E	R	Y	L	L	K	Q	L	Q	D	I	K	A	G	50
A. vinelandii	A	P	N	F	P	K	L	A	G	Q	G	E	R	Y	L	L	K	Q	M	Q	D	I	K	A	G	
Ps. stutzeri	S	T	P	G	A	P	E	G	V	G	R	K	V	L	E	M	T	G	M	L	D	P	L	S	D	75
A. vinelandii	T	K	P	G	A	P	E	G	S	G	R	K	V	L	E	M	T	G	M	L	D	N	F	S	D	
Ps. stutzeri	Q	D	L	E	D	I	A	A	Y	F	S	S	Q	K	G	S	V	G	Y	A	D	P	A	L	A	100
A. vinelandii	Q	D	L	A	D	L	A	A	Y	F	T	S	Q	K	P	T	V	G	A	A	D	P	Q	L	V	
Ps. stutzeri	K	Q	G	E	K	L	F	R	G	G	K	L	D	Q	G	M	P	A	C	T	G	C	H	A	P	125
A. vinelandii	E	A	G	E	T	L	Y	R	G	G	K	L	A	D	G	M	P	A	C	T	G	C	H	S	P	
Ps. stutzeri	N	G	V	G	N	D	L	A	G	F	P	K	L	G	G	Q	H	A	A	Y	T	A	K	Q	L	150
A. vinelandii	N	G	E	G	N	T	P	A	A	Y	P	R	L	S	G	Q	H	A	Q	Y	V	A	K	Q	L	
Ps. stutzeri	T	D	F	R	E	G	N	R	T	N	D	G	D	T	M	I	M	R	G	V	A	A	K	L	S	175
A. vinelandii	T	D	F	R	E	G	A	R	T	N	D	G	D	N	M	I	M	R	S	I	A	A	K	L	S	
Ps. stutzeri	N	K	D	I	E	A	L	S	S	Y	I	Q	G	L	H											190
A. vinelandii	N	K	D	I	A	A	I	S	S	Y	I	Q	G	L	H											

Figure 2: Amino acid sequences of cytochrome c_4 from *Pseudomonas stutzeri*[22] and *Azotobacter vinelandii*[30].

been grown anaerobically the cells have been inoculated aerobically [23]. Another possibility might therefore be that the synthesis of cytochrome c_4 is induced under these conditions. In any case the relatively high reduction potentials[1] of cytochrome c_4 suggest that the protein is located close to a terminal electron acceptor. The di-heme nature of cytochrome c_4 could be a device insuring co-ordinated transfer of two electrons. It could also be that cytochrome c_4 is bound to both a cytochrome reductase and a cytochrome oxidase involving intramolecular electron transfer.

In the work presented here the bacterium *Pseudomonas stutzeri* was grown aerobically following a procedure [27] which is somewhat modified compared with the procedure in reference [21]. The modified procedure is based on factorial design experiments performed to optimise the growth yield. The yield is almost 20 g of wet cell paste per liter of growth medium. In the program to isolate and purify cytochrome c_4, 200 g of cells are suspended in 400 ml butanol, blended and centrifugated to release the protein from the membrane. This is followed by ion-exchange (where the proteins are separated according to charge) on a DE-23 anion exchange column, and gel filtration (where the proteins are separated according to size) on a Sephadex-G75 column. Finally cytochrome c_4 was isolated from remaining proteins on a Hiload 16/10 Q Sepharose (Pharmacia) column connected to a FPLC apparatus. Yields of cytochrome c_4 were 20-27 mg per 200 g wet cell paste [27].

2   Amino acid sequence and crystal structure for cytochrome c_4

2.1   Amino acid sequence

With a recent determination of the amino acid sequence for *Pseudomonas stutzeri* cytochrome c_4 by cDNA-techniques [22], sequences for cytochrome c_4 from *Pseudomonas stutzeri*, *Azotobacter vinelandii* [30] and *Pseudomonas aeruginosa* [31] are now available. A comparison of the *Ps. stutzeri* and *A. vinelandii* sequences is shown in figure 2.

---

[1]241 and 328 mV *vs.* SHE for *Pseudomonas stutzeri* cytochrome c_4, *vide infra*.

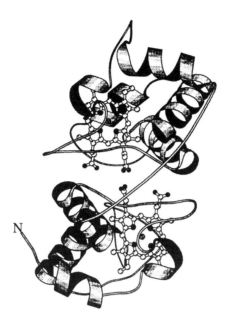

Cytochrome c4

Figure 3: X-ray diffraction structure of cytochrome c_4 from *Pseudomonas stutzeri*[35].

The comparison reveals that there is high conservation. For example — the sequences of *Pseudomonas stuzeri* and *Azotobacter vinelandii* are 79% strictly identical and 88% with a conservative substitution included. However, the sequence resemblance between the domains within one single species is minor ($\approx 30\%$) compared to the overall sequence similarity between species ($\approx 80\%$). This means that if the two domains of cytochrome c_4 are an outcome of gene duplication, this must have taken place a long time ago.

Pseudomonas stutzeri cytochrome c_4 consists of a single polypeptide chain of 190 amino acid residues which form two domains. In each domain is a set of heme-attachment cysteine residues at positions 14/17 and 119/122. A bridge region links the two domains.

In all three cytochromes c_4 the axial ligands are histidine No. 18 and 123 together with methionine No. 66 and 167. Based on the amino acid composition and estimated pK_a-values for the heme propionate groups the net charge of *Pseudomonas stutzeri* cytochrome c_4 has been calculated to -22. For *Azotobacter vinelandii* the pI values for oxidised and reduced cytochrome c_4 have been determined to 4.7 and 4.4 respectively [32].

2.2 Crystal structure

Crystallisation of cytochrome c_4 from *Pseudomonas aeruginosa* was reported as early as 1981 together with a low-resolution X-ray electron density map on two heavy-atom derivatives [33]. Furthermore, in the book of Moore and Pettigrew [12] additional details have been published (referred to as: unpublished crystallographic data kindly provided by L. Sawyer).

Table 1:

	$[Co(terpy)_2]^{2+/3+}$	$[Co(bipy)_3]^{3+}$	$[Co(phen)_3]^{3+}$	$[Fe(CN)_6]^{3-}$
$E°$ (mV)	260	310	370	410
$k_{-1}(M^{-1}s^{-1})$	$0.7 \cdot 10^5$	$2.4 \cdot 10^5$	$1.2 \cdot 10^5$	$3.5 \cdot 10^5$
$k_{-2}(M^{-1}s^{-1})$		$1.1 \cdot 10^6$		
$k_2(M^{-1}s^{-1})$	$1.1 \cdot 10^5$			
Ref.	[37]	[38]	[37]	[37]

From these data it can be seen that cytochrome c_4 from *Pseudomonas aeruginosa* is constituted of two helical domains of approximately 80 amino acids and that each domain accommodates one heme group. The two domains are connected by an extended polypeptide chain. The two heme groups are seen to be almost co-planar with the propionates pointing towards each other within hydrogen-bonding distance.

Cytochrome c_4 from the bacterium *Pseudomonas stutzeri* has been crystallised [34] and X-ray diffraction data been collected to 2.2 Å resolution [34, 35]. The structure of cytochrome c_4 can be seen in Color plate 8 (page xxii). From figure 3 [35] it can be seen that cytochrome c_4 has two symmetric domains, each accommodating one heme group (with an axial His-Met co-ordination), and that the propionate groups from each heme are oriented towards each other, and are within hydrogen-bonding distance. Furthermore, the hemes are not co-planar but tilted almost 30° (See Color plate 8, page xxii). Figure 4 reveals that the axially co-ordinated methionine has an unusual orientation [35]. It "takes off" almost vertically from the heme plane. Cytochrome c_4 has been studied by Nuclear Magnetic Resonance (NMR) [36]. The 1D NMR spectrum of oxidised cytochrome c_4 has resonance shifts out to almost 50 ppm [36]. This is quite unusual since oxidised low-spin heme proteins normally have shifts out to 30 ppm, whereas high-spin proteins have shifts out to 70 ppm or more [36]. The NMR spectrum of oxidised cytochrome c_4 is thus something between these two cases.

Furthermore, a temperature study of oxidised cytochrome c_4 shows that most low field resonances are shifted toward lower field with increasing temperature. This is in line with the crystallographic data (Fig. 4). Figure 5 [35] shows that there is a hydrogen-bond network in the proximity of the hemes and in the area between the two domains (not least between one of the propionate groups from each heme). This could be of importance for the reaction kinetics of cytochrome c_4. It seems to open the possibility for electrons to enter and leave cytochrome c_4 not only at the heme edges at each end of the molecule but also in the "groove" between the domains. Intramolecular ET between the two hemes might not be facile since the hydrogen-bond network could need reorganisation upon ET, thereby contributing to the reorganisation Gibbs free energy or work terms. It is therefore understandable that neither the kinetic data nor 1D NMR data indicate that intramolecular ET occurs on these time scales. From the crystal structure of *Pseudomonas stutzeri* cytochrome c_4 the distribution of surface charges can be obtained. This reveals that even though cytochrome c_4 has a net negative charge it is a dipolar protein with a charge distribution from which a difference in reduction potentials between the two hemes would be expected.

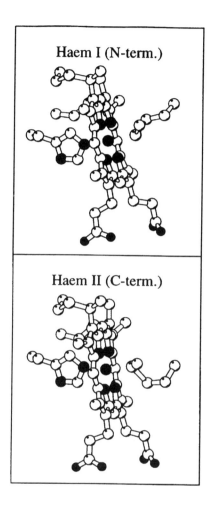

Figure 4: X-ray structure[35] showing the heme groups and axial ligands of the two hemes in cytochrome c_4.

3   Reaction kinetics of cytochrome c_4

Studies of the reaction kinetics of cytochrome c_4 with different reaction partners have been described in the literature [37, 38]. The kinetic data have been described by the following two equations (assuming no intramolecular ET in cytochrome c_4):

$$H_1^{III} H_2^{III} + [Red] \underset{k_{-1}}{\overset{k_1}{\leftrightarrow}} H_1^{III} H_2^{II} + [Ox]$$

$$H_1^{III} H_2^{II} + [Red] \underset{k_{-2}}{\overset{k_2}{\leftrightarrow}} H_1^{II} H_2^{II} + [Ox] \tag{1}$$

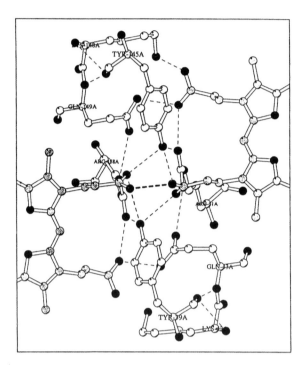

Figure 5: See reference [35].

H_1 and H_2 are the two heme groups and the superscripts indicate the oxidation state. Some of the rate constants above have been reported for different reaction partners and are listed in table 1.

In the present investigation kinetic data for cytochrome c_4 $H_1^{II}H_2^{II}$ oxidation and cytochrome c_4 $H_1^{III}H_2^{III}$ reduction with the inorganic redox couples $[Co(terpy)_2]^{2+/3+}$ and $[Co(bipy)_3]^{2+/3+}$ were recorded on a Hi-Tech SF-53 stopped-flow instrument. Data were acquired and treated with OLIS 4300S software (On-Line-Instrument-Systems, Jefferson, Georgia, USA). The compounds $[Co(terpy)_2]Cl_2 \cdot 5H_2O$, $[Co(terpy)_2](ClO_4)_3 \cdot H_2O$, and $[Co(bipy)_3]$ $(ClO_4)_3 \cdot 3 H_2O$ were prepared according to the procedures in [39], [40], and [41], respectively. $[Co(bipy)_3]^{2+}$ were prepared merely by mixing $CoCl_2 \cdot 6H_2O$ and 2,2'-bipyridine in the mol ratio 1 to 3.5[2]. The cytochrome c_4 concentration in the range 0.1-2.0 μM was followed at 420 nm. The inorganic reaction partners were always in at least 25-fold excess. All experiments were performed at 25 °C in 20 mM Tris-HCl buffer, pH=7.6 and I=0.1 M (NaCl). The choice of inorganic redox couples were based on their reduction potential values ($E° =260$ mV and 310 mV for $[Co(terpy)_2]^{2+/3+}$ and $[Co(bipy)_3]^{2+/3+}$, respectively ([42] and [43]). These values are close to the reduction potentials of the two heme groups and will enable rate constant investigations in both directions.

The kinetic data could not be fitted to mono-phasic kinetics but very well to both bi-

---

[2]For each preparation of $[Co(bipy)_3]^{2+}$ the ratio between $[Co(bipy)_3]^{2+}$ and $[Co(bipy)_2(H_2O_2)]^{2+}$ was calculated assuming that $[Co(bipy)_2(H_2O)_2]^{2+}$ does not react (because of its high reduction potential). These calculations yielded the "effective" concentration of $[Co(bipy)_3]^{2+}$.

and tri-phasic kinetics. This offers various mechanistic options, which are discussed in the following.

    1. Parallel ET of each heme group and no inter-heme interaction. This mechanism is described by eq.(1) and is the mechanism implicit in reported ET data [37, 38]. Using this mechanism the rate constants shown in table 2 are obtained from bi-exponential fits to the data.

Table 2:

	$k_{-1}(M^{-1}s^{-1})$	$k_1(M^{-1}s^{-1})$	$k_{-2}(M^{-1}s^{-1})$	$k_2(M^{-1}s^{-1})$
$[Co(terpy)_2]^{2+/3+}$	$0.478 \cdot 10^5$	$7.35 \cdot 10^5$	$2.19 \cdot 10^5$	$0.903 \cdot 10^5$
$[Co(bipy)_3]^{2+/3+}$	$1.32 \cdot 10^4$	$2.46 \cdot 10^4$	$8.64 \cdot 10^4$	$0.700 \cdot 10^4$

With the rate constants (table 2) the reduction potentials for cytochrome c_4 were calculated by the following two equations as exemplified for $[Co(terpy)_2]^{2+/3+}$:

$$E^{\circ}_{cytc_4} = E^{degr}_{[Co(terpy)_2]^{2+/3+}} - 0.059\log\frac{k_{-1}}{k_1}$$

$$E^{\circ}_{cytc_4} = E^{degr}_{[Co(terpy)_2]^{2+/3+}} - 0.059\log\frac{k_{-2}}{k_2} \qquad (2)$$

The two reduction potentials of cytochrome c_4 were calculated to 242 and 328 mV *vs.* SHE (the data for $[Co(terpy)_2]^{2+/3+}$ and $[Co(bipy)_3]^{2+/3+}$ are quite similar). These values correspond to macroscopic midpoint potentials. There is an (apparent) difference in reduction potential of 86 mV between the two heme groups. A larger separation of 110 mV has been obtained by redox titration [26] at low ionic strength on a different strain of *Pseudomonas stutzeri*.

The mechanism should give bi-exponential kinetics with approximately equal (and temperature-independent) amplitudes. However, the amplitudes are notably different in both bi- and tri-exponential modes, the faster phases having the smaller amplitudes[3]. Rate constants and amplitude ratios also depend significantly on temperature. This has led to consideration of other mechanisms:

    2. Parallel ET of each heme group and fast intramolecular redox equilibrium. Bi-exponential kinetics with different, temperature-dependent amplitudes emerge where the time constants and amplitudes incorporate the rate and equilibrium constants. A problem here is, however, that fast intramolecular ET is not sustained by other evidence.

    3. The cytochrome c_4 molecule is strongly dipolar (at pH=7.6) [35] and might cause positively charged reaction partners to be repelled from the C-terminal heme group and ET to take place only at the N-terminal heme. Such a mechanism gives tri-exponential kinetics [27] where the time constants directly coincide with the intramolecular and two intermolecular ET rate constants. The observed

---

[3]Observed inverse rates are always well above the instrumental time limits and significant loss of amplitude due to partial conversion prior to initiation of data recording is not likely.

[Co(III)]/[Co(II)]-dependence of all the three phases is, however, at variance with this mechanism.

4. Parallel, co-operative ET of each heme group. Co-operativity is now a key additional feature and implies that the intermolecular ET rate constant of a given heme group is different depending on whether the other heme group is oxidised or reduced. The mechanism is described by the following scheme (for oxidation):

$$H_1^{II} H_2^{II} + Co(III) \xrightarrow{k_{1a}} H_1^{III} H_2^{II} + Co(II)$$
$$H_1^{II} H_2^{II} + Co(III) \xrightarrow{k_{2a}} H_1^{II} H_2^{III} + Co(II)$$
$$H_1^{II} H_2^{III} + Co(III) \xrightarrow{k_{1b}} H_1^{III} H_2^{III} + Co(II)$$
$$H_1^{III} H_2^{II} + Co(III) \xrightarrow{k_{2b}} H_1^{III} H_2^{III} + Co(II)$$

$$(3)$$

The rate of oxidation of heme No. 1 is thus different ($k_{1a} \neq k_{1b}$) depending on whether heme No. 2 is oxidised or reduced (electrostatic effect). The same applies to oxidation or reduction of heme No. 2 ($k_{2a} \neq k_{2b}$). This mechanism gives tri-exponential kinetics where all the three time constants are proportional to the Cobalt-complex concentration [27]. At present this mechanism appears to be the one best in line with the data.

5. Parallel, co-operative ET as in mechanism No. 4 *and* intramolecular ET between the two heme groups. This mechanism is also represented by tri-exponential kinetics, but the time constants now include [Co(III)]/[Co(II)]-independent terms. This is not in line with the data.

Using mechanism No. 4 the rate constants in tables 3 and 4 for oxidation and reduction using [Co(terpy)$_2$]$^{2+/3+}$ and [Co(bipy)$_3$]$^{2+/3+}$ are obtained.

Table 3: Rate constants k ($M^{-1}s^{-1}$) and amplitude (A) ratios from tri-exponential resolution of data for the reaction of cytochrome c_4 with [Co(terpy)$_2$]$^{2+/3+}$ and [Co(bipy)$_3$]$^{2+/3+}$ in 20 mM Tris/HCl buffer, pH=7.6, I=0.1 M (NaCl) and T=25°C. The three phases are distinguished by subscripts, I being the fastest and III the slowest phase.

Reactant	k_I	k_{II}	k_{III}	A_{III}/A_I	A_I/A_{II}
[Co(terpy)$_2$]$^{2+}$	$(7.2 \pm 0.7) \cdot 10^5$	$(1.6 \pm 0.1) \cdot 10^5$	$(0.9 \pm 0.1) \cdot 10^5$	0.8 ± 0.2	0.7 ± 0.1
[Co(terpy)$_2$]$^{3+}$	$(3.0 \pm 0.3) \cdot 10^5$	$(0.7 \pm 0.3) \cdot 10^5$	$(0.6 \pm 0.1) \cdot 10^5$	1.9 ± 0.6	1.3 ± 0.2
[Co(bipy)$_3$]$^{2+}$	$(1.7 \pm 0.5) \cdot 10^4$	$(0.8 \pm 0.1) \cdot 10^4$	$(0.5 \pm 0.3) \cdot 10^4$	1.4 ± 0.4	0.8 ± 0.1
[Co(bipy)$_3$]$^{3+}$	$(1.0 \pm 0.1) \cdot 10^5$	$(2.7 \pm 0.6) \cdot 10^4$	$(1.0 \pm 0.2) \cdot 10^4$	1.4 ± 0.4	0.8 ± 0.1

By combining the forward and reverse rate constant ratios k_{1a}/k_{-1a}, k_{1b}/k_{-1b}, k_{2a}/k_{-2a}, k_{2b}/k_{-2b} with the reduction potentials of the Co-complexes one can obtain a set of microscopic reduction potentials and inter-heme interaction potentials. These are summarised in tables 5 and 6. It can be noted that the microscopic reduction potential of a given heme group is shifted by 30-50 mV when the oxidation state of the other heme group is changed. The interaction potentials are all negative and must therefore have a dominating electrostatic component.

Table 4: Microscopic rate constants ($M^{-1}s^{-1}$) calculated from tri-exponential kinetic resolution and the scheme in eq. (3). Same conditions as in table 3.

Reactant couple	k_{1a}	k_{1b}	k_{2a}	k_{2b}	k_{-1a}	k_{-1b}	k_{-2a}	k_{-2b}
$[Co(terpy)_2]^{2+/3+}$	$1.8 \cdot 10^5$	$0.7 \cdot 10^5$	$1.4 \cdot 10^5$	$0.6 \cdot 10^5$	$0.9 \cdot 10^5$	$4.7 \cdot 10^5$	$1.6 \cdot 10^5$	$4.2 \cdot 10^5$
$[Co(bipy)_3]^{2+/3+}$	$0.7 \cdot 10^5$	$2.7 \cdot 10^4$	$0.4 \cdot 10^5$	$1.0 \cdot 10^4$	$0.5 \cdot 10^4$	$0.6 \cdot 10^4$	$0.8 \cdot 10^4$	$0.8 \cdot 10^4$

Table 5: Microscopic reduction potentials of the two heme groups in cytochrome c_4 calculated from the rate constants in table 3 and 4 using the standard reduction potentials of $[Co(terpy)_2]^{2+/3+}$ and $[Co(bipy)_3]^{2+/3+}$. The reduction potentials are denoted by the letter e and are in mV *vs.* SHE. Subscripts "1" and "2" refer to the low- and high-potential heme group, respectively. Superscript "ox" and "red" denote the oxidation state of the heme group complementary to the one indicated by the subscript.

Reaction Partners	e_1^{red}	e_2^{red}	e_1^{ox}	e_2^{ox}
$[Co(terpy)_2]^{2+/3+}$	243	263	307	309
$[Co(bipy)_3]^{2+/3+}$	245	267	273	304

The two interaction potentials should ideally coincide. Lack of numerical coincidence is due to the separate experimental determination of the forward and reverse rate constants and the uncertainty of the four-parameter analysis in the tri-exponential kinetic traces. Imposing the constraint of numerical coincidence would modify the values of the interaction potentials but not their sign or order.

4   Concluding remarks

The kinetic ET pattern and data analysis for the di-heme protein cytochrome c_4 indicate that rather detailed resolution of inter- and intramolecular ET networks is accessible. This extends in principle to the individual microscopic rate constants and reduction potentials, and to the interaction potentials. In this respect two-centre proteins are central as they are probably the only composite proteins for which complete resolution is possible. Proteins with more than two centres are too complex in this respect.

The data analysis is, however, presently not unique. Fast intramolecular ET (on the stopped-flow time scale) and co-operative intermolecular ET with no intramolecular ET are both formally in line with the data. The formal di-phasic and tri-phasic time evolution associated with these two mechanisms should offer a way of resolving this difference if combined with kinetic recording at multiple wave lengths and global data fitting. Another way would be to focus on cytochrome c_4 reaction partners with intermolecular ET in other time ranges (either notably slower or notably faster than for the cobalt-complexes used in the present investigation). This could bring the intermolecular ET time ranges closer to the time ranges for possible intramolecular electron exchange in the two alternative mechanisms presently most likely.

Table 6: Interaction potentials, Δe_{12} and Δe_{21} (mV), between the two heme groups, calculated from the rate constants and microscopic reduction potentials in tables 3 - 5. Δe_{12} is the increase in the microscopic reduction potential of the low-potential heme group ("1") when the high-potential heme group ("2") goes from the reduced to the oxidised form. Δe_{21} is, similarly, the increase in the microscopic reduction potential of the high-potential heme group when the low-potential heme group goes from the reduced to the oxidised form.

Reaction Partners	Δe_{12}	Δe_{21}
$[Co(terpy)_2]^{2+/3+}$	64	46
$[Co(bipy)_3]^{2+/3+}$	27	37

The kinetic data suggest that the interaction potentials in the tri-phasic co-operative intermolecular ET mechanism are dominated by electrostatic interactions between the "excess" electrons on the two heme groups. This is in line with expectations based on the two-domain structure of cytochrome c_4 and the single-string inter-domain contact, even though the latter is reinforced by the hydrogen-bond network between the heme groups. This is different from the co-operativity pattern in cytochrome c_3 where non-electrostatic co-operativity features are also observed [6]. Different, non-electrostatically based co-operativity patterns might also be expected for di-heme cytochromes of the b-type. The two heme groups are here attached to the *same* α-helices and likely to be more intimately coupled by conformational interactions along the α-helix structures.

We are presently pursuing co-operative inter-heme functionality in di-heme proteins by kinetic, electrochemical and in situ scanning tunnel microscopy approaches, and by UV/VIS, resonance Raman, NMR, and circular dichroism spectroscopy.

Acknowledgements

We acknowledge financial support from The Danish Natural Science Research Council. Professor A.V. Xavier and Dr. I. B. Coutinho, ITQB, Portugal, and Dr. H.E.M. Christensen are thanked for co-operation and information of pre-published data.

References

[1] H. B. Gray and B. Malmström, *Biochemistry*, 28, p. 7499-7505, 1989.

[2] G. Tollin and J. J. Hazzard, *Arch. Biochem. Biophys.*, 287, p. 1-7, 1991.

[3] H. Sigel and A. Sigel (eds.), *Metal Ions in Biological Systems*, vol. 27, Marcel Dekker, New York, 1991.

[4] N. Murata (ed.), *Research in Photosynthesis*, vol. I-IV, Klüwer, Dordrecht, 1992.

[5] A. V. Xavier, *J. Inorg. Biochem.*, 28, p. 239-243, 1986.

[6] M. Colette, T. Catarino, J. Legall and A. V. Xavier, *Eur. J. Biochem*, 202, p. 1101-1106, 1991.

[7] H. Santos, J. J. G. Moura, I. Moura, J. Legall and A. V. Xavier, *Eur. J. Biochem.*, 141, p. 283-296, 1984.

[8] I. B. Coutinho and A. V. Xavier, *Meth. Enzymol.*, in press 1994.

[9] H. E. M. Christensen, L. S. Conrad, I. Coutinho, J. M. Hammerstad-Pedersen, G. Iversen, M. H. Jensen, J. J. Karlsson, J. Ulstrup and A. V. Xavier, *J. Photochem. Photobiol. A. Chem.*, 82, p. 103-115, 1994.

[10] C. W. Jones and E. R. Redfearn, *Biochem. Biophys. Acta.*, 142, p. 340-353, 1967.

[11] T. Kodama and S. Shidara, *J. Biochem.*, 65, p. 351-360, 1969.

[12] G. R. Moore and G. W. Pettigrew, *Cytochromes c. Evolutionary, Structural and Physicochemical Aspects*, Springer-Verlag, Berlin, 1990.

[13] M. C. Liu, W. J. Payne, H. D. Peck, Jr. and J. Legall, *J. Bacteriol.*, 154, p. 278-286, 1983.

[14] T. Yamanaka and M. Shiara, *J. Biochem.*, 75, p. 1265-1273, 1974.

[15] K. K. Andersson, G. T. Babcock and A. B. Hooper, *FEBS Lett.*, 170, p. 331-334, 1984.

[16] M. A. Carver and C. W. Jones, *FEBS Lett.*, 155, p. 187-191, 1983.

[17] N. Ellfolk, M. Rönnberg, R. Aasa, L. -E. Andreasson, and T. Vanngård, *Biochem. Biophys. Acta.*, 743, p. 23-30, 1983.

[18] I. Moura, M. C. Liu, J. Legall, H. D. Peck, Jr., W. J. Payne, A. V. Xavier and J. J. G. Moura, *Eur. J. Biochem.*, 141, 297-303, 1984.

[19] M. D. Esposito, M. Crimi, C. Kortner, A. Kroger and T. Link, *Biochem. Biophys. Acta.*, 1056, p. 243-249, 1991.

[20] H. Pelletier and J. Kraut, *Science*, 258, 1748-1754, 1992.

[21] D. J. B. Hunter, K. R. Brown and G. W. Pettigrew, *Biochem. J.*, 262, p. 233-240, 1989.

[22] H. E. M. Christensen, *Gene*, 144, p. 139-140, 1994.

[23] G. W. Pettigrew and K. R. Brown, *Biochem J.*, 252, p. 427-435, 1988.

[24] A. Tissiéres and R. H. Burris, *Biochem. Biophys. Acta.*, 20, p. 436-437, 1956.

[25] A. Tissiéres, *Biochem. J.*, 64, p. 582-589, 1956.

[26] F. A. Lietch, K. R. Brown and G. W. Pettigrew, *Biochem. Biophys. Acta.*, 808, p. 213-218, 1985 .

[27] L. S. Conrad, J. J. Karlsson and J. Ulstrup, *Eur. J. Biochem.*, submitted for publication 1995.

[28] R. P. Ambler and S. Murray, *Biochem. Soc. Trans.*, 1, p. 162-164, 1973.

[29] S. Shidara, *J. Biochem.*, 87, p. 1177-1184, 1980.

[30] R. P. Ambler, M. Daniel, K. Melis and C. D. Stout, *Biochem. J.*, 222, p. 217-227, 1984.

[31] R. P. Ambler, in *From Cyclotrons to Cytochromes*, A. R. Robinson and N. O. Kaplan (eds.), p. 263-280, Academic Press, New York, 1982.

[32] W. H. Campell, W. H. Orme-Johnson and R. H. Burris, *Biochem. J.*, 135, p. 617-630, 1973.

[33] L. Sawyer and C. L. Jones, *J. Mol. Biol.*, 153, p. 831-835, 1981.

[34] A. Kadziola, S. Larsen, H. E. M. Christensen, J. -J. Karlsson and J. Ulstrup, *Acta Crystallographica*, in press 1995.

[35] A. Kadziola and S. Larsen, in preparation 1995.

[36] I. B. Coutinho, J. -J. Karlsson and A. V. Xavier, unpublished data, 1994.

[37] R. T. Hartshorn and A. G. Sykes, *Rec. Trav. Chim. Pays-Bas.*, 106, p. 293, 1987.

[38] L. S. Conrad, *Electron Transfer Behaviour of Single- and Multi-centre Metalloproteins*, Ph. D. thesis, Chemistry Department A, The Technical University of Denmark, Denmark, 1992.

[39] R. Hogg and R. G. Wilkins, *J. Chem. Soc.*, p. 341-350, 1962.

[40] A. G. Sykes *et al.*, *Biochem. Biophys. Acta.*, 994, p. 37, 1989.

[41] B. Martin and G. M. Waind, *J. Chem. Soc.*, 4284, 1958.

[42] E. L. Yee, R. J. Cave, K. L. Guyer and M. J. Weaver, *J. Am. Chem. Soc.*, 101, p. 1131-1137, 1979.

[43] A. M. Kjær and J. Ulstrup, *Inorg. Chem.*, 25, 644-651, 1986.

Profile Methods for Protein Structure and Fold Determination

Sequence Matching in Homology Modeling

Michael Gribskov

San Diego Supercomputer Center, P.O. Box 85608-20, San Diego, CA 92186-9784, U. S. A.

Abstract

Homology-based modeling, or more simply homology modeling, is becoming increasingly important. Models accurate to within 1-2 Å RMS deviation from the actual three-dimensional structure can be produced by homology modeling in favorable cases. With the number of known three-dimensional structures projected to grow to more than ten thousand structures by the end of the decade, it will be possible to model a significant fraction of all sequences using these approaches.

In homology modeling, a known three-dimensional structure is used as a template from which a three-dimensional model of a novel sequence is calculated. In the first stages of this procedure, the critical steps are the location of an appropriate homologous structure to use as the template, and the correct mapping of the novel sequence onto the known structure. The detection of a homologous structure involves the inference that the structure is indeed homologous based on a sequence or structure-based comparison. This inference is based on the assumption that if the sequence and structure are, by some measure, significantly similar, they are homologous. Unfortunately, for many extant methods, the influence of various parameters on the significance of the similarity is not well understood. In particular, the influence of variables such as the scoring system, and penalties for insertions and deletions in dynamic programming based approaches are still not theoretically understood and can only be determined by empirical approaches. This work examines the effects of scoring system and affine gap penalties on the ability of a local-similarity dynamic programming algorithm to discriminate between homologous and unrelated sequences.

1 Introduction

The prediction of the three-dimensional structure of proteins based on the known structure of homologous proteins is becoming increasingly successful, often producing modeled structures accurate to within 1-2 Å RMS deviation from the actual three-dimensional structure (for a recent comprehensive review see [1]). The continuing exponential growth of both sequence and structural databases makes it increasingly likely that a homologous protein with known three-dimensional structure can be found for a novel sequence. Homology-based modeling, or more simply homology modeling, will therefore increase in importance over the next several years as the increasing data makes it more practical. This will be especially true as the Human Genome Projects around the world begin producing completed sequences.

Homology modeling involves a series of steps, with each step depending on the success of the preceding one. A simple outline of the homology modeling process is:

1. Find a template structure, a sequence with known structure that is significantly similar to the target sequence.
2. Align the target sequence with the template structure to maximize the structural similarity.
3. Replace amino acid sidechains in the template with the corresponding ones from the target sequence.
4. Model regions of insertions/deletions between the target and template sequences, and other weakly conserved regions such as loops.
5. Minimize the calculated energy of the entire structure.

The first two steps in this scheme deal with the location and alignment of the target sequence with the template structure. Similar or identical algorithms are often used for steps 1 and 2. When the matching is based on sequences, the method of choice is usually a local-similarity dynamic programming approach (Smith-Waterman algorithm) [2], or a fast approximation to it [3, 4]. More recently, approaches that attempt to match the target and template based on the local structural environment of the template structure [5] or an empirical energy function [6, 7, 8] have been developed. These methods can also be used in both step 1 and step 2.

Because the same algorithms can be used for both steps, the differences between steps 1 and 2 are not always clearly distinguished. For instance, it has often been implicitly assumed that the conditions that give a correct matching of the target and template (step 2) are the same conditions that should be used in step 1 to find the template.

2 Methods

2.1 MPSRCH

Sequence comparisons were performed using a local similarity dynamic programming algorithm [2], as implemented in the MPSRCH program (IntelliGenetics, Inc., Mountain View CA). Results were normalized for systematic dependence on sequence length using the "ranking function" method implemented in this package. MPSRCH was used in the affine gap scoring mode in which a length independent (gap initiation) and a length dependent (gap extension) penalty are used. Query sequences were compared to the Swiss-Prot database release 28.0 [9] which contains 1.25×10^7 residues in 36,000 sequences.

2.2 Receiver Operating Characteristic (ROC)

The receiver operating characteristic is widely used in clinical fields to evaluate both treatments and the predictive success of clinical tests (for a review see [10]). It is the latter use that concerns us here. An example of a clinical use of ROC analysis might be to evaluate the success of a test, for instance serum cholesterol level, in predicting the future presence of a disease condition, for instance heart attack. In this case, the easily performed test acts as a surrogate for the physically impossible examination of the heart itself. Similarly, in sequence comparisons the determination of sequence similarity is an easily performed test that acts as a surrogate for the more difficult process of determining actual homology.

ROC analysis has several advantages over other approaches: it is a function of both sensitivity and specificity of the test, it is insensitive to threshold, and it is simple to calculate. It may be contrasted with other approaches such as simply counting the number of true positives in a fixed number of the top scores from a database search [11] which measures the sensitivity of the search but doesn't measure the specificity, or examination of the fractions of true positive and true negatives above a specified threshold [12, 13] which measures both sensitivity and specificity, but is very sensitive to the threshold. The sensitivity of the latter method to the threshold is particularly important since an appropriate threshold value is usually not known in advance.

2.2.1   Construction of the ROC plot

The ROC plot compares the sensitivity (fraction of true positives) and specificity (1-fraction of true negatives) of the test at all possible threshold levels. Before constructing the plot, the test results are sorted in order of decreasing score. This is the normal ordering for the results of database searches. Each result is then classified, based on the identity of the database sequence, as either a positive (i.e., homologous to the query sequence) or negative (i.e., not homologous to the query sequence). The ROC plot is then constructed by plotting the fraction of positives (ordinate) and fraction of negatives (abscissa) found above each successive entry in the ordered list of results. In other words, the sensitivity and 1-specificity are plotted for a continuously varying decision threshold.

   The area under the ROC plot provides a simple quantitative measure of the accuracy of a test. A test in which all of the positives score above all of the negatives will have an area of 1.0 and a test in which the positives and negatives are completely undistinguished will have an area of 0.5. The area under the ROC plot is related to the rank-sum test for two independent samples (Mann-Whitney or Wilcoxon test), and can be regarded as the probability that a randomly selected positive case (homologous sequence) will score above a randomly selected negative case (unrelated sequence).

2.2.2   Calculation of ROC_{50}

The area under the ROC plot is very close to 1.0 for most query sequences when database searches are performed using the Smith-Waterman algorithm. This is mostly because, for any particular query sequence, there are generally a hundred to a thousand times more negatives in the database than positives (homologous sequences). Any search in which the positive sequences are found within the top 1800 (5% of 36,000) scores will have an area of at least 0.95. Since most sequence queries are capable of this level of discrimination, the differences in the areas under the ROC plot will be quite small when calculated over the complete database. Realistically however, it is common to investigate only the highest scoring results from a database search, typically less than one hundred. I therefore define the ROC_{50} as the area under the ROC plot constructed using the results of the search only to the point at which 50 true negative (unrelated) sequences have been found. The ROC_{50} value is thus the probability that a homologous sequence will have a comparison score higher than one of the highest scoring false positives.

2.3   Definition of positives

Initial groups of positive sequences were defined based on the entries in the PROSITE database [14]. A group of five to ten sequences were picked from this initial group that, based on the sequence annotation, did not appear to be closely related. These sequences were then used as queries in database searches using both MPSRCH and BLAST, and the results inspected for sequences that had high but not significant comparison scores with most of the queries. These represent sequences that may be very distantly related members of the sequence family (or they could be matching by chance). Each of these candidate family members was then used as a query in a further database search using MPSRCH. The results of this search were evaluated and the candidate sequence included in the family if the ROC_{50} was greater than 0.4.

3   Results and discussion

In this study I investigate the affect of scoring table, and affine gap penalties on the sensitivity and specificity of the Smith-Waterman algorithm, using query sequences from three homologous protein families. For each family, four to six sequences representative of the range of sequences in the entire family were selected as queries based on initial database searches. The ROC_{50} was then determined for each query sequence using four different PAM scoring tables [15] and a range of both gap initiation and gap extension values. These results therefore represent a condensation of approximately 5400 complete searches of the protein sequence database.

3.1   4Fe-4S Ferredoxins

The 4Fe-4S ferredoxins are small proteins involved in electron transfer[16]. Ferredoxin-like molecules are also function in photosynthesis, and are found as independent domains in a variety of enzymes involved in oxidation-reduction reactions. These ferredoxins bind a 4Fe-4S cluster at a highly conserved 26 residue sequence. The core of the conserved region has the consensus pattern C-X-X-C-X-X-C-X-X-X-C-[PEG] and generally insertions or deletions are not required to align this region. The core of the pattern is notably rich in cysteine, an amino acid residue that is relatively rare and immutable, and which therefore receives high comparison scores in scoring tables based on the Dayhoff model. Most of the members of this family have two copies of the characteristic 26 residue repeat and bear two 4Fe-4S centers. Figure 1a shows that the optimal PAM distance varies with the probe sequence, but is generally about 150 to 200 PAM. Figure 1b shows the best ROC_{50} obtained at different values of the gap initiation penalty. This is clearly an important variable, but shows a broad peak in the 16 - 26 range. Finally Figure 1c shows the best ROC_{50} obtained for various settings of the gap extension parameter. This plot is striking in its flatness, implying that this parameter is essentially irrelevant. This lack of dependence on the gap extension penalty is not surprising given the nature of the conserved core region in this family.

3.2   LysR family

The LysR family of bacterial transcriptional regulatory proteins [17, 18]. These proteins can be either activators or repressors of the transcription of suites of genes, and are often found to control their own transcription as well. In this case, the sequence similarity is expected to comprise the entire DNA binding domain which spans roughly 65 - 100 residues in the N-terminus of these proteins. Correct alignment over the entire DNA binding domain should require a number of gaps generally in the range of one to three residues long. Figure 1d-f show the results of the parameter screening for this group of sequences. Again there is some variation in the optimal PAM scoring table depending on the probe sequence. The effect of the gap initiation parameter is similar to that seen in the ferredoxins with a broad plateau (Fig. 1e) and rapid drop off at lower values (not shown). The plot (Fig. 1f) for the gap extension penalty is again nearly flat suggesting the relative irrelevance of this parameter.

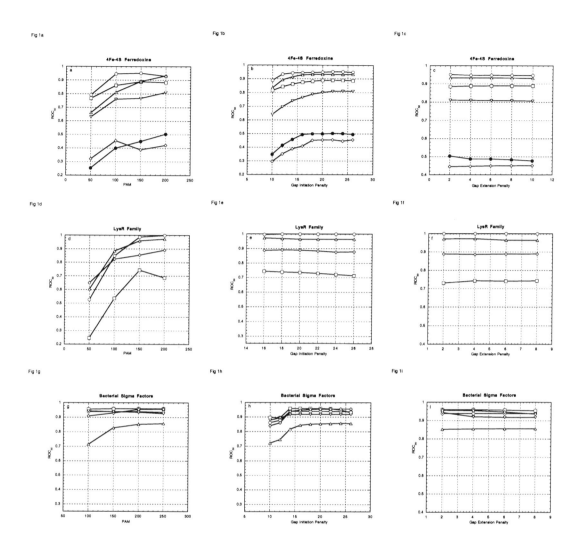

Figure 1: Effect of Scoring System, and gap Penalties on Database Discrimination. Panel a) shows the best ROC_{50} for any tested combination of gap initiation and gap extension penalty. Panels b) and c) show the best ROC_{50} at the best PAM distance for each query sequence for the specified values of gap initiation penalty and gap extension penalty respectively. Query sequences are FER_ENTHI (open circle), FER_THETH (open square), ASRC_SALTY (open diamond), DCMA_METSO (filled circle), FRXB_WHEAT (open triangle, point down) and PSAC_CHLRE (open triangle, point up). Panels d)-f) are the same as panels a)-c) but represent query sequences from the LysR family: METR_SALTY (open circle), BLAA_STRCI (open square), GLTC_ECOLI (open diamond), and AMPR_RHOCA (open triangle). Panels g)-i) are the same as panels a)-c), but represent query sequences from the bacterial sigma factor family: 46LIA_PSEAE (open circle), RP32_ECOLI (open square), RP70_ECOLI (open diamond), RPSH_BACSU (open triangle, point up), RPSK_BACSU (open triangle, point down).

3.3   Bacterial sigma factors

Bacterial sigma factors are a widespread group of proteins with a distinctive pattern of conserved and variable regions (for a recent review see [19]). The proteins vary greatly in length, from approximately 280 residues to more than 600. This variation in length is both due to variation in the length of the variable regions and to the lack of some of the conserved regions in the smaller proteins. Some of these sequences require very large insertions and deletions, up to nearly 300 residues, to produce the known homologous matching. More commonly, variations of the spacings between conserved regions of about 40 residues are seen. This requirement for large insertions and deletions is the type of situation wherein one expects to get the greatest benefit from the affine gap penalties used with the Smith-Waterman algorithm. Figure 1g-i show the results of the parameter screening for this group of sequences. Again there is some variation in the optimal PAM scoring table to use depending on the probe sequence, and a clear dependence on the gap initiation parameter. Figure 1i shows a more pronounced dependence of the best ROC_{50} on the gap extension penalty than in the previous two groups, especially for the RP70_ECOLI and RPSK_BACSU queries. However, the effect is still relatively minor, amounting to a difference of approximately 0.03 in the ROC_{50}. This amount of difference corresponds to roughly 1 sequence difference in sensitivity.

3.4   Alignment versus database searching

The results of Figure 1a-i suggest that less is gained from the explicit affine gap model used in most implementations of the Smith-Waterman algorithm than might be expected. To a large extent, this is due to the fact that the discrimination found in a database search depends as much on the score for the negatives one wishes to discriminate against, as on the comparison score for the positives one wishes to find. The overall effect of scoring systems and gap penalties on discrimination is a complex function of the effects of each of these parameters on individual positive and negative sequences.

Figure 2 shows a comparison of the effect of varying the gap extension penalty at a constant value of the gap initiation penalty. Figure 2a clearly shows that, in the case of RPSH_BACSU, increasing the gap extension penalty affects the comparison scores for unrelated sequences much more than those of sigma factors. This leads to an increase in ROC_{50} from 0.714 at a gap extension penalty of 2, to 0.736 at a gap extension penalty of 12. This increase, while small, is due to the relatively larger effect of increasing the gap extension penalty on decreasing the scores of the unrelated sequences compared to those of homologous sequences. In comparison, figure 2b shows a similar plot for searches using RPSK_BACSU as a query. In this case, due to the particulars of the comparisons between RPSK_BACSU and the rest of the sigma factors, there is a large effect of increasing the gap extension penalty on both unrelated and homologous sequences. In this case the ROC_{50} decreases from 0.897 at a gap extension penalty of 2 to 0.871 at a gap extension penalty of 14.

Because the discrimination obtained in a database search depends on comparisons to both related and unrelated sequences, it is clear that the optimal conditions for a database search are in no way tied to the conditions used to get the best homologous matching between two particular sequences. A dramatic example of this can be seen in figure 3. As with most 4Fe-4S ferredoxins, both FER_THETH and 46RXB_MARPO contain two Fe-S binding sites. Figure 3a shows the alignment between FER_THETH and 46RXB_MARPO under conditions that optimize the discrimination between ferredoxins and non-ferredoxins. This alignment is a 16 residue segment that comprises the amino-terminal copy of the Fe-S binding site in FER_THETH and the carboxyl-terminal copy in FRXB_MARPO. Using lower gap initiation and gap extension penalties, an alignment that shows the similarity between the amino-terminal

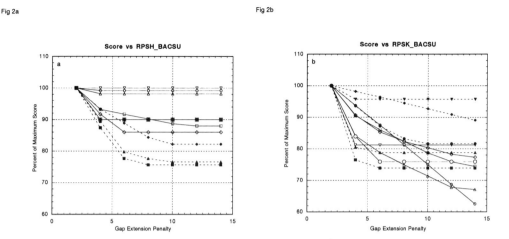

Figure 2: Effect of gap extension penalty of homologous and unrelated sequences a) Comparison score for database sequences using RPSH_BACSU as the query. Open symbols represent homologous sequences selected by choosing. approximately every 10th sequence: RPSH_BACLI (open circle), RPSP_STAAU (open square), RP80_MYXXA (open diamond), RPSB_BACSU (open triangle, point up), RPSF_BACSU (open triangle, point down), 46LIA_PAEAE (open large square), YAD2_CLOAB (filled circle), CH60_GALSU (filled square), TPM_SCHPO (filled diamond), VMP_SOCMV (filled triangle). b) Comparison score for database sequences using RPSK_BACSU as the query. Open symbols represent homologous sequences selected by choosing approximately every 10th sequence: RP28_BACTK (open circle), RPSG_BACSU (open square), HRDB_STRCO (open diamond), RP70_BUCAP (open triangle, point up), RP32_CITRFR (open triangle, point down), HRDC_STRCO (open circle with dot), BCNA_CLOPE (filled circle), GLB1_SCAIN (filled square), IMMF_BPPH1 (filled diamond), HLYD_ACTPL (filled triangle, point up), ACON_LEGPN (filled triangle, point down).

and carboxyl-terminal copies of the Fe-S binding site in both sequences can be found. Since the presence of two Fe-S binding sites is a widespread conserved feature in this family, it is likely that the alignment in figure 3b more closely represents the homologous matching between these sequences than does the one in figure 3a.

A close inspection of the ROC_{50} results shows that there is a distinct interplay between the effects of the gap initiation and gap extension penalties. When the ROC_{50} values are plotted versus the gap initiation and gap extension penalties, the optimal conditions often lie in a line along which the sum of the two penalties remains approximately equal (not shown), with long tails extending along increasing gap initiation penalty and increasing gap extension penalty. The main effect of the gap penalty, in the context of database searching, is thus to suppress high comparison scores with unrelated sequences, with only a secondary and smaller effect on the subset of comparisons to homologous sequences whose alignments require fairly long gaps to reach a significant score. At the penalty levels required to suppress matches to unrelated sequences, long insertions in homologous sequences are also suppressed and the gap extension penalty, in particular, becomes irrelevant. It may therefore be possible to achieve near optimal discrimination in a database search using an implementation of the algorithm that does not support full affine gap costs. Such an implementation can be considerably faster on

a) under optimal database searching conditions

```
FER\_THETH    37 EECIDCGACVPACPVN 52
                 :  || |  ||  ||:|
46RXB\_MARPO  62 DKCIACEVCVRVCPIN 77
```

b) under better alignment conditions

```
FER\_THETH     5 CQPCIGVKDQSCVEVCPVE.CIYD.........GGDQFYIHPEECIDCGACVPACPVN 52
                 | :|      :  || |||::  : |            : |    || || ||  || |
46RXB\_MARPO  64 CIAC.....EVCVRVCPINLPVVDWELKKTIKKKQLKNYSIDFGVCIFCGNCVEYCPTN 117
```

Figure 3: Comparison of alignments under optimal database searching and alignment conditions. Both alignments were of the complete sequences using the PAM 150 scoring table. a) gap initiation penalty = 20, gap extension penalty = 20. b) gap initiation penalty = 12, gap extension penalty = 0.8. Vertical bars indicate identical residues in the aligned sequences, colons indicate mutationally similar residues.

some architectures, e.g., the MasPar.

3.5   General Conclusions

- The scoring table has biggest effect on database discrimination Scoring tables representing evolutionary distances of 150-200 PAM seem best.
- The gap initiation is the second largest effect on database discrimination There is a broad plateau at values of approximately 16 - 20.
- The gap extension penalty is almost irrelevant.
- The optimal search conditions do not correspond to best alignment conditions.

Acknowledgements

This work was supported by the National Science Foundation through cooperative agreement ASC-8902825 with the San Diego Supercomputer Center, and by NIH grant P41 RR08605. Any opinions, findings, and conclusions or recommendations expressed in this publication are those of the author and do not necessarily reflect the views or policies of the National Science Foundation, the National Institutes of Health, or other supporters of the San Diego Supercomputer Center. I thank IntelliGenetics for access to the MPSRCH software prior to its offical release.

References

[1] M. S. Johnson , N. Srinivasan, R. Sowdhamini, and T. L. Blundell, Knowledge-based protein modeling, *Critical Rev. in Biochem. and Mol. Biol.*, 29, 1-68, 1994.
[2] T. F. Smith and M. S. Waterman, Identification of common molecular subsequences, *J. Mol. Biol.*, 147, 195-7, 1981.
[3] W. R. Pearson and D. J. Lipman, Improved tools for biological sequence comparison, *PNAS* , 858, 2444-8, 1988.

[4] S. F. Altschul, W. Gish, W. Miller, E. W. Myers and D. J. Lipman, Basic local alignment search tool, *J. Mol. Biol.*, 215, 403-10, 1990.

[5] J. U. Bowie, R. Luthy and D. Eisenberg, A method to identify protein sequences that fold into a known three-dimensional structure, *Science*, 253, 164-70, 1991.

[6] M. J. Sippl, Calculation of conformational ensembles from potentials of mean force. An approach to the knowledge-based prediction of local structures in globular proteins, *J. Mol. Biol.*, 213, 859-83, 1990.

[7] D. T. Jones, W. R. Taylor and J. M. Thornton, A new approach to protein fold recognition,*Nature*,358, 86-9, 1992.

[8] S. H. Bryant and C. E. Lawrence, An empirical energy function for threading protein sequence through the folding motif, *Proteins*, 16, 92-112, 1993.

[9] A. Bairoch and B. Boeckmann, The SWISS-PROT protein sequence data bank: current status, *NAR*, 22, 3578-80, 1994.

[10] M. H. Zweig and G. Campbell, Receiver-operating characteristic ROC plots: a fundamental evaluation tool in clinical medicine, *Clinical Chemistry*, 39, 561-77, 1993.

[11] D. L. Brutlag, J.-P. Dautricourt, R. Diaz, J. Fier, B. Moxon and R. Stamm, BLAZE: an implementation of the Smith-Waterman sequence comparison algorithm on a massively parallel computer, *Computers & Chemistry*, 17, 203-7, 1993.

[12] W. R. Pearson, Searching protein sequence libraries: comparison of the sensitivity and selectivity of the Smith-Waterman and FASTA algorithms, *Genomics*, 11, 635-50, 1991.

[13] S. Henikoff and J. G. Henikoff, Amino acid substitution matrices from protein blocks, *PNAS* , 89, 10915-9, 1992.

[14] A. Bairoch and P. Bucher, PROSITE: recent developments, *NAR*, 22, 3583-9, 1994.

[15] M. O. Dayhoff, R. M. Schwartz and B. C. Orcutt, Chapter 22: A model of evolutionary change in proteins, in *Atlas of Protein Sequence and Structure*, Vol. 5, Supp. 3, M. O. Dayhoff, (ed.), National Biomedical Research Foundation, Washington D.C., 1978.

[16] H. Beinert, Recent developments in the field of iron-sulfur proteins, *FASEB*, 4, 2483-91, 1990.

[17] S. Henikoff,G. W. Haughn, J. M. Calvo and J. C. Wallace, A large family of bacterial activator proteins, *PNAS*, 85, 6602-6606, 1988.

[18] M. A. Schell, Molecular biology of the LysR family of transcriptional regulators, *Ann. Rev. Microbiol.*, 47, 597-626, 1993.

[19] M. Lonetto, M. Gribskov and C. A. Gross, The σ^{70} family: sequence conservation and evolutionary relationships, *J. Bacteriology*, 174, 3843-9, 1992.

Screening Genome Sequences for Known Folds

Michael Braxenthaler and Manfred J. Sippl[1]

Center for Applied Molecular Engineering, Institute for Chemistry and Biochemistry,
University of Salzburg, Jakob Haringer Straße 1, A-5020 Salzburg, Austria

Abstract

Genome sequencing projects produce large numbers of new sequences. Previous
experience has shown that for approximately half of the new genes discovered
a biological role or function can be assigned by sequence comparison. The biological information contained in the remaining sequences is not accessible. Fold
recognition might have the potential to supplement the information accessible on
the sequence level. By combining sequences with known structures it should be
possible to recognize structural features of the unknown native folds of several
uncharacterized gene products. We perform a large scale fold recognition study
on the 483 genes found in the central gene cluster of *Caenorhabditis elegans*
chromosome III [1], using a data base of 263 crystal structures. We correctly
identify the three dimensional folds of 12 gene products whose structures were
previously inferred from sequence homology, and we obtain putative models
for the unknown folds of 20 sequences, demonstrating that fold recognition
retrieves valuable biological information and that large scale applications are
computationally feasible.

Current genome projects produce sequence information on an astonishing rate. The
recently completed sequence of the central gene cluster of *Caenorhabditis elegans* chromosome
III [1], for example, contains 483 putative reading frames. For roughly one third of these
sequences functional and/or structural information can be obtained by sequence comparison
techniques. Hence at present, a major part of the sequence information acquired cannot be
interpreted in terms of functional role or biological significance.

It is well established that proteins frequently adopt similar folds, even in cases where no
similarity is recognizable on the sequence level (for recent reviews see [2, 3]), and it is likely
that several protein products of the uncharacterized putative genes resemble some known fold.
The question we address here is whether or not fold recognition techniques are able to reveal
some of these coincidences.

---

[1] Corresponding author.

Table 1: Significant sequence homologies ($>$ 25% amino acid identity) found between the sequence and structure databases.

Rank	Alignment Name	Length Seq	Str	Ident. [%]
1	CELF54H12_1:1aco	788	753	73
2	CELC29E4_2:1ake-a	248	214	47
3	CEF55H2_1:2sod-b	184	151	45
4	CER107_7:1gsr-a	208	207	42
5	CEF58A4_9:1aak	164	150	38
6	CEF54C8_5:121p	207	166	33
7	CEZK637_10:2tpr-b	499	481	30
8	CELC30C11_3:1ats	776	382	29
9	CEF59B2_6:121p	205	166	28

Intensive research by several groups [4, 5, 6, 7, 8, 9, 10] over the last years have identified important features necessary to implement fold recognition techniques. Necessary ingredients are

1. force fields, parameter sets, or energy functions providing a reasonable description of protein solvent systems,
2. techniques to produce useful alignments between sequences and structures, and
3. strong criteria for the identification of native like sequence structure combinations.

In addition, computational efficiency is required to permit large scale applications on genome sequence data.

Here we investigate the performance of our current implementation of fold recognition which uses a knowledge based mean field [10, 11, 12, 13]. We focus on the large scale applicability of this technique using the 483 putative genes of C.elegans as an example. These sequences are combined with 263 X-ray structures resulting in $483 \times 263 = 127,029$ models. A crucial step is to identify native-like models among these $\approx 10^5$ combinations. Evaluation of the quality of each model [14, 15] requires 10^3 conformational energy calculations so that the total computational complexity of this study is in the order of 10^8 energy calculations.

The 483 genes can be classified in three categories, according to the information that can be deduced from similarities between sequences:

1. structural
2. functional, or
3. none.

A particular gene is characterized structurally if its sequence is homologous to the sequence of a protein with known structure, and it is characterized functionally if its sequence is similar [16] to a protein of known function. It is clear that a successful fold recognition technique has to be able to identify and confirm those cases where a structure of a protein can be inferred by sequence comparison techniques. For nine genes of the *C. elegans* chromosome III the structure can be inferred in this way (Table 1).

Table 2: The models of sequences for which significant scores were found are grouped according to the type of information available from sequence comparison.
[a] Sequences are identified by their codes in GenPept, a database of conceptual translations of GenBank genes.
[b] Structures are identified by their Brookhaven code with an optional chain identifier separated by a dash.
[c] Score is the geometric mean of an alignment factor and a scoring factor. The alignment factor reflects the formal completeness of the alignment, i.e. when sequence and structure have the same length and are fully aligned without gaps this factor is 1.0. The scoring factor becomes 1.0 when the energetic quality of the model (Z-score) is identical to the average quality of correct models of the same length.
[d] Sequence identities between the sequence and the structure on amino acid level.
[e] The column 'structure' gives a short description of the structure found to provide the best template for the correlated sequence, compared to the result of sequence homology searches in the last column.

```
------------------------------------------------------------------------------
GenBank      PDB     Score^c Ident^d Structure^e               Sequence homology with^e
locus name^a code^b          [%]
------------------------------------------------------------------------------
Direct structural information available:
CELF54H12_1  1aco    1.06    73    ACONITASE                   aconitase
CER107_7     1gsr-a  1.05    42    GSH S-TRANSFERASE CLASS PI  GSH S-transferase P subunit
CELC29E4_2   1ake-a  1.02    47    ADENYLATE CYCLASE           adenylate cyclase
CEF58A4_9    1aak    0.97    38    UBIQUITIN CONJUGTG. ENZYME  ubiquitin conjugating enzymes
CEF59B2_6    121p    0.93    28    ONCO RAS P21                ras-related GTP-bdg proteins
CEZK637_10   2tpr-b  0.92    30    TRYPANOTHIONE REDUCTASE     gluthatione reductase
CELC30C11_3  1ats    0.92    29    HSP70 (YEAST)               Msi3p (HSP70 protein family)
CEF54C8_5    121p    0.91    33    ONCO RAS P21                ras protein family
CEF55H2_1    2sod-b  0.90    45    CU,ZN SUPEROXIDE DISMUTASE  superoxide dismutase
------------------------------------------------------------------------------
Indirect structural information available:
CEZK637_12   1mbd    0.91    .     MYOGLOBIN (DEOXY)           globin-like antigen homologue
CER08D7_5    5cpv    0.90    .     CA-BINDING PARVALBUMIN B    caltractin, Ca-bdg proteins
CELC50C3_8   1sas    0.90    .     SARCOPLASM. CA-BDG. PROTEIN calmodulin
------------------------------------------------------------------------------
Functional information available:
CEZK632_8    121p    0.99    .     ONCO RAS P21                ADP ribosylation factor
CEZK637_3    2msb-a  0.94    .     MANNOSE-BINDING PROTEIN A   HSV11 IE110 homologue
CELB0303_4   1guh-a  0.92    .     GSH S-TRANSFERASE A1-1      phenylethanolamine-N-methyl-TF
CELF44B9_2   1ndk    0.91    .     NUCLEOSIDE DI-P KINASE      protein phosphatase
CEC15H7_2    4gst-a  0.91    .     GSH S-TRANSFERASE (ISO 3-3) tyrosine kinases
------------------------------------------------------------------------------
No information available:
CELC08C3_4   2rsl-c  0.94    .     GAMMA-DELTA-RESOLVASE           --
CELZC262_4   2mhr    0.93    .     MYOHEMERYTHRIN                  --
CEZK632_12   1ndk    0.92    .     NUCLEOSIDE DIPHOSPHATE KINASE   --
CELC30A5_2   1fha    0.92    .     FERRITIN (H-CHAIN)             --
CELZK652_2   1hyp    0.91    .     HYDROPHOBIC PROTEIN FROM SOYBEAN --
CEF02A9_2    2fbj-l  0.91    .     IG*A FAB FRAGMENT              --
CEC40H1_5    2aza-a  0.91    .     AZURIN (OXIDIZED) (E-TRANSPORT) --
CEC40H1_4    1tbp-b  0.91    .     TATA-BINDING PROTEIN (YEAST)   --
CELZK652_4   1ubq    0.90    .     UBIQUITIN                      --
CELZK370_6   2fxb    0.90    .     FERREDOXIN (E-TRANSPORT)       --
CELZK353_7   1hst-a  0.90    .     HISTONE H5                     --
CELZC97_2    2rsl-c  0.90    .     GAMMA-DELTA-RESOLVASE          --
CELZC262_2   1crn    0.90    .     CRAMBIN                        --
CELR05D3_5   2trx-a  0.90    .     THIOREDOXIN (E-TRANSPORT)      --
CELF09G8_5   2scp-a  0.90    .     SARCOPLASMIC CA-BINDING PROTEIN --
CELC29E4_4   1guh-a  0.90    .     GSH S-TRANSFERASE A1-1         --
------------------------------------------------------------------------------
```

Table 2 summarizes the most significant models out of 10^5 obtained in the alignment production stage. The significance is expressed by a score incorporating information about the energy distribution in conformation space [14, 15] and the fraction of residues matched between sequence and structure. All nine genes whose three dimensional structure can be assigned (Table 1) score among the most significant models. Therefore, the technique produces reasonable alignments, and the results obtained in these nine cases indicate the range of significant scores for native like sequence structure pairs to be ≥ 0.90.

Additional clues on the performance of the technique are obtained from those genes where structural information can be inferred indirectly. For example, gene CEZK637_12 has been shown to be homologous to some globin sequence, but this sequence has no significant homology to any of the globins in the structure database used in this study. This sequence combined with the myoglobin structure (1mbd) results in a model whose score of 0.91 is significant. In this case the technique successfully identifies the correct fold in the absence of sequence homology. Two further examples of indirect structural information are CER08D7_5 and CELC50C3_8 whose folds are also correctly identified as calcium binding proteins.

For the sequences discussed so far the folds retrieved by fold recognition agree with the available structural information. For the remaining genes with significant scores assembled in Table 2 the fold recognition technique predicts structures. It is clear that these are putative and approximate models of the native folds of these gene products. Here we can distinguish between sequences which are homologous to some known sequence and genes whose biological role is unknown. In the first case the results indicate that the gene product and its related protein adopt native folds which are both similar to the template structure. One such example is CEZK632_8 whose structure is here predicted to be related to onco RAS p21, 121p. By the above argument ADP ribosylation factors are also predicted to have a RAS p21 related structure. For the remaining gene products in Table 2, where no information is available from sequence comparison, fold recognition predicts a structural template for the unknown native fold.

To summarize, in all cases where structural information is available the applied fold recognition technique yields correct results, and the respective scores provide an estimate for the confidence limits. In all other cases the models obtained are necessarily putative. Presently we can judge their quality mainly with respect to the confidence limits defined above. Interpreted in this way the technique reveals additional structural information for 20 gene products of the *C. elegans* chromosome III using a database of 263 known folds. Clearly the amount of information retrievable depends on the number of structures used.

Often even sparse structural information on proteins has triggered considerable progress in understanding biological phenomena on a molecular level. Since the putative models obtained here are blind predictions the accuracy of individual models is unknown. If the quality of the predictions is comparable to those cases where structural information is available then most of the models should be useful starting points for further structural or biochemical studies. Alignments and coordinates of the models listed in Table 2 are available via anonymous FTP from gundi.came.sbg.ac.at (IP 141.201.27.11).

Alignment production and score calculation for one sequence structure combination require 30 CPU seconds on a single R4400 processor. Over all 1000 CPU hours were needed to complete this study, demonstrating the feasibility of fold recognition as a routine tool for sequence analysis in genome projects.

Acknowledgements

We are indebted to Hannes Flöckner for technical assistance, Jiri Novotny and Bob Bruccoleri for their support in using the Bristol-Myers Squibb computing facilities, and Colombe Chappey and Jim Ostell for helpful discussions. This work was supported by the Fonds zur Förderung der wissenschaftlichen Forschung (Austria) and the Jubiläumsfonds der Österreichischen Nationalbank.

References

[1] R. Wilson *et al.*, *Nature*, 368, p./ 32-38, 1994.

[2] C. Orengo, *Curr. Opp. Struc. Biol.*, 4, p. 429-440, 1994.

[3] J. P. Overington, *Curr. Opp. Struc. Biol.*, 2, p. 394-401, 1992.

[4] J. U. Bowie, R. Lüthy and D. Eisenberg, *Science*, 253, p. 164-170, 1991.

[5] M. J. Sippl and S.. Weitckus, *Proteins*, 13, p. 258-271, 1992.

[6] C. Ouzounis, C. Sander, M. Scharf and R. Schneider, *J. Mol. Biol.*, 232, p. 805-825, 1993.

[7] J. U. Bowie and D. Eisenberg, *Curr. Opp. Struc. Biol.*, 3, p. 437-444, 1993.

[8] A. Godzik, A. Kolinski and J. Skolnick, *J. Comp. Aid. Mol. Des.*, 7, p. 397-438, 1993.

[9] D. T. Jones and J. M. Thornton, *J. Comp. Aid. Mol. Des.*, 7, p. 439-456, 1993.

[10] M. J. Sippl, *J. Comp. Aid. Mol. Des.*, 7, p. 473-501, 1993.

[11] M. J. Sippl, *J. Mol. Biol.*, 213, p. 859-883, 1990.

[12] M. Hendlich *et al.*, *J. Mol. Biol.*, 216, p. 167-180, 1990.

[13] M. J. Sippl, S. Weitckus and H. Flöckner, in *The protein folding problem and tertiary structure prediction*, S. LeGrand and K. M. Merz (eds.), p. 353-407, 1994.

[14] M. J. Sippl and M. Jaritz, in *Protein structure by distance analysis*, H. Bohr and S. Brunak (eds.), p. 113-134, 1994.

[15] M. J. Sippl, *Proteins*, 17, p. 355-362, 1993.

[16] S. F. Altschul *et al.*, *Nat.Genet.*, 6, p. 119-129, 1994.

[17] F. C. Bernstein *et al.*, *J. Mol. Biol.*, 112, p. 535-542, 1977.

Protein Fold Determination Using a small Number of Distance Restraints

A. Aszódi*, M. J. Gradwell[†] and W. R. Taylor*

* Laboratory of Mathematical Biology and [†] Laboratory of Molecular Structure, National Institute for Medical Research, The Ridgeway, Mill Hill, London NW7 1AA, UK

Abstract

We have designed a distance geometry-based method for obtaining the correct global fold of proteins from a limited number of structure-specific distance restraints and the secondary structure assignment. Unknown interresidue distances were predicted from patterns of conserved hydrophobic amino acids deduced from multiple alignments. A simple model chain was then folded by projecting its distance matrix into Euclidean spaces with gradually decreasing dimensionality until a final 3-dimensional embedding was achieved. Tangled conformations produced by the projection steps were eliminated using a novel filtering algorithm. The robustness of the method was increased by incorporating background information on various aspects of protein structure such as accessibility and chirality. The correct folds of three small proteins were successfully identified from a small number of restraints, indicating that the method could serve as a useful computational tool for determining protein structures from NMR data.

1 Introduction

The molecular conformation of small proteins can now be determined in solution, thanks to the rapid development of NMR spectroscopy techniques. Experimental structural information is supplied in the form of distance restraints (*i. e.* interatomic distance ranges flanked by lower and upper bounds), obtained from NOE (Nuclear Overhauser Effect) spectra. A wide variety of computer programs can then be used to generate plausible conformations which satisfy the distance restraints [17, 13, 15]. Most methods are based on restrained molecular dynamics or distance geometry techniques, the latter being natural candidates for NMR structure determination since they provide an elegant way to satisfy the distance restraints and the stereochemical constraints (bond lengths, angles etc.) imposed upon the structure simultaneously. Often a hybrid approach is applied whereby a set of candidate conformations, generated by the distance geometry program, are subsequently refined by molecular dynamics simulations.

The distance restraints obtained from NMR spectra may not be sufficient to define a unique 3-dimensional conformation. Robust algorithms are needed which can utilise the experimental data effectively and are able to incorporate general stereochemical information as well in order to produce adequate global folds. The theoretical minimum number of restraints was determined by [12], based on statistical mechanics considerations. Computer experiments [14, 22] also suggest that it is possible to design reliable methods which can generate the correct conformation using a small amount of distance information. Theoretical structure prediction studies led to similar conclusions [26, 11].

We have designed the programs DRAGON and DRAGON-2 which folded model polypeptide chains into compact three-dimensional conformations possessing a hydrophobic core and secondary structure using distance geometry techniques [3, 4]. The choice of interresidue distances was guided by the hydrophobicity of the monomers and the general stereochemical restraints of main-chain hydrogen bonding imposed upon the chain. The DRAGON programs were originally intended for the theoretical study of structure forming factors in polypeptides and although the chains were folded into protein-like conformations, they could not be regarded as models of any particular protein. In order to perform proper molecular modeling, external distance restraints had to be supplied to the projection algorithm, coupled with additional background information about various aspects of protein structure such as topological constraints and chirality. The built-in stereochemical knowledge was expected to increase the robustness of the algorithm which was tested on simulated sparse distance restraint sets.

2   Methods

The molecular modeling method presented here is implemented as the program DRAGON-3, an extension of the distance geometry program DRAGON-2 [4]. Only a brief overview of the techniques applied in DRAGON-3 can be given below; a detailed description will be published elsewhere [1].

The objective of the present study was to simulate the determination of the correct folds of monomeric proteins by NMR. This is a crucial step in the elucidation of protein structure especially if the set of distance restraints are too sparse or inconsistent in which cases several different folding topologies might be found. Once the correct topology is known, the researcher can rely on various methods to refine the details of the conformation; however, it is quite unlikely that he can obtain the correct structure starting from an incorrect global fold.

DRAGON-3 was designed to generate a small number of plausible folds corresponding to a sparse set of distance restraints quickly. The program operates on a reduced representation of the polypeptide chain using just two atoms per amino acid: a C_α atom making up the backbone connections and a pseudo-C_β atom having the same van der Waals volume as the corresponding side chain. This low-resolution representation, while retaining the essential geometric features of the polypeptide chain, was crucial in reducing computer time requirements.

2.1   External information

DRAGON-3 relied on two sources of input, NMR data and sequential homology (Fig. 1). Instead of using experimental information, simulated data were generated from high-resolution protein structures deposited in the Protein Data Bank [6]. This approach enabled us to retain full control over the input data and also the quality of the results could be easily assessed by comparing the model conformations to the corresponding target PDB structure.

2.1.1   NMR-derived data

Distance restraints between amino acids separated by more than 5 residues in sequence (henceforth referred to as "long-range" interactions) were supposed to have been obtained from NOEs in 2D NMR experiments. These long-range restraints were simulated from the target PDB

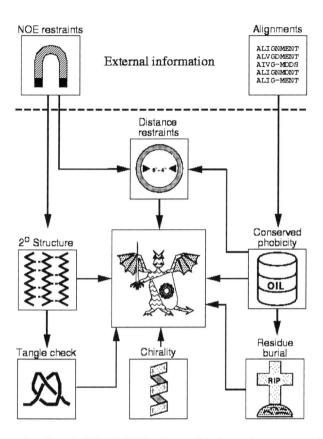

Figure 1: Information flow in DRAGON-3. External information was supplied in the form of NOE distance restraints and multiple sequence alignments.

structures by collecting the centroid distances between side chain pairs closer together than 5.0 Å . Lower and upper bounds were obtained by adding ± 2 Å to these centroid distances (Fig. 2). The number of restraints were varied by removing randomly selected items to create sparse data sets. These restraints were applied to the pseudo-C_β atoms representing side chains. "Short-range" NOE data between close sequential neighbours were not used directly but we assumed that a full secondary structure assignment could be obtained from these. The assignment procedure itself was not carried out; instead, the secondary structure information in the target PDB entry was used.

2.1.2   Sequence information

Interresidue distances, for which no NMR-derived information was available, were predicted from the pairwise conserved hydrophobicity score [25]. The underlying assumption was that conserved *and* hydrophobic pairs of residues are likely to be close together in the core of the molecule. Sequences from a range of evolutionarily distant organisms which showed a moderate homology to the target sequence were obtained from the SwissProt database [5] and the conserved hydrophobicity scores were calculated from multiple alignments generated by the MULTAL algorithm [24]. The pairwise scores were then transformed into interresidue

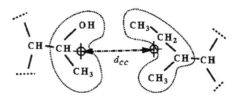

$\oplus$: side chain centroid

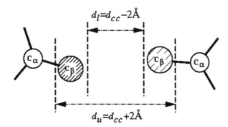

Figure 2: The calculation of simulated NOE distance restraints. Pairs of side chains closer together than a preset limit were chosen and the lower and upper distance limits (d_l and d_u) were obtained from the centroid—centroid distance d_{cc} by subtracting and adding 2 Å respectively. Variable fractions of randomly chosen restraints were then removed from the initial set to produce more and more sparse sets.

distance estimates by an appropriate nonlinear function so that their distribution matched the observed distance distribution in monomeric proteins [2]. However, individual interresidue distances cannot be predicted accurately from general features such as hydrophobicity, therefore the estimates obtained from the prediction were used only as guidelines in the course of the iteration.

In addition to the calculation of conserved hydrophobicity scores, the hydrophobicity values of the amino acids in the target sequence were also used in the adjustment of residue accessibilities. During iteration, accessibilities were monitored by the "cone" algorithm [4] and residue positions were adjusted so that hydrophobic amino acids became buried and hydrophilics exposed.

2.2   Secondary structure and stereochemical information

The formation of regular secondary structure drastically reduces the number of available conformations of the polypeptide chain, due to the strict distance restraints imposed upon the backbone by the main-chain hydrogen bonds. Since the full secondary structure assignment of the target molecule was assumed to be known (cf. above), DRAGON-3 could utilise the interresidue distance information from the geometry of ideal α-helices and β-sheets [19, 20, 27]. Secondary structure also enabled the incorporation of additional stereochemical knowledge about chirality and tangles.

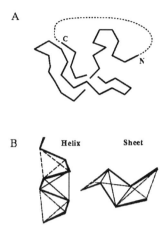

Figure 3: Tangle detection. A, The topological definition of tangled polypeptide chains is difficult since even if the termini are connected to form a closed loop, the resulting object may not be knotted. B, Tangles were detected by checking whether a part of the chain penetrated the tetrahedra on secondary structure elements.

2.2.1   Chirality

Since the distance matrices of a point set and its mirror image are identical, distance geometry-based methods cannot distinguish between enantiomers without extra information. Furthermore, N-dimensional chiral objects become achiral in $N + 1$ dimensions and consequently handedness consistency cannot be maintained in the gradual projection method [4]. Since the simplified chain representation used by DRAGON-3 is made up of asymmetric monomers, correct 3D chirality had to be imposed upon them in a separate refinement stage. This was accomplished through the adjustment of the torsion angle about the main chain H-bonds as described in [4].

2.2.2   Tangles

Tangled conformations are frequently generated by distance geometry projections although such structures are very few, if not completely absent, among proteins [9]. We designed a fast and efficient algorithm that filtered out the tangled conformations after every projection step. The method was based on the elimination of crossings between segments of the polypeptide chain (Fig. 3). Crossings were detected by placing tetrahedra onto secondary structure elements and checking for other segments penetrating these tetrahedra. Tangle elimination was accomplished by moving interlocked segments away from each other until no more violations were observed.

2.3   Controls

The performance of DRAGON-3 was compared to that of X-PLOR Version 3.1 [8], a popular tool frequently used for NMR structure determination. Although X-PLOR is capable of performing all-atom energy minimisations, the simulations were carried out on model chains containing just two pseudo-atoms per monomer (cf. above) to facilitate comparison with

DRAGON's reduced representation. Pseudobond lengths and angles were maintained by appropriate "hard" potential functions, while secondary structure geometries were adjusted by imposing suitable distance restraints enforced by a soft asymptotic square-well potential [18]. These potentials were also used to impose the NOE-derived long-range distance restraints to the pseudo-C_β atoms. Starting from an extended chain, conformational search was carried out by using a simulated annealing protocol (for details, see [1]).

For each target structure, several distance restraint sets were defined and 25 model structures were generated from every restraint set by DRAGON-3 and X-PLOR. Modeling precision and accuracy were assessed by calculating coordinate root mean square (RMS) deviations between the target and model C_α backbones. Model topologies were evaluated by visual inspection and were classified as "correct", "slightly incorrect" (i. e. one secondary structure segment misplaced), "incorrect" or "mirror image".

2.4   Target structures

Three well resolved small monomeric proteins (Brookhaven codes given in parentheses) were chosen for analysis representing the major structural classes.

1. bovine vitamin D-dependent Ca^{2+}-binding protein (3ICB): This protein represented the all-α structural class. It is 75 residues long and contains four α-helices and a small irregular helix. The X-ray structure was determined at 2.3 Å resolution [23]. The multiple sequence alignment was constructed from eight other calcium-binding proteins containing EF-hand motifs.
2. Tendamistat (3AIT): This 74-residue long protein, an α-amylase inhibitor from *Streptomyces tendae*, is a sandwich of two 3-strand antiparallel β-sheets and contains two disulfide bonds. The structure of the PDB entry was determined by constrained energy minimisation from solution NMR measurements using the AMBER 3.0 protocol [7]. The multiple alignment was constructed from six α-amylase inhibitor sequences from other *Streptomyces* species.
3. Thioredoxin (2TRX): Thioredoxin is an electron transport protein from *Escherichia coli*. The PDB entry contains two chemically identical chains in the unit cell designated "A" and "B" among which chain "A" was chosen as the target structure. The molecule is 108 amino acids long and contains a 5-strand mixed β-sheet in the core, shielded by five helices in a fold similar to that of flavodoxin (4FXN). The structure was determined at a resolution of 1.68 Å [16]. The multiple alignment was constructed from twelve other thioredoxin and S—S isomerase sequences.

2.5   Implementation

DRAGON-3 was implemented as an ANSI C program by A.A. The models presented in this paper were produced by running DRAGON-3 in batch mode on various SGI computers. Execution time for a 3ICB model (75 residues) was about 2 mins on a SGI Challenge S equipped with a R4400/150 MHz processor. X-PLOR was run on a Sun Sparcstation 10 model 41 and a 3ICB model with 86 long-range restraints was generated in about 35 mins. The corresponding execution time for DRAGON on the same machine was about 4 mins.

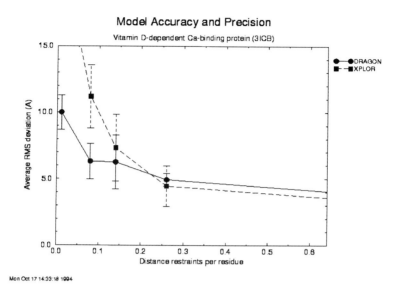

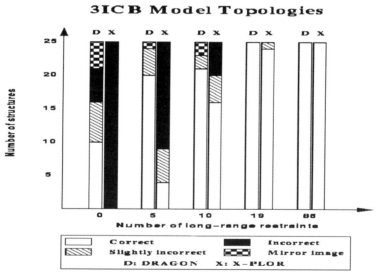

Figure 4: Simulation results for the bovine vitamin D-dependent Ca^{2+}-binding protein (3ICB). A, Average RMS deviation of the models from the PDB structure as a function of the number of long-range distance restraints per residue. Circles and squares represent the models generated by DRAGON-3 and X-PLOR, respectively. B, Results of the visual topology checks. White, striped and black bars symbolise correct, slightly incorrect and seriously incorrect topologies, respectively. Chequered bars symbolise mirror images. For every restraint set, the left and right bars represent DRAGON (D) and X-PLOR (X) models, respectively.

3   Results

3.1   Bovine vitamin D-dependent Ca^{2+}-binding protein

Five sets of simulated NOE restraints were generated for the models, containing 86, 19, 10, 5 and 0 long-range restraints, respectively. With 86 and 19 long-range restraints, both

DRAGON-3 and X-PLOR identified the correct fold, and the average RMS deviations of the X-PLOR structures were slightly better than those of produced by DRAGON-3. The DRAGON structures generated from 10 or 5 restraints still had essentially correct topologies (apart from an occasional misplaced helix), while the X-PLOR models became increasingly inaccurate (Fig. 4 and Color plate 9, page xxiii, respectively). In the no-restraints case, DRAGON-3 correctly identified the native fold in 40% of the runs and even the incorrect folds were globular and compact, whereas X-PLOR failed to pack the helices together at all.

3.2   Tendamistat

The datasets for tendamistat contained 120, 46, 10, 5 and 0 long-range simulated NOE restraints. For this protein, DRAGON-3 always performed much better than X-PLOR, the latter producing a large number of mirror-image topologies and tangled structures. The DRAGON-3 folds were correct down to the 5 long-range restraint case, where packing became loose but the native topology was still preserved (Figs. 5 and Color plate 10, page xxiv, respectively). Without any long-range restraints, 20% of the model conformations became slightly incorrect.

3.3   Thioredoxin

The NOE distance datasets for thioredoxin contained 161,48,30,20 and 0 simulated restraints. Starting from the two largest restraint sets, DRAGON-3 always found the correct fold, while X-PLOR produced several mirror-image conformations and tangled structures even for the largest dataset. With 30 restraints, DRAGON-3 produced two distinct families of solutions. Half of the models were still correct with RMS deviations around 4.5 Å, while the other half possessed incorrect topologies. The corresponding X-PLOR models were of comparable quality but with a higher number of mirror images and seriously incorrect topologies (Fig. 6 and Color plate 11, page xxv respectively). When the number of restraints were further reduced, both programs generated models with high RMS deviations and only about one-third of the folds were correct. Similarly to the case of 3ICB, X-PLOR had difficulties with packing the helices when only a small number of long-range restraints were available and therefore the models had much larger RMS deviations than the corresponding compact DRAGON-3 structures. However, neither program could produce useful conformations from less than 20 long-range restraints.

4   Discussion

4.1   Accuracy and precision

In an NMR structure determination problem, the attainable accuracy is limited by the quality of the experimental data which is influenced by the number of restraints, the ranges spanned by the lower and upper bounds and by the distribution of restraints between main-chain and side-chain atoms. These factors contribute to the overall accuracy and precision in a complicated way and for the sake of tractability we focused on just one of them, *viz.* the number of distance restraints. The simplifications consisted of generating simulated distance restraints so that the lower and upper bounds were always separated by 4 Å and the restraints were applied only to the pseudo-C_β atoms. Under these circumstances DRAGON-3 generally produced more accurate results than X-PLOR. The gradual projection algorithm coupled to high-dimensional structural optimisation could often find the correct topology even from sparse datasets. This correlates with the observation that local minima can be avoided by performing energy minimisation in

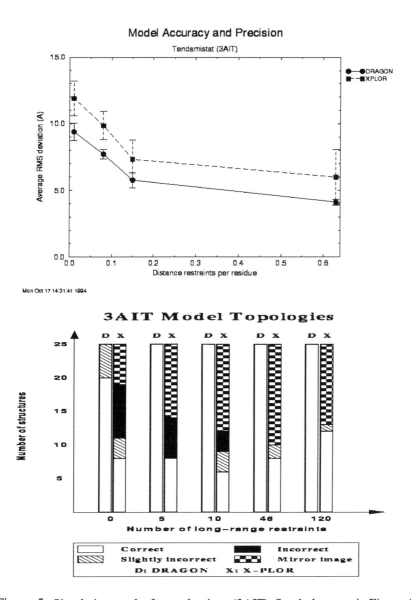

Figure 5: Simulation results for tendamistat (3AIT). Symbols are as in Figure 4.

four or more dimensions [10, 21]. Judging from the results obtained with very sparse distance data, the minimal number of restraints per residue necessary for successful fold identification grows with the chain length in a non-linear fashion.

The precision of the DRAGON models was almost always significantly better than those generated by X-PLOR, as indicated by the RMS deviation values of the individual models from the corresponding average structures. From our previous studies [3] it was known that the self-consistent triangle inequality smoothing performed before each projection step in the DRAGON algorithm generated a wide variety of conformations in the absence of external structural information, indicating that the algorithm sampled the conformational space

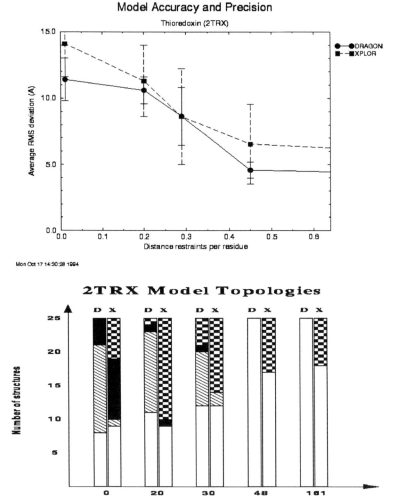

Figure 6: Simulation results for thioredoxin (2TRX). Symbols are as in Figure 4.

adequately [13]. The low standard deviation of model RMS values obtained with external distance restraints indicates that the algorithm delivered high precision and good sampling at the same time.

4.2 Robustness

In the context of NMR structure determination, a program is considered robust if it is capable of producing satisfactory conformations (i.e. correct global folds) from scarce sets of interresidue distances. Robustness can be achieved if the program is equipped with heuristic knowledge about the stereochemistry of proteins. The most important of the heuristics employed by DRAGON-3 were the modeling of the hydrophobic effect, the elimination of tangled conformations and chirality checks.

4.2.1   Compactness and the hydrophobic effect

The hydrophobic effect was modeled by reducing the distances between hydrophobic residues and by adjusting the accessibility of every side chain in the molecule. In the absence of external distance restraints this approach still succeeded in producing compact structures, often with the correct topology. However, DRAGON-3 was more successful with α-helices which usually provide clear structural orientation in the form of their hydrophobic moments.

The hydrophobic core building heuristics forced exposed hydrophobic residues towards the centre of the molecule. This approach could fail on small proteins which might lack a compact hydrophobic core. In many cases the function of the protein in question requires that apolar residues occupy exposed positions on the surface, thus being exceptions to the rule of hydrophobic burial. A good example is tendamistat, one of the target proteins used in this study, a small enzyme inhibitor which had these inconvenient features from the modeling point of view. Indeed, with just 5 long-range distance restraints DRAGON-3 could not pack the constituent β-sheets together.

4.2.2   Tangles

Native folded polypeptides rarely, if ever, contain tangles but unfortunately they are quite easy to generate in models. Distance geometry projection techniques are also not immune from this artifact especially when larger molecules are modeled. Since tangles may trap the chain in incorrect conformations, their elimination is highly desirable. However, the detection of tangling by computer is difficult due to the lack of a reliable topological definition. The tangle elimination heuristic employed in DRAGON-3 was not universal since it hinged on the topology of secondary structures and could not be used on chains without any secondary structure. Nevertheless, most tangles were successfully eliminated, indicating that a practical compromise was found between generality and practicality.

4.2.3   Chirality

All distance geometry-based methods must handle chirality separately since the distance matrix does not contain any handedness information. While the ultimate source of chirality in polypeptides is the handedness of the C_α-atoms of the amino acids, the simplified chain representation in DRAGON-3 enabled us to monitor handedness at a higher structural level. By adjusting the chirality of the secondary structure elements [4], incorrect mirror image folds could be filtered out since these became energetically slightly unfavourable diastereomers compared to the correct topology.

4.3   Concluding remarks

Our aim has been to show that correct overall folds are more easily obtained from sparse distance data when general properties of proteins are incorporated, producing compact, untangled conformations with well-defined hydrophobic cores. Although the algorithm presented above was based on Distance Geometry, the stereochemical heuristics could have been built into other optimisation methods operating in three-dimensional Euclidean space. The main application of our method could be the generation of a family of good starting conformations which could then be further refined by a suitable program such as X-PLOR, thus helping the experimental scientists to obtain more reliable structures from sparse NMR data.

Acknowledgments

The authors wish to thank Dr. J. Feeney and Dr. A. Šali for their helpful comments and suggestions.

References

[1] A. Aszódi, M. J. Gradwell, and W. R. Taylor, Global fold determination from a small number of distance restraints, *J. Mol. Biol. (submitted)*.

[2] A. Aszódi and W. R. Taylor, Estimating polypeptide alpha-carbon distances from multiple sequence alignments, *J. Math. Chem. (in press)*.

[3] A. Aszódi and W. R. Taylor, Folding polypeptide alpha-carbon backbones by distance geometry methods, *Biopolymers*, 34, 489–505, 1994.

[4] A. Aszódi and W. R. Taylor, Secondary structure formation in model polypeptide chains, *Protein Engng.*, 7, 633–644, 1994.

[5] A. Bairoch and B. Boeckmann, The SWISS-PROT protein sequence data bank, *Nucleic Acids Res.*, 19, 2247–2249, 1991.

[6] F. C. Bernstein, T. F. Koetzle, G. J. B. Williams, E. F. Meyer, M. D. Brice, J. R. Rodgers, O. Kennard, T. Shimanouchi, and M. Tasumi, The protein databank, a computer-based archival file for macromolecular structures, *J. Mol. Biol.*, 112, 535–542, 1977.

[7] M. Billeter, T. Schaumann, W. Braun, and K. Wüthrich, Restrained energy refinement with two different algorithms and force fields of the structure of the alpha-amylase inhibitor tendamistat determined by NMR in solution, *Biopolymers*, 29, 695–706, 1990.

[8] A. T. Brünger, *XPLOR Manual*, Yale University, New Haven, Connecticut, 1992.

[9] M. L. Connolly, I. D. Kuntz, and G. M. Crippen, Linked and threaded loops in proteins, *Biopolymers*, 19, 1167–1182, 1980.

[10] G. M. Crippen, Conformational analysis by energy embedding, *J. Comp. Chem.*, 3, 471–476, 1982.

[11] T. Dandekar and P. Argos, Folding the main-chain of small proteins with the genetic algorithm, *J. Mol. Biol.*, 236, 844–861, 1994.

[12] A. M. Gutin and E. I. Shakhnovich, Statistical mechanics of polymers with distance constraints, *J. Chem. Phys.*, 100, 5290–5293, 1994.

[13] T. F. Havel, An evaluation of computational strategies for use in the determination of protein structure from distance constraints obtained by nuclear magnetic resonance, *Prog. Biophys. Mol. Biol.*, 56, 43–78, 1991.

[14] J. C. Hoch and A. S. Stern, A method for determining overall protein fold from NMR distance restraints, *J. Biomol. NMR*, 2, 535–543, 1992.

[15] T. L. James Computational strategies pertinent to NMR solution structure determination, *Current Opin. Struct. Biol.*, 4, 275–284, 1994.

[16] S. K. Katti, D. M. LeMaster, and H. Eklund, Crystal structure of thioredoxin from Escherichia coli at 1.68 Å resolution, *J. Mol. Biol.*, 212, 167–184, 1990.

[17] I. D. Kuntz, J. F. Thomason, and C. M. Oshiro, Distance geometry, *Meth. Enzymol.*, 177, 159–204, 1989.

[18] M. Nilges, A. M. Gronenborn, A. T. Brünger, and G. M. Clore, Determination of three-dimensional structures of proteins by simulated annealing with interproton distance

restraints. Application to crambin, potato carboxypeptidase and barley serine protease inhibitor 2. *Prot. Engng.*, 2, 27–38, 1988.

[19] L. Pauling and R. B. Corey, The pleated sheet, a new layer configuration of polypeptide chains, *Proc. Natl. Acad. Sci. U. S. A.*, 37, 251–256, 1951.

[20] L. Pauling and R. B. Corey, The structure of synthetic polypeptides, *Proc. Natl. Acad. Sci. U. S. A.*, 37, 241–250, 1951.

[21] E. O. Purisima and H. A. Scheraga, An approach to the multiple-minima problem by relaxing dimensionality, *Proc. Natl. Acad. Sci. U. S. A.*, 83, 2782–2786, 1986.

[22] M. J. Smith-Brown, D. Kominos, and R. M. Levy, Global folding of proteins using a limited number of distance constraints, *Protein Engng.*, 6, 605–614, 1993.

[23] D. M. E. Szebenyi and K. Moffat, The refined structure of vitamin D-dependent calcium-binding protein from bovine intestine. Molecular details, ion binding and implications for the structure of other calcium-binding proteins, *J. Biol. Chem.*, 261, 8761–8777, 1986.

[24] W. R. Taylor, A flexible method to align large numbers of biological sequences, *J. Molec. Evol.*, 28, 161–169, 1988.

[25] W. R. Taylor, Towards protein tertiary fold prediction using distance and motif constraints, *Protein Engng.*, 4, 853–870, 1991.

[26] W. R. Taylor, Protein fold refinement, Building models from idealised folds using motif constraints and multiple sequence data, *Protein Engng.*, 6, 593–604, 1993.

[27] H. Wako and H. A. Scheraga, Distance-constraint approach to protein folding. I. Statistical analysis of protein conformations in terms of distances between residues, *J. Prot. Chem.*, 1, 5–45, 1982.

How many protein fold classes
are to be found?

Per-Anker Lindgård and Henrik Bohr*

Department of Condensed Matter Physics, Risø National Laboratory, DK-4000 Roskilde,
Denmark
* Center for Biological Sequence Analysis, The Technical University of Denmark, DK-2800
Lyngby, Denmark

Abstract

A new, unique representation for folds is presented in terms of a chiral spin
model. It allows a systematic classification of protein folds. It is employed
to yield an estimate of how many protein fold classes there can exist in nature
using arguments from statistical mechanics and polymer physics. The final
answer comes out to be around 4000, which is in the same range as Chothia's
estimate made on the basis of the growth rate in the experimental protein structure
database.

1   Introduction

Along with the rapid expansion of sequence data from the worlds genome projects it is
interesting to asses how many radically new protein structures which are yet to be discovered.
This has remained an important and open question in micro biology. Remarkably one can
obtain an upper bound of ≈ 4000 fold classes, from simple physical arguments. Recently
Chothia [1] addressed the question of how many protein families or fold classes there might
be from a very different point of view than the present. Based on the pace of discovery and the
presently known number Chothia estimated a total of one thousand families. More interesting
yet would be if that number was contained in the information provided by the amino acid
sequence of the proteins themselves. A simple model for super structures of secondary protein
structures is here shown to give approximately that number just from the linear sequence
information and the constraint that the useful proteins are densely packed. A fold means
[2, 3, 4, 5, 6, 7, 8] a particular structure with a specific topology that a folded protein, or part
of it, can assume in its native state. We have represented folds on a lattice where it is easy
to define, by symmetry and lattice link replacements, when structures belong to the same or
a different fold class. However, contrary to previous lattice models which consider lattices
of monomers [9, 10], we project the full secondary structures onto lattice animals. It is a
new paradigm to classify proteins by their structural topology rather than their sequence or, as
usual, their function.

Proteins appear to belong to families, like plants, with specific characteristics. The
families contain many variants. Linné [11] in the 18th century succeeded in the field of
botany to identify the important classification parameters. It gives a systematic, although not
natural classification. The dense fold patterns for proteins may be such characteristics and

we shall identify a class of similar folds with families in agreement with Chothia (and with the qualifications mentioned that the fold classes need not be the natural families, a problem already encountered by Linné in his classification). Chothia gave a good review of the present knowledge of the protein families, which need not be repeated here.

2   Schematization of protein folds

A major puzzle has been how nature can fold a long protein into its dense form in a short time without trying all possibilities. This can be elucidated by well-known problems in condensed matter physics. In many cases in physics of highly degenerate problems it is the weak symmetry breaking forces which determine the major structure, whereas it is the strong forces which determine the details. An example is the Heisenberg magnet for which an infinitesimal anisotropic field will determine the overall direction of the ordering vector, whereas all other properties are determined by the exchange interaction. Consider now an extended protein, already composed of its secondary structures, with elements such as (1) α-helices [12], β-strands for potential β-sheets and (2) the intervening strands (e.g. representing turns). Let us then suppose that the linear amino acid information provides a very weak preference for a particular bending at each junction. This would break the symmetry, which gives rise to the enormous "random walk" degeneracy, and thus determines essentially the final folds, the fold classes, and to a certain extent removes the Levinthal paradox [13]. He pointed out, that the space of possible configuration, i.e. the number of local minima that a medium size protein can attain, is enormous ($\sim 20^{100}$) judged just from the linear sequence information. Our hypothesis is that nature solves the paradox and reduces the number of possibilities drastically by breaking the proteins up into building blocks, secondary structures, domains etc., with specific rules of connections. Finkelstein *et al.* [14] have discussed a selected set of prototypical protein folds from a simplified structural point of view. To describe the α-helical globule they introduced a close packing rule of linear α-helix elements. In another paper about β-sheets [15] they discuss various sequential stackings using a different schematic model. We wish to introduce an even simpler model, which simultaneously is able to describe these two essential fold types. We have analysed the discussed structures and found that for the β-sheets a rectangular description of course is very natural - with elements of different lengths. However, even in the case of the α-helix globule a mapping can be made to a rectangularized representation (which can be demonstrated by wire models and by direct computer mapping of the coordinates). The realistic, more 'closed packed angles' may be thought of having arisen after a twisting of the rectangular structures. Neglecting this (in analogy to considering the simpler cubic high temperature phase of complicated closed packed solid state structures in for example metals) both the α-helix globule and the β-sheets can be described in the same framework. A direct mapping for all the structures discussed by Finkelstein *et al.* [14, 15] can be demonstrated to be possible. On the other hand is it not possible from the idealized, rectangular structures to predict the actual detailed twisted structure - these belong to a sub class of the folding classes in which we are interested.

3   A chiral spin model

Let us introduce a highly simplified model. Suppose the above mentioned elements are essentially linear of various lengths, the direction is given by a unit vector $\hat{e}$. To describe the junctions consider for example at site P a vertical α-helix ($\hat{e}_z^P$) with a strand entering at the bottom in the direction north. Suppose the α-helix can transfer the information that the strand going out at the top is approximately in the same direction ≈north, opposite ≈south, or ≈east, or ≈west. The situation can be described by the hinge variables S_p as spins giving the hinge direction and sense of turn. The information along the element is then reduced to a set of interaction constants J_p, K_p within a total of four values ($\pm J, \pm K$) which favors one of the four relative spin directions. The same can be done for the other elements (J_p, K_p for element (1) and j_p, k_p for element (2)). Thus one could characterize a given fold configuration (here a four-helix-bundle beginning at the dark open arrow) by a linear string of e.g. the following content: $(\updownarrow -J) \updownarrow j \updownarrow K \updownarrow j \updownarrow K \updownarrow j \updownarrow (-J \updownarrow)$,

where $\updownarrow$ represents one of the arrow symbols in figure 1, which also shows a more realistic representation of the four-helix bundle 1hmq. The reduced information giving the spin directions can be furnished by many amino acid sequences. This provides in fact the basis for the classification, i.e. many variants having the same fold. In order to be able to describe the energy cost for violating the optimum fold we write the argument as a Hamiltonian

$$\mathcal{H} = - \sum_{P=2n+1} (J_P S_P \cdot S_{P+1} \quad + \quad K_P S_P \times S_{P+1} \cdot \hat{e}^P_\alpha)$$
$$- \sum_{p=2n} (j_p\, S_p \cdot S_{p+1} \quad + \quad k_p\, S_p \times S_{p+1} \cdot \hat{e}^p_\alpha). \tag{1}$$

This simple model is more general than a lattice model because we are allowing for both a variable length of the elements and for a flexibility in angles. From a specific sequence of j_p, k_p and J_p, K_p we can find the corresponding spin directions and construct the protein structure given the lengths of the elements. We have thus constructed a unique name for a fold class. If we neglect the orientations of the first and last of the type (2) strand elements (which are not particularly well defined) we can describe the four-helix-bundle fold simply by the five letters $jKjKj$. This name is (i) invariant under rotations of the structure as a name of course must be. However, it is (ii) dependent on the sense of direction. Thus if one starts at the light open arrow the name is $j\bar{K}j\bar{K}j$, where $\bar{K} = -K$. These two properties (i) and (ii) are essential for defining unique fold classes. By Monte Carlo computer simulations the model can be shown to exhibit known folds amongst a wealth of other structures such as non-compact and loosely packed structures and structures that are too densely entangled in one another. After randomly varying the linear representation and permuting the coupling constants one can search for the minima of the energy function given above. In that way one can obtain members from different folding classes and in principle traversing the whole space of possible folds. A phase diagram can easily be extracted from such an analysis based on the energy function $\mathcal{H}$ and we already know from previous analysis [16, 17, 18] that this type of energy function exhibits an ordered phase at low temperature corresponding to folded structures of proteins and disordered phases at higher temperature corresponding to unfolded or misfolded patterns.

4   Estimate of the number of fold classes

Here we shall demonstrate that the model is amenable to a simple estimate of the number of dense protein fold classes. For a random sequence of interaction parameters it is most likely that the structure is extended. The number of such structures is very large and can be estimated as $\mathcal{N}_{random} \propto z^N = 4^N \approx 10^{12}$, where $N = 20$ (taken as the average number of structural elements in proteins times two, counting the intervening strands too) is a typical number of junctions (spins) and $z = 4$ the turn possibilities. The problem is to find those sequences which result in dense structures. This problem is closely related to that of self avoiding random walks (SAW), see e.g. de Gennes [19]. The end-to-end square distance R_f^2 can be shown to scale

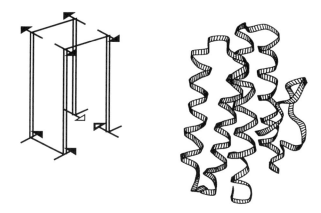

Figure 1: Chiral spin model representation of the four helix bundle protein $1hmq \equiv jKjKj$ (to the left) and the $1hmq$ protein in a ribbon representation rotated $90°$ (to the right).

with N as $R_f \propto N^\nu$, $\nu = 3/5$, for dimension $d = 3$. For the protein to be dense, R_f must be small, and that reduces the number of possibilities drastically to $\mathcal{N}_{SAW,close} \propto \bar{z}^N / R_f^d$. For self avoiding walks $\bar{z} = z - 1 - \epsilon$, where the -1 corrects for the direct return and where $\epsilon = 0.32$, for $d = 3$, is a small correction for possible later crossings. By construction of the model we have no direct returns and thus $\bar{z} = 4$ or better $\bar{z} \approx 4 - \epsilon$. However, we want to require that the proteins are still denser. The root-mean-square radius scales as $< r^2 > \propto N$. Therefore the number of proteins with extent being of the order of the length of the elements is further reduced by a factor $N^{\frac{d}{2}}$. Hence one obtains the following estimate of the number of proteins which are dense and self avoiding

$$\mathcal{N}_{SAW,dense} \propto \bar{z}^N / N^{d(\nu+\frac{1}{2})} = \bar{z}^N / N^{3.3}. \tag{2}$$

For a typical protein consisting of 10 α-helices or β-strands there are $N = 18$ junctions; and the number of distinct structural folds is computed from (2) to be $\mathcal{N} = 10^6$. This number is vastly reduced from that of the free random walk estimation ($\approx 10^{11}$). It must further be reduced considerably by requiring that the potential β-strands are close together in space in order to form β-sheets. Assuming n α-helices and m β-strands the restriction gives a reduction factor $\propto n!m!/(n+m)!$, which for $n \approx m$ gives a reduction factor 250 and brings the estimated number down to

$$\mathcal{N}_{foldclasses} \approx 4000 \tag{3}$$

for the typical proteins. This is very close to the estimate made by Chothia, who obtained his estimate in a totally different way. It is still a bit higher and allows therefore both for more possible findings than foreseen by Chothia, and for the possibility that nature in the course of the evolution has not used all the statistically possible options, or rather that some folded protein configurations were discarded because of lack of functionality. Clearly a further reduction is arising if the structures must in addition fulfill certain functional demands.

5   Conclusion

We have introduced a simple chiral spin model, which allows a unique description of schematized protein folds. Real folds can be mapped onto this representation. The model allows us to make an estimate of the expected number of existing protein fold classes. The argument given here has been to estimate the number, or upper bound, (≤ 4000) of the final structures. In these the strong forces between the elements can equally well be included, probably distorting the structures somewhat. However, the more important aspect in our model is that the proteins already in their linear amino acid combination have the fold class impregnated within them, allowing the fold to be much more well determined and self-organized than that conceivable from a totally random trial and error method. It is clear from the argument that a given fold cannot be used to determine the amino acid sequence, whereas the reverse is possible. In our model the folds are coded in a decimating code. We have only discussed relatively small proteins, but as discussed by Chothia, the larger proteins produced at the recent stages of evolution are generally combinations of the elementary ones. This will not increase the number of possibilities drastically!

Acknowledgement

The authors wish to thank P. G. Wolynes and G. M. Crippen for enlightening discussions. Furthermore The Danish National Research Foundation and RISOE National Laboratory are acknowledged for support.

References

[1] C. Chothia, *Nature*, 357, p. 543, 1992.
[2] J. W. Ponder and F. M. Richards, *J. Mol. Biol.*, 193, p. 775, 1987.
[3] S. T. Rao and M. G. Rossmann, *J. Mol. Biol.*, 76, p. 241, 1973.
[4] J. S. Richardson, *Adv. Protein Chem.*, 34, p. 167, 1981.
[5] D. J. Jones, W. R. Taylor and J. M. Thornton, *Nature*, 358, p. 86, 1992.
[6] T. L. Blundell and M. S. Johnson, *Protein Science*, 2, p. 877, 1993.
[7] S. Pascarella and P. Argos, *Protein Engineering*, 5, p. 121-137, 1992.
[8] C. Sander and L. Holm, *J. Mol. Biol.*, 225, p. 93, 1992.
[9] C. J. Camacho and D. Thirumalai, *Phys. Rev. Lett.*, 71, p. 2505, 1993.
[10] E. I. Shaknovich, *Phys. Rev. Lett.*, 72, p. 3907, 1994.
[11] C. von Linné, *Fundamenta Botanica*, p. 1738, *Species Plantarum*, p. 1753.
[12] Nature only uses α-helices with one handedness, therefore we only assign one element to an α-helix.
[13] C. J. Levinthal, *Chem. Phys.*, 65, p. 99, 1968.
[14] A. G. Murzin and A. V. Finkelstein, *J. Mol. Biol.*, 204, p. 749, 1988.
[15] A. V. Finkelstein and B. A. Reva, *Nature*, 351, p. 497, 1991.
[16] T. Castán and P. A. Lindgård, *Phys. Rev. B*, 40, p. 5069, 1989.
[17] M. Sasai and P. G. Wolynes, *Phys. Rev. Lett.*, 65, p. 2740, 1990.
[18] H. Bohr and P. G. Wolynes, *Phys. Rev. A*, 46, p. 5242, 1992.
[19] P. G. de Gennes, *Scaling Concept in Polymer Physics*, Cornell University Press, Ithaca, 1979.

Distance-Based Protein Structure
Prediction and Evaluation

The Effect of a Distance-Cutoff on the Performance of The Distance Matrix Error when used as a Potential Function to drive Conformational Search

Scott Le Grand, Arne Elofsson and David Eisenberg

UCLA-DOE Laboratory of Structural Biology and Molecular Medicine, Molecular Biology Institute, and Department of Chemistry and Biochemistry, University of California Los Angeles, Box 951570, Los Angeles, CA 90095-1570, USA

Abstract

Several recent papers have argued that the main obstacle to the prediction of the three-dimensional structures of proteins is less the difficulty of exhaustively searching the possible conformations of a protein, and more the difficulty of developing a useful potential energy function to score the relative stabilities of protein conformations. Conformational searches of proteins driven by many currently available potential functions locate non-native conformations which are scored as more stable than their experimentally determined structures. To gain insight into the failure of a simple potential energy function to score the experimental structure as most stable, we investigate the behavior of a simple but artificial potential function: the distance matrix error (DME), described below, which measures the difference between any protein conformation and its experimental structure in terms of interatomic distances. The DME is an artificial potential function because it requires *a priori* knowledge of the interatomic distances in the protein's experimental structure. We study the power of this function to drive a conformational search to the experimental structure, subject to a distance-based cutoff, c, of the interatomic distances derived from the experimental structure. The resulting function is called the cutoff-DME or cDME. We find that cDME-driven conformational searches fail to locate the experimental structure if c is small (< 10 Å) and converge to structures with increasing similarity to the experimental structure as c increases to 24 Å, where the cDME becomes approximately equivalent to the DME. That is, for the DME, long distance information is required to drive a conformational search to the experimental structure. However, at any given c value, the cDME of any final conformer of a conformational search is approximately the global minimum cDME, that of the experimental structure. These results indicate that the absence of long range structural information in the DME causes the experimental structure to be degenerate: there are multiple conformations with global minimum cDMEs, but with high DMEs relative to the experimental structure.

0-8493-4009-8/96/$0.00+$.50

1   Introduction

1.1   The problem

Several recent papers have argued that the main obstacle to predicting protein tertiary structures by computer is less the difficulty of exhaustively searching the conformational space of a
protein's conformation space [1], and more the accuracy of the potential functions used to estimate the energy difference between arbitrary protein conformations and their experimentally
determined structure [2, 3, 4]. Conformational searches using stochastic optimization techniques such as Monte Carlo methods or genetic algorithms can locate near global optimum
conformations of proteins if given an artificial, essentially unambiguous potential function
such as the root mean square deviation (RMSD) or distance matrix error (DME) [5, 6]. Of
course, both the RMSD and related functions such as the DME require *a priori* knowledge of
a protein's experimental structure.

1.2   Folding funnels

Successful conformational searches for the native structure require the existence of an unambiguous attractor to the experimental structure or what has been termed a "folding funnel" [7] in
the potential function. This folding funnel guides a conformational search to the experimental
structure rather than to alternative structures with comparable or lower energies. Unfortunately, little is known about how to design a potential function to contain folding funnels. This
paper presents an attempt at understanding how a folding funnel arises in a simple potential
function which is calculated from interatomic distances. Our simplified potential function is
based on the DME, Eq. (1),

$$DME = \frac{2}{n(n-1)} \sqrt{\sum_{i<j} (d_{ij} - e_{ij})^2} \tag{1}$$

where n is the number of atoms in a protein, d_{ij} is the distance between atoms i and j in
an arbitrary conformation, and e_{ij} is the distance between atoms i and j in the experimental
structure. The DME contains a folding funnel to the experimental structure in the sense that
conformational searches which use the DME as a potential function will converge to near
native structures with DMEs < 1.0 Å Å [8]. Unfortunately, the DME's requirement of *a priori*
knowledge of the native structure of the target protein gives this function no predictive value.

1.3   How much information is enough to fold a protein?

Our focus is to investigate the amount of accurate information about the experimental structure
of a protein which is required for a conformational search, utilizing the DME as a potential
function, to converge consistently to the native structure, thus implying the existence of a
folding funnel to the native structure. The extent of experimental structure information in
the DME is controlled by introducing a distance-based cutoff into its components. We call
this modified functional form of the DME the cutoff-DME or cDME (defined below). The
amount of information about the experimental structure of a protein in the cDME decreases
with decreasing distance cutoff and conversely increases with increasing distance cutoff.

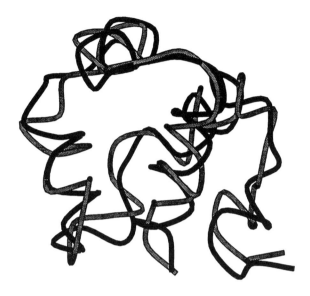

Figure 1: α-carbon trace of the best fit of the lattice model, in gray, to the experimental structure of 434 repressor (PDB entry 1r69), in black. The α-carbon DME between the lattice model and the experimental structure is 1.3 Å.

2 Methods

2.1 Target protein

The 434 repressor (PDB entry 1r69) [9] was represented as an α-carbon trace of 63 atoms on a body centered cubic lattice, all other backbone and sidechain atoms of this protein are ignored. The lattice spacing was set to 3.8 Å between each lattice point and its 12 nearest neighbors. This interresidue distance is close to the average real space distance between adjacent α-carbons in proteins. The best fit of the α-carbon trace of 434 repressor to this lattice is 1.3 Å DME (Fig. 1).

Therefore, any conformational search which converges to a final conformation with a DME close to 1.3 Å is considered to have located the experimental structure. Since both the α-carbon model and the DME are insensitive to chirality, there is a mirror image of every conformation with the same DME and for the purposes of this paper, these mirror images are considered the same conformation.

2.2 Conformational search

The algorithm for conformational search consisted of iterated rearrangements of segments of the lattice protein chain from 3–5 residues in length, subject to the constraint of having the same beginning and endpoint Cα positions. Moves were accepted or rejected on the basis of *threshold accepting* [10]; if the rearrangement lowered the cDME, the move was automatically accepted. If the rearrangement increased the cDME, it was accepted if a random number was less than or equal to $T \cdot (1\text{-step})/\text{steps}$ where T is the threshold, set to 2.0 Å for all

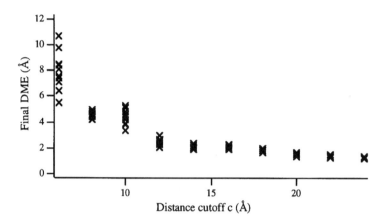

Figure 2: Convergence of cDME conformational searches with respect to the DME. This figure plots the Distance Matrix Error (DME) of the final conformations produced by 100 independent conformational searches of the Cα trace of 434 repressor (PDB entry 1r69) under the cDME potential function versus distance cutoff c. Each X represents the DME of a final conformation produced by a conformational search. At low c values, the final DMEs are those of random, non-native conformations but which have mostly correct secondary structure. As c increases, the final conformations collapse into increasingly native-like conformations until c reaches a value of 24 Å where all the final conformations are as close to the native structure as the lattice model allows. Overall, this figure demonstrates that the DME requires knowledge of long range interactions in order to drive conformational searches to the native structure. Knowledge of local interactions alone is not sufficient.

conformational searches reported here, step is the current iteration, and steps is the total number of iterations, set to 300,000 for all runs reported here. For each conformational search, 100,000 subsequent steps of hillclimbing (T=0.0 Å) were performed in order to increase the probability that the final conformer was at a local minimum in the potential energy surface. Hence, each conformational search consists of 400,000 attempted conformational rearrangements.

2.3   Potential function

The cutoff-DME (cDME) Eq. (2) was used as the potential function for all conformational searches reported here where c is a pre-specified distance cutoff which limits the cDME to m interatomic distances, as described below, rather than $n(n-1)/2$ as in the DME, d_i is interatomic distance i (out of m) in an arbitrary protein conformation, and e_i is interatomic distance i in the experimental structure of that protein.

$$cDME = \frac{1}{m}\sqrt{\sum_{i=1}^{m}\begin{cases} c^2 & \text{if } d_i > c \\ (d_i - e_i)^2 & \text{if } d_i \leq c \end{cases}} \qquad (2)$$

Specifically, the cDME differs from the DME in that it utilizes a distance cutoff c in two ways. First, all components of the DME arising from interatomic distances $> c$ Å in the native structure are ignored. Second, the errors of each of the m interatomic distances $\leq c$

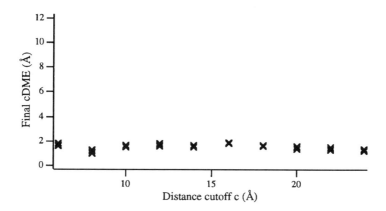

Figure 3: Convergence of cDME conformational searches as function of distance cutoff. This figure plots the Cutoff-Distance Matrix Error (cDME) of the final conformations produced by 100 independent conformational searches of the $C\alpha$ trace of 434 repressor (PDB entry 1r69) under the cDME potential function versus distance cutoff c. Each X represents the cDME of a final conformation produced by a conformational search, many of which superimpose. At each value of c, the cDMEs are close to that of the global minimum. Therefore, all of these conformational searches have converged to global optimum conformations. However, the information from figure 2 above indicates that at low values of c, these global optimum conformations are significantly different from the native structure of 434 repressor. This indicates that in the absence of long range interaction information, the native structure is not the unique global optimum conformation of the cDME.

Å in the native structure are the same as in the DME if the interatomic distance $\leq c$ Å in the current conformation being measured relative to the native structure, or they are each set to c if the interatomic distance is $> c$ Å in the current conformation. This potential function monotonically decreases with increasing numbers of correct interatomic contacts within the cutoff c. The global optimum conformation will minimize the error of the m interatomic distances $\leq c$ Å in the native structure, subject to the constraints imposed by the lattice model, and will not be influenced by the error in any of the other interatomic distances.

The value of c determines the value of m which in turn determines the amount of native structure information in the cDME. Our results explore the effect of varying c from 6.0 to 24.0 Å in 2 Å intervals, gradually increasing the level of native structure information in the cDME. Ten independent conformational searches were performed at each distance cutoff value.

3 Results

3.1 DME versus cDME

Figure 2 shows the effect of the distance cutoff c on the final DME of conformational searches: it plots the final DMEs of 100 independent conformational searches driven by the cDME versus distance cutoff c ranging from 6.0 to 24.0 Å. This figure illustrates that in the absence of information about long range interactions, conformational searches converge to final conformations with high DMEs. That is, even though the cDME function supplies perfect information about interatomic distances in the experimental structure of 434 repressor, the longer interatomic distances are required to drive a conformational search to an experimental-like final conformation.

3.2   Behavior of the cDME

Figure 3 shows the effect of the distance cutoff c on the final cDME of conformational searches, it plots the average final cDME of the same 100 conformational searches versus the distance cutoff c. This figure illustrates that these final conformations all have near global optimum cDMEs, close to that of the best fit of the Cα trace to the body-centered cubic lattice model. The close fit of the cDME values of the conformations which have high DMEs to those which have low DMEs indicates that the native structure is not uniquely determined in the absence of long range information in the DME. That is, there are multiple distinct conformations which have cDME values close to the cDME of the native structure. At low c values, these conformations have random DME values relative to that of the experimental structure. These conformational searches have failed to locate the native state because the cDME potential function cannot distinguish the native state from the many equivalent structures with low cDMEs.

3.3   Effect of the cutoff on conformational searches

The nature of the final conformations that result from the conformational searches changes with increasing distance cutoff. Starting at $c = 6.0$ Å, the final conformers are extended random coils (Fig. 4) with intermittent segments of correct secondary structure. This indicates that many close range contacts involving residues which are also close in sequence have been located while few or no close contacts involving widely separated residues have been located. At a low distance cutoff, most of the components of the cDME involve contacts between residues close in sequence, therefore long range contacts have less impact on the value of the cDME than close range contacts and are not worth satisfying relative to maximizing the content of correct sequentially close range contacts. As the distance cutoff increases, the number of long range contacts counted in the cDME increase. The increasing presence of these long range contacts first cause the final conformers to become compact with correct secondary structure, then compact with both correct secondary structure and the approximate correct fold, and finally approximate the best fit of the native structure to the lattice model (Fig. 5) as the cDME becomes approximately equivalent to the DME.

3.4   Distance cutoff and the folding funnel

These results indicate that the folding funnel of the DME potential function appears gradually with increasing distance cutoff and that the existence of the folding funnel in the DME requires the inclusion of long range interaction information.

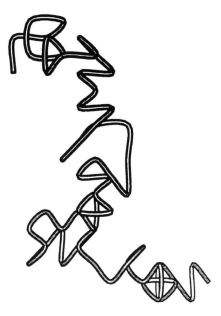

Figure 4: α-carbon trace of a global minimum cDME conformer of 434 repressor when c is 6.0 Å. There are some correct local interresidue contacts, which lead to intermittent segments of correct secondary structure, but few correct long-range contacts, and hence little correct tertiary structure.

4   Discussion

4.1   The right cutoff

Distance cutoffs are a common feature of potential functions used for molecular mechanics as well as for tertiary structure prediction. This paper demonstrates that the use of too small a distance cutoff can destroy the uniqueness of the native structure under the DME, making the function an inaccurate indicator of the difference between an arbitrary protein conformation and its experimental structure. In effect, a small distance cutoff destroys the folding funnel which drives a conformational search to the native structure. Since it is likely that the exact cutoff value for the preservation of the folding funnel is potential function-dependent, the only general conclusion to draw from this work is that potential functions should be evaluated with numerous distance cutoffs to check for the existence of incorrect global optimum conformations that are influenced by the distance cutoff.

4.2   Uniqueness

This work illustrates the existence of numerous, equivalent, non-experimental conformations which all have approximately global minimum cDMEs in the presence of a short distance cutoff. This indicates that there is no folding funnel to the native structure at low values of c. In a real potential function, the existence of these alternative conformations with seemingly experimental-like character would doom the function to failure because there is no way to

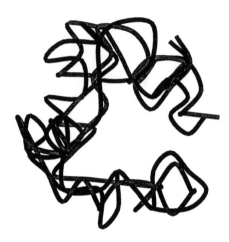

Figure 5: α-carbon trace of a global minimum conformer when c is 24.0 Å, in gray, super-imposed on the best fit of the experimental structure to the lattice model, in black. These two conformers have the same DME relative to the experimental structure, 1.3 Å, and therefore both represent global minimum conformations of 434 repressor on the body-centered lattice model.

distinguish them from the experimental structure. There must be a folding funnel to the experimental structure for the potential function to properly drive a conformational search. If instead there are n such conformations with potential energies which are close to the global minimum value, all of them are equally likely to be located by a single conformational search. This means that each individual conformational search has a $1/(n+1)$ chance of converging to the experimental structure. If n is large ($\gg 100$), then location of the experimental structure by conformational search is impractical. If n is small (<100), then the experimental structure could possibly be picked out from the n alternative incorrect structures by a criteria independent from that used to drive the conformational search such as a 3D-1D profile (Bowie *et al.*, 1991), or a different potential function.

4.3   Model dependence?

The influence of the distance cutoff is not limited to the cDME. We have observed similar behavior in an off-lattice model using a full atom-atom potential function. The interatomic potential function utilized 26 atom classes (20 β carbon classes plus carbon, charged and uncharged nitrogen, charged and uncharged oxygen, and sulfur atom classes to represent all other backbone and side chain atoms). The potential energy of a protein conformation was calculated as the absolute difference from the experimental structure of all atom-atom nonbonded interactions between pairs of atoms from different residues in 1 Å bins out to a cutoff of c Å. The use of 6, 8, 10, and 12 Å nonbond cutoffs allowed for the existence of numerous non-native states which had approximately the same nonbond distribution as the native structure (<100 interactions difference). The use of a 20 Å distance cutoff made the native structure almost unique and caused some conformational searches to converge to near-native conformations. Therefore, the errors introduced by too low a distance cutoff can occur with multiple potential functions and may be one of the reasons for the difficulty in generating a potential function for tertiary structure prediction.

Acknowledgements

S.L. was supported by NSF Postdoctoral Research Fellowship in Chemistry CHE- 9302860, and A.E. was supported by Swedish Research Council for Engineering Sciences Postdoctoral Scholarship # 282-94-775. This work was supported by the DOE cooperative agreement DE-FC03-8TER60615.

References

[1] C. Levinthal, In *Mossbauer spectroscopy in biological systems*, P. Debrunner, J. C. M. Tsibris and E. Münck (eds.), Urbana, University of Illinois Press, p. 22-24, 1969.

[2] S. Le Grand, and K. Merz, The application of the genetic algorithm to the minimization of potential energy functions, *J. Global Opt.*, 3, p. 49-66, 1993.

[3] S. Le Grand and K. M. Merz, Jr., The application of the genetic algorithm to the conformational search of polypeptides and proteins, *Mol. Simul.*, 13, p. 299-320, 1994.

[4] A. Šali, E. Shakhnovich and M. Karplus, How does a protein fold?, *Nature*, 36919, p. 248-251, 1994.

[5] J. U. Bowie and D. Eisenberg, An evolutionary approach to folding small α-helical proteins that uses sequence information and an empirical guiding fitness function, *Proc. Natl. Acad. Sci. USA*, 91, p. 4436-4440, 1994.

[6] A. Elofsson, S. Le Grand and D. Eisenberg, Local moves, an efficient algorithm for simulation of protein folding, in press, 1995.

[7] P. E. Leopold, M. Montal and J. N. Onuchic, Protein folding funnels, a kinetic approach to the sequence-structure relationship, *Proc. Natl. Acad. Sci. USA*, 8918, p. 8721-8725, 1992.

[8] A. Elofsson and S. Le Grand, unpublished data, 1994.

[9] F. C. Bernstein, T. F. Koetzle, G. J. D. Williams, E. F. Meyer, D. W. Rice, G. W. Hardy, M. Merrett and A. W. Phillips, The protein data bank, A computer-based archival file for macromolecular structures, *J. Mol. Biol.*, 112, p. 535-542, 1977.

[10] L. N. Morales, R. Garduno-Juarez and D. Romero, The multiple minima problem in small peptides revisited. The threshold accepting approach, *J. Biomolecular Struct. Dyn.*, 5, p. 951-957, 1992.

Protein Structure Prediction:
How Self-misleading can be avoided

Azat Ya. Badretdinov, Alexander M. Gutin* and Alexei V. Finkelstein

Institute of Protein Research, Russian Academy of Sciences, 142292, Pushchino, Moscow
Region, Russian Federation
* Present address: Department of Chemistry, Harvard University, Cambridge, MA 02138,
U.S.A.

Abstract

An effect on protein structure prediction caused by inevitable energy function
errors is considered. We show that a search for a single conformation of minimal
energy usually gives a misleading prediction when errors exceed some small
threshold. We have estimated the number of low-energy folds containing among
them the native fold.

1   Introduction

Energy-based prediction of 3D protein structure involves models always somewhat simplified,
and energy functions which inevitably contain some errors. Nonetheless, after CPU time-
consuming computations, researchers hope to get a result which is usually imagined as a
single protein structure (or fold) which must be the native one.

This poses the question: at what minimal precision of energy calculations can this approach
(search for one fold) yield an actual native structure?

To answer this question, we shall assume (as it is usually done) that protein folding is
under thermodynamic control, i.e. the native protein fold occupies the very bottom level of
the protein energy spectrum. Thus, the task of the theorist seems to be voluminous[1], but very
simple: to calculate the energies[2] of all the protein chain folds[3](see the right part of Fig. 1
for a typical spectrum) and to choose the fold with energy at the very bottom of the calculated
spectrum.

However, due to the inevitable errors in the energetic parameters, all the *computed* energies
are known with some error. If the exact knowledge of *actual* energies of all the folds is godsend,
we will then see that part of the computed energy levels shift downwards from their actual
positions, and that some of the computed energy levels shift upwards.

Since the number of high-energy folds is large, one of them has a good chance (when the
error in energetic parameters is not negligible) to have the *computed* energy below that of the

---

[1]Here we do not consider formidable computational difficulties in searching for the lowest-energy
fold!

[2]The term "energy" is used here only for simplicity; strictly speaking, the term "mean force potential"
must be used, because hydrophobic and electrostatic forces are solvent-mediated ones.

[3]One can assume that all the chain conformations are divided into a great but finite number of "folds",
which can be compared to the local energy minima and their vicinities.

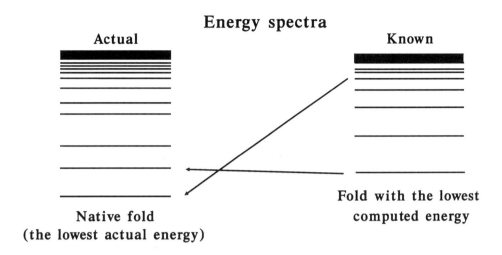

Figure 1: Schematic representation of the "actual" and "known" energy spectra of a heteropolymer chain. Each line corresponds to the energy of some chain fold. For two folds, taken as examples, arrows show the correspondence between their positions in both spectra.

fold which *actually* has the lowest energy (i.e., of the native fold); therefore, the prediction based on energy minimization fails when the errors are not small enough.

To find out what this "enough" is, we pose the following question: Let us assume that we have the energy parameters with a given precision. Does a fold with the lowest calculated energy have a good chance to be indeed the actually lowest-energy (native) fold? How many low-energy folds must one collect in order to have the native one among them? In other words: what is the expected *ranking* of the native fold in the computed energy spectrum depending on the precision of the energy parameters?

It is possible to answer this question irrespective of any particular model of protein structure prediction. Our answer is grounded on the basic properties of protein energy spectra. This answer depends only on the precision of energetic parameters and on the energy gap separating the native fold from the continuous part of the actual energy spectrum.

2   Theory

Let us start with a short summary of the present understanding of protein energy spectra [1, 2, 3].

2.1   Energy spectra of protein chains

In essence two phenomena determine the form of a typical energy spectrum of a heteropolymer like protein.

First, a protein chain is composed of various amino acids which interact in many different ways. Therefore, the energy of each chain fold is the sum of many virtually independent microscopic energy terms. Second, the chain can fold in numerous ways [4, 5], the number of these ways is exponentially high, and, as a rule, different chain folds have very few common interactions [6]. Thus, the Random Energy Model [7] is applicable to the energy spectra of a protein chain [6]. This means that the energy levels have a random Gaussian distribution (Fig. 2) and that the spectrum consisting of M lines (corresponding to M folds) typically has a density

$$m(E) = M \left(2\pi\sigma^2\right)^{-1/2} \exp\left(-\frac{E^2}{2\sigma^2}\right) \tag{1}$$

where E is the fold energy and σ is the standard deviation of a fold energy from the mean fold energy $\langle E \rangle$ which is taken as zero.

The similarity region of different spectra is limited to the range of high density where $m(E) > 1/\sigma$; this part is called the "continuous spectrum". The most probable point of its beginning $E^{\mathrm{cr}} = -\sigma\sqrt{2\ln M}$ (also referred to as the "critical energy") follows from the condition $m(E^{\mathrm{cr}}) = 1/\sigma$.

The individuality of the heteropolymer chain depends on the gap Δ between E^{cr}, the edge of the continuous energy spectrum, and E^N, the energy of the native (the lowest-energy) fold [1, 3]. Unlike random heteropolymers which have a very small gap and gradual melting [6], proteins must have a significant gap Δ (Fig. 2) [1, 3], since they undergo an "all-or-none" transition during denaturation [8]. Thus, the native fold energy is

$$E^{\mathrm{N}} = E^{\mathrm{cr}} - \Delta \tag{2}$$

where $\Delta \gg RT$, T being the melting temperature. In principle, the value of Δ can be estimated from thermodynamic experiments [9].

2.2   Precision of energy functions

Assume that one uses a set of parameters to evaluate various interactions in proteins (including interactions with the solvent) and computes the energies[4] of different folds[5] of a protein chain. Then each fold ω ($\omega = 1, 2, ..., M; M$, the number of folds) has a "computed" energy E_c^ω, while its actual energy is E_a^ω. The correlation coefficient C between those two sets of values can be found from a conventional equation

$$C = \frac{\langle (E_c - \langle E_c \rangle)(E_a - \langle E_a \rangle) \rangle}{\left[\langle (E_c - \langle E_c \rangle)^2 \rangle \langle (E_a - \langle E_a \rangle)^2 \rangle\right]^{1/2}} \tag{3}$$

where $\langle \cdots \rangle$ means averaging: $\langle E \rangle = \frac{1}{\mathrm{M}} \sum_{\omega=1}^{M} E^\omega$, etc.

For a given protein the correlation coefficient can be estimated from a comparison of the calculated energy and the entropy of melting obtained in experiments. A more accurate estimate of the precision of the parameter set can be obtained from a comparison of the experimental and computed stabilities of many proteins.

In summary, this correlation coefficient C is the generalized measure of precision of the energy functions used for computation.

---

[4]See footnote 2.
[5]See footnote 3.

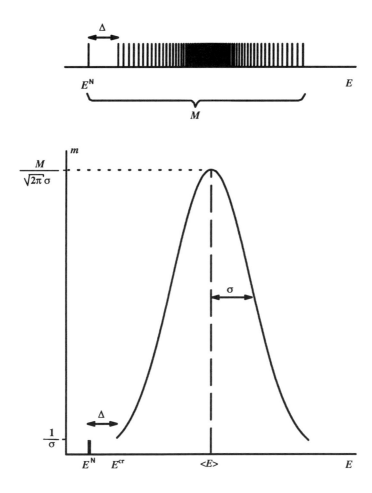

Figure 2: (Above) Energy spectrum of a typical protein. The position of the native fold energy (E^N) is separated from the dense ("continuous") part of the spectrum by gap Δ. (Below) The density of the spectrum shown above. The density m of the continuous part of the spectrum is determined by three parameters: the total number of folds (spectrum lines) M, the standard energy deviation σ, and the mean energy $\langle E \rangle$ (which is assumed to be zero in this study). E^{cr} is the energy of the beginning of the continuous spectrum. The position of the native fold energy (E^N) is shown by the black rectangle.

2.3 Actual energy and its "known" part

"Actual" fold energy can be represented as a "known" energy and a random error:

$$E_a^\omega = E_k^\omega + \delta E^\omega$$

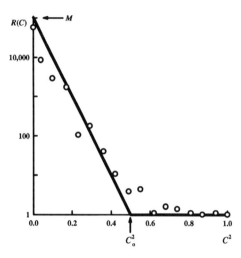

Figure 3: Positions of the native fold in the computed ("known") spectrum (circles) averaged over 20 sequences with the gap $\Delta_a \approx 8$ (one of the corresponding energy spectra is shown in Fig. 5b). The theoretical estimate (see eq. (12)) is shown by the bold line with a bend in the analytically estimated point (eq. (11)) $C_o = (1 + \Delta_a/(-E^{cr}))^{-1} = (1 + 8/20)^{-1} = 0.71$ (the values of Δ_a and E^{cr} correspond to the same values in Fig. 5b).

"Known" energy $E_k^\omega = \lambda E_c^\omega + b$ corresponds to the best possible fit of computed energies E_c^ω to the actual ones. This fit has the form

$$E_a^\omega = \lambda E_c^\omega + b + \delta E^\omega \qquad (4)$$

where λ and b are adjustable coefficients. The best fit corresponds to the minimal (over λ and b) error $\langle \delta E^2 \rangle$ (in practice this best fit of λ and b can be obtained from a systematic comparison of experimental and computed stabilities of proteins). It is readily seen that when $\langle \delta E^2 \rangle$ is minimal, $\langle \delta E \rangle = 0$ and δE does not correlate with E_c, i.e. $\langle \delta E \cdot E_c \rangle = 0$.

The value $E_k^\omega = \lambda E_c^\omega + b$ is called the "known" energy of the fold ω. Its mean value $\langle E_k \rangle = 0$ because $\langle \delta E \rangle = 0$, and $\langle E_a \rangle$ is taken as zero (see above). As $\langle \delta E \cdot E_c \rangle = 0$ and $\langle \delta E \rangle = 0$, $\langle \delta E \cdot E_k \rangle = 0$ as well.

It is apparent that the coefficient of correlation between E_k and E_a is the same as between E_c and E_a (see eq. (3)), i.e. $C = \langle E_k E_a \rangle / [\sigma_k \sigma_a]$, where $\sigma_k = \langle E_k^2 \rangle^{1/2}$ and $\sigma_a = \langle E_a^2 \rangle^{1/2}$ are the standard deviations for energies E_k and E_a.

Moreover, as $\langle \delta E \cdot E_k \rangle = 0$, then $\langle E_k \cdot E_a \rangle = \sigma_k^2$ and consequently the correlation coefficient C can be expressed through the dispersions of "known" and "actual" energies:

$$C = \sigma_k / \sigma_a \qquad (5)$$

Lastly, as $\langle \delta E \cdot E_k \rangle = 0$ and $\langle \delta E \rangle = 0$, the standard deviations σ_a, σ_k, and $\sigma_e = \langle \delta E^2 \rangle^{1/2}$ are related by the equation

$$\sigma_a^2 = \sigma_k^2 + \sigma_e^2. \qquad (6)$$

2.4   Native fold ranking in the computed spectrum

Now the problem can be posed as follows: It is given that the actual fold energy consists of the "known" part and the unknown error, $E_a^\omega = E_k^\omega + \delta E_e^\omega$, and that there is a correlation coefficient C between the actual energy and its known part as well as a gap Δ_a dividing the lowest-energy fold from the edge of the continuous part of the actual spectrum (this gap determines protein stability, see [1, 3]).

The questions are:

1. What is the most probable value of the "known" energy E_k^N for the native fold; and
2. What is the most probable ranking of this E_k^N in the list of "known" energies of the folds?

If $m_k(E_k)$ is the number of folds with known energy E_k, and $P_e(E_a - E_k)$ is a probability to have the error δE equal to $E_a - E_k$, the expected number of folds having actual energy E_a and known E_k is

$$\overline{m}(E_a, E_k) = m_k(E_k) \cdot P_e(E_a - E_k) \tag{7}$$

The most probable value of E_k for a given E_a is $E_k = \overline{E}_k(E_a)$ where

$$\frac{\partial}{\partial E_k} \overline{m}(E_a, E_k) = 0 \tag{8}$$

Since both known fold energies E_k and errors δE (as well as actual energies E_a) are composed of many independent terms, E_k and δE (as well as E_a) must have similar Gaussian distributions given above by eq. (1). The characteristic widths of these distributions are σ_k for $m_k(E_k)$, and $\sigma_e = \sqrt{\sigma_a^2 - \sigma_k^2}$ for $P_e(\delta E)$. Substituting $m_k(E_k)$ and $P_e(E_a - E_k)$ into eq. (7), it is seen that eq. (8) results in

$$E_a \cdot \sigma_k^2 - \overline{E}_k(E_a) \cdot (\sigma_e^2 + \sigma_k^2) = 0$$

Using eqs. (6) and then (5), one obtains that the most probable E_k value for a given E_a is

$$\overline{E}_k(E_a) = E_a \cdot [\sigma_k^2/\sigma_a^2] = E_a \cdot C^2$$

In particular, when E_a is the native fold energy $E_a^N = E_a^{cr} - \Delta_a$ (see eq. (2)), the most probable value of the "known" native fold energy reads as

$$\overline{E_k^N} \equiv {}_=E_k(E_a^N) = (E_a^{cr} - \Delta_a) \cdot C^2$$

The average native fold ranking from the bottom of the known energy spectrum is

$$\overline{R} = 1 + \int_\infty^{\overline{E_k^N}} \overline{m_k}(E)dE \tag{9}$$

where the integral is the average number of folds with the known energy below that of the native fold, and $\overline{m_k}(E)$, a typical distribution of "known" fold energies, is given by eq. (1) with $\sigma = \sigma_k$.

Taking the integral at $\overline{E_k^N} \langle -\sigma_k$, one obtains

$$\overline{R} \approx 1 + M \cdot \exp\left(-\frac{\left(\overline{E_k^N}\right)^2}{2\sigma_k^2}\right) = 1 + M \cdot \exp\left(-\frac{[E_a^{cr}]^2[1 - \Delta_a/E_a^{cr}]^2 C^4}{2\sigma_k^2}\right) =$$

$$= 1 + M \cdot \exp\left[-\ln M \cdot [1 - \Delta_a/E_a^{cr}]^2 \cdot C^4 \cdot (\sigma_a^2/\sigma_k^2)\right] = 1 + M^{1-C^2/C_o^2} \tag{10}$$

Here we use eq. (5), and define C_o as

$$C_o = \left[1 + \frac{\Delta_a}{(-E_a^{cr})}\right]^{-1} = \left[1 + \frac{\Delta_a}{\sigma_a\sqrt{2\ln M}}\right]^{-1} \tag{11}$$

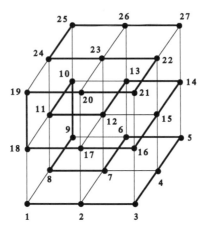

Figure 4: One of the 103,346 possible pathways of a chain of 27 monomers on a 3x3x3 fragment of simple cubic lattice. Two monomers are assumed to be in contact if they are separated by one rib (e.g., 3 and 16).

Here we use eq. (5), and define C_o as

$$C_o = \left[1 + \frac{\Delta_a}{(-E_a^{cr})}\right]^{-1} = \left[1 + \frac{\Delta_a}{\sigma_a\sqrt{2\ln M}}\right]^{-1} \tag{11}$$

As a result, the $\overline{R}$ dependence on C can be represented as

$$\overline{R}(C) \simeq \begin{cases} 1 & \text{when } C > C_o \\ M^{1-C^2/C_o^2} & \text{when } C_o > C \end{cases} \tag{12}$$

Thus, the number of candidates for the native fold role (solid line in Fig. 3) depends only on the total number of folds M (according to protein melting entropy [8], $M \sim 10^{\text{number of chain residues}}$), on the energy gap Δ_a dividing the native fold from the continuous part of the actual energy spectrum and on the correlation of the known and actual energies.

The list of candidates for the role of the native fold is shorter for the sequences which form more stable 3D native folds, because of a larger gap Δ_a between the native fold and the continuous part of the spectrum; it is shorter for those generalized models of protein structures (e.g. "folding patterns") where the variety of conformations is not so large; and, of course, it is shorter for accurate sets of energetic parameters.

When the correlation between the actual and known energies is good enough, i.e. when $C > C_o$, there is, in essence, only one candidate — the native fold itself.

3   Computer experiments with a simple model of a protein globule

It is worthwhile to illustrate (and test!) the above described general theory by computer experiments with a simplified model of protein. The model is taken from [10]: the protein

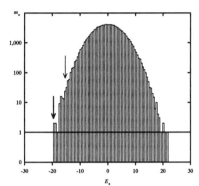 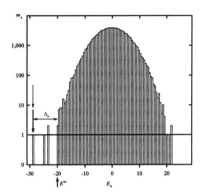

Figure 5: Logarithmic representations of the density histograms of the "actual" energy spectra: (a) for one of the 20 stochastically generated sequences, and (b) for the same sequence after adding $\Delta\varepsilon = -0.4$ to each contact energy ε_{ij}^a, corresponding to the native contacts of links. For both spectra, the mean fold energy is taken as zero. The energy gap Δ_a between the native fold energy and the energy E^{cr} of the beginning of the continuous spectrum is shown only for the "edited" sequence (horizontal arrow in (b)); for the random sequence, this gap is negligible (and therefore not shown in (a)). In each spectrum the position of the fold with the lowest *actual* energy (native fold) is shown by the bold arrow, and the position of the fold with the lowest *known* (computed on the basis of only 61% of the terms ε_{ij}^a, see the text) energy is shown by the thin arrow.

molecule is represented as a chain of 27 links of different kinds; it can form self-avoiding folds on a 3x3x3 fragment of the cubic lattice (Fig. 4). The actual energy E_a^ω of fold ω is a sum of the energies of all contacts between links:

$$E_a^\omega = \sum_{i<j} \sum_{-1} \delta_{ij}^\omega \varepsilon_{ij}^a$$

Here the sum is taken over all the monomers not adjacent along the chain; $\delta_{ij}^\omega = 1$, if monomers i and j are in contact in fold ω, and $\delta_{ij}^\omega = 0$ if not; ε_{ij}^a is the energy of contact between monomers i and j.

The energies ε_{ij}^a, are generated randomly with a Gaussian distribution

$$P(\varepsilon_{ij}^a) = (2\pi)^{-1/2} \exp\left(-\frac{(\varepsilon_{ij}^a)^2}{2}\right)$$

In this way 20 different $\{\varepsilon_{ij}^a\}$ matrices ("sequences") were generated. For all these 20 sequences the energies of all $M = 103,346$ folds were computed, the energy spectra were obtained (see, e.g., Fig. 5a) and the native (the lowest-energy) folds were found.

To model proteins with an energy gap in a spectrum, we slightly edited each obtained random sequence: we added a negative value Δ_ε to all the contact energies present in the native fold (so that the new energies $\widetilde{\varepsilon}_{ij}^a = \varepsilon_{ij}^a + \delta_{ij}^N \Delta\varepsilon$).

In the spectra of the edited chains the native fold energies are shifted downwards, while most of the other spectrum lines virtually do not shift (Fig. 5b).

Thus, now we had the "actual" spectra of 20 edited sequences, all of which had virtually equal energy gaps between the native fold and the continuous energy spectrum and we found the "actual" native folds of these 20 chains.

To simulate the "errors of computation", one can "forget" (replace by zeros) some of the "actual" energies $\tilde{\varepsilon}_{ij}^a$, and then calculate the "known" energies E_k^ω only on the basis of the preserved $\tilde{\varepsilon}_{ij}^a$. This action is similar to the mutation of some part of the protein residues to an "average" amino acid like alanine. To have a correlation C between the "known" and "actual" energies, one has to preserve the C^2 part and "forget" the other $1 - C^2$ part of the $\tilde{\varepsilon}_{ij}^a$ values (see eq. (5) and keep in mind that both σ_a^2 and σ_k^2 are proportional to the number of terms, contributing to the "actual" and "known" energy, respectively).

In this way we obtained the "known" energies for a given level of correlation, and then found (again by exhaustive enumeration) the fold with the lowest "known" energy and a ranking of the actual native fold from the bottom of the "known" energy spectrum. The results presented in figure 3 are in a good concordance with the theoretical estimates given in this paper.

4   Conclusion

Thus, to avoid self-misleading in protein structure prediction the following two values must be known.

1. The correlation coefficient C between the computed and the actual energies. This can be estimated, in particular, from a comparison of the computed and measured changes in the stabilities of mutated proteins.
2. The minimal correlation coefficient C_o appropriate for unambiguous protein structure prediction; the value $1 - C_o$ can be found (see section ß3) as the fraction of the residues that destroy native protein when randomly chosen and mutated to an "average" amino acid like alanine.

A comparison of these two values, C and C_o, shows can the native protein structure be predicted unambiguously, or one must give a list of candidates for the native fold role. In the last case, the size of this list can be estimated from eq. (12).

Acknowledgements

AVF and AYB acknowledge the financial support of the International Science Foundation (grant MTU000).

References

[1] E. I. Shakhnovich and A. M. Gutin, Ground state of random copolymers and the discrete random energy model, *J. Chem. Phys.*, 98, p. 8174–8177, 1993.

[2] A. V. Finkelstein, A. M. Gutin and A. Ya. Badretdinov, Why are the same protein folds used to perform different functions, *FEBS Lett.*, 325, p. 23–28, 1993.

[3] A. V. Finkelstein, A. M. Gutin and A. Ya. Badretdinov, Boltzmann-like statistics of protein architectures: origins and consequences, In *Subcellular Biochemistry: structure, function and protein engineering* B. B. Biswas and S. Roy (eds.), Plenum Press, New York, 34, p. 1–26, 1995.

[4] D. G. Covell and R. L. Jernigan, Conformations of Folded Proteins in Restricted Spaces, *Biochemistry*, 29, p. 3287–3294, 1990.

[5] H. S. Chan and K. A. Dill, Compact Polymers, *Macromolecules*, 22, p. 4560–4573, 1989.

[6] E. I. Shakhnovich and A. M. Gutin, Formation of unique structure in polypeptide chains. Theoretical investigation with the aid of replica approach, *Biophys. Chem.*, 34, p. 187–199, 1989.

[7] B. Derrida, Random-energy model: an exactly solvable model of disordered systems, *Phys. Rev. B.*, 24, p. 2613–2626, 1981.

[8] P. L. Privalov, Stability of Proteins. Small Globular Proteins, *Adv. Prot. Chem.*, 33, p. 167–241, 1979.

[9] A. V. Finkelstein, A. M. Gutin and A. Ya. Badretdinov, Perfect Temperature for Protein Structure Prediction and Folding, *Proteins: Structure, Function, Genetics*, in press 1995.

[10] E. I. Shakhnovich and A. M. Gutin, Implication of thermodynamics of protein folding for evolution of primary sequences, *Nature*, 346, p. 773–775, 1990.

Sequence Space Analysis: Identification of Functionally or Structurally important Residues in Protein Sequence Families

Georg Casari[1], Chris Sander and Alfonso Valencia

EMBL, Protein Design Group, Meyerhofstrasse 1, D-69012 Heidelberg, Germany

Abstract

Multiple sequences in a protein family reflect the history of the evolutionary process of mutations and selection. This process causes functionally important residues to be conserved while other residues can vary in residue type. However, members of most protein families share only some aspects of their function and do not all have identical constraints on sequence. This diversity makes it non-trivial to identify those key positions in the family. Here, we describe a method that can detect and exploit such subtle patterns of conservation for the prediction of functional residues. In its algorithmic nature it is a distance geometry method applied to sequences in an abstract high dimensional sequence space. The quality of derived predictions is demonstrated with examples.

1 Introduction

Protein and DNA sequence databases are growing with accelerating speed leaving us with a wealth of information that is buried in the massive quantity of these data. Very efficient database search tools have been developed that enable researchers to find proteins of the same protein family in those databases by their homologous sequence [1, 2]. The probability that a new protein can be classified as a member of a sequence family is already near 50% [3]. All these proteins in a family are related by a common ancestor and derived by evolutionary events. Evolutionary constraints are imposed by requirements of three-dimensional structure and of biological function. In general, functional requirements are known to be more pronounced and cause residue types to be kept identical throughout the functionally equivalent proteins. Completely conserved residues in a dispersed protein family usually have a direct role in function. Given a multiple sequence alignment, it is generally straightforward to spot the

---

[1]To whom correspondence should be addressed.

most conserved residues and predict their involvement in function. Mutation of such residues typically causes loss of protein function.

Sequence conservation is less obvious for residues that modulate the specificity of biological function. Such residues change as a protein evolves to satisfy modified functional constraints, while the basic biochemical mechanism and the overall three-dimensional fold remain unaltered. Mostly proteins within a family cover a variety of different specificities and make it difficult to find those functional residues that play distinct roles in each subgroup, especially by mere inspection of a multiple sequence alignment.

Here we describe a method to identify residues that are likely to be responsible for functional differences between protein subfamilies by their subtle conservation patterns [4]. The approach requires only a multiple sequence alignment as input and provides an experimentally testable prediction in the form of likely functional residues. The analysis is illustrated with examples in which there is a proven correlation between prediction and experiment.

The method is based on analysis of protein multiple sequence alignments that can be generated using well-tested algorithms [5]. Typically, the sequences are retrieved by scanning the protein sequence databases for homologues of a search sequence [2, 1]. The quality of the multiple alignment is crucial, as all further results depend on it.

The novelty of the approach comes from a mathematically convenient representation that allows grouping of protein families and identification of characteristic sequence patterns in a unified fashion. We represent each sequence as a vector (point) in a multi-dimensional space, called "sequence space", with residue types at each position as the basic dimensions. The formalism of principal component analysis [6] can then be applied to determine the directions in sequence space most strongly populated by the proteins in the family. We generally display a graph showing the positions of all sequences in the subspace of the first most prominent directions. At the same time the vector representation of sequences enables us to trace the principal components back to the individual residues and positions that are characteristic of the different subfamilies.

2   The algorithm

The whole Sequence Space approach relies on a vector representation of sequences that is simple but effective and permits application of an arsenal of vector analysis tools on sequences. Sequence vectors used in this approach are analogous to conventional sequence profiles derived from multiple alignments. Profiles give a tabular summary of the amino acid content at each position in an alignment. The same way sequence vectors consist of 1's for the sequence's residue type and 0's for all other residue types at each position in the alignment (Fig. 1). For each sequence k all these numbers constitute a long row vector $\bar{\mathbf{F}}^k$, corresponding to a point in $20l$-dimensional space. (l is the length of the sequence alignment and k is the index for the protein). An alignment $\mathcal{F}$ of n sequences is a matrix of n rows of length $20l$, each row holding the components of a single sequence vector.

$$\mathcal{F} = \begin{pmatrix} \bar{\mathbf{F}}^1 \\ \vdots \\ \bar{\mathbf{F}}^k \\ \vdots \\ \bar{\mathbf{F}}^n \end{pmatrix} \tag{1}$$

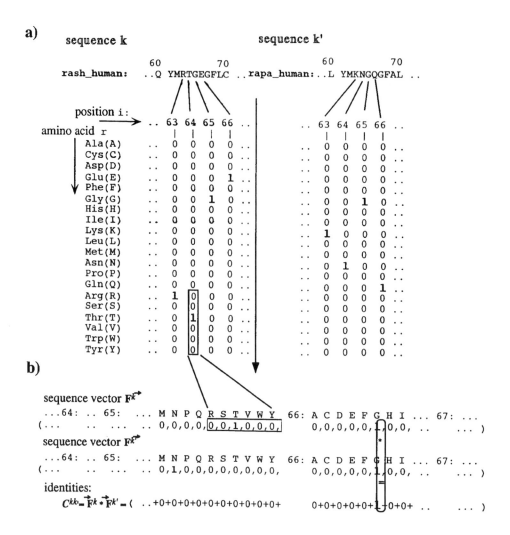

Figure 1: Representation of two protein sequences as vectors in sequence space: a) Translation of two sequences k and k' (shown at the top) into tables with cells for each residue type at each position (profiles). 1's are entered for residue types at positions found in the sequence, 0's in all other cells. Rearranging the entries of the table results in sequence vectors as shown in b). These vectors point to the location of the corresponding sequences in sequence space. b) The number of identities $C^{kk'}$ between sequence k and k' can be calculated as the vector product of the sequence vectors $\vec{F}^{k}$ and $\vec{F}^{k'}$. A box highlights an identity between sequences k and k' corresponding their common G residue at position 66.

All possible sequences of length up to l residues can be represented as points in the $20l$-dimensional sequence space. Members of a protein family are somewhat similar and typically populate only a small region of this space. Therefore, the main features of a family can be described in a subspace of a far smaller number of dimensions. The subspace most suitable for the description of a particular family can be found by principal component analysis, an algorithm related to the embedding in distance geometry calculation:

As the first step in this analysis all sequences of a family are compared and their similarities are calculated. The number of identities $C^{kk'}$ between sequences k and k' can be expressed as the inner product of the sequence vectors (Fig. 1b).

$$C^{kk'} = \bar{\mathbf{F}}^k \cdot \bar{\mathbf{F}}^{k'} = \sum_{i,r} \mathbf{F}_{ir}^k \mathbf{F}_{ir}^{k'} \tag{2}$$

A comparison matrix C holding the number of identities for all pairs of sequences can thus be expressed as matrix product between alignment $\mathcal{F}$ and its transpose $\mathcal{F}^{\mathrm{T}}$:

$$\mathbf{C} = \mathcal{F}\mathcal{F}^{\mathrm{T}} \tag{3}$$

In more sophisticated comparisons identities are replaced by similarities and calculated using a mutation matrix M. This matrix takes care of the fact that some amino acid replacements are easily accepted, others are quite drastic. Therefore, harmless changes are scored almost as high as identities, whereas drastic mutations are more heavily penalised. The similarities $C^{kk'}$ between sequence k and k' are then computed as

$$C^{kk'} = \sum_{i} M(r_i^k, r_i^{k'}) \tag{4}$$

where $M(r_1, r_2)$ is the similarity score for an amino acid exchange from type r_1 to r_2 as defined in the mutation matrix and r_i^k is the actual residue type in sequence k at position i.

In a second step we search for those regions (dimensions) in sequence space most populated by the sequence family. These dimensions are defined by axes in sequence space, corresponding to the most prominent sequence patterns in the alignment and are found by minimising the differences between each axis and all sequences using least squares. Successive axes are maintained orthogonal and provide independent information. This criterion can be formulated as an eigenvalue problem where the principal axes $\bar{u}_p$ defining the maximal fitting subspace are the eigenvectors corresponding to the largest eigenvalues λ_p of the comparison matrix C.

$$\mathbf{C}\,\bar{u}_p = \lambda_p\,\bar{u}_p \tag{5}$$

The p-th coordinate x_p^k of protein in this subspace is calculated as:

$$x_p^k = \sqrt{\lambda_p}\,u_p^k \tag{6}$$

Representation of the family members in a lower-dimensional subspace, e.g., as points in a two-dimensional graph, illustrates the main similarity relationships (Fig. 2). Subfamilies are revealed as clusters, analogous to major branches in a tree representation. Higher dimensions, in order of decreasing eigenvalues, describe increasingly finer details in the similarity relationships, analogous to sub-branches in a tree.

The conceptual advantage of the vector representation of sequences becomes evident when vectors of individual residues (columns in alignment $\mathcal{F}$), rather than those of entire sequences (rows in $\mathcal{F}$), are projected along the principal directions. The principal axes $\bar{v}^p$ defined by contributions of each individual residue $v_{i,r}^p$ as components can be directly calculated from the eigenvectors $\bar{u}^p$ of the comparison matrix C, their corresponding eigenvalues λ_p and the original set of sequence vectors $\mathcal{F}$:

$$\bar{v}^p = \mathcal{F}^{\mathrm{T}}\,\bar{u}_p\,\lambda_p^{-1/2} \tag{7}$$

Analogous to equation (6) coordinates $y_p^{i,r}$ of residue r at position i in the sequence are computed as [6]:

$$y_{i,r}^p = \sqrt{\lambda_p v_{i,r}^p} \qquad (8)$$

This way individual residues can be placed in the same space as the full-length protein sequences. This unified representation emphasises links between sequence subfamilies and their corresponding characteristic residues.

3   Reading sequence space diagrams

Proteins as well as individual residues can now be represented as points in low dimensional subspaces of sequence space, e.g. 2D plots, that depict the similarity relationships within the protein family. When coupled to an interactive graphics program, one can explore sequence families and their specific residue patterns through the most important dimensions in sequence space and can identify likely functional residues.

The geometric origin of sequence space as defined here is the central point of reference. Relative to the origin, both direction and length of the vectors have a biological meaning. *Directions* in sequence space represent specific sequence *patterns* (profiles), i.e., combinations of specific residue types at specific sequence positions. The directions of the principal axes can be interpreted as the sequence patterns that best discriminate between members of the protein family. Typically, the direction of the first principal axis (largest eigenvalue) corresponds to the consensus pattern of the entire family. Preferred directions in this space reveal which residue types at which sequence positions best distinguish a subfamily. The resulting concept is simple: proteins of a particular subfamily as well as residues characteristic for the function of this subfamily point to the same direction in sequence space.

The *lengths* of vectors represent the *degree of conservation*. A protein more distant from the origin (Fig. 2A) is more representative in that it contains a larger fraction of residues characteristic for this direction in the subspace. Similarly, the most strongly conserved residues take the most distant positions (Fig. 2B) and form edges of the region occupied by all residues. Residues conserved in only one subfamily form the distant edge in the direction of this subfamily. Residues conserved in two subfamilies occupy the corner where the two corresponding edges meet (Fig. 2D). Clear clusters of residues on these corners and edges can reflect strong evolutionary selection and their member residues are predicted to be directly involved in function. In short, by representing both single residues and proteins in the principal dimensions of sequence space, protein subfamilies are evident as clusters and characteristic residues as corners and edges.

4   Summary and prospects

The sequence space method developed here identifies functional residues by exploiting evolutionary information in a set of related sequences — the "fossil record" of evolution under selective pressure. As has been proven in control examples the new method picks up subtle patterns of conservation and is capable of accurate predictions. Beyond the mere identification of functional residues, such residues can be subclassified according to subtasks they perform depending on the proteins in the groups and subgroups that contain these characteristic residues. For example, residues conserved in all proteins are required for the overall function of the family (e.g., nucleotide binding in the Ras superfamily) whereas specific residues characteristic for subgroups define the interactions with specific molecular partners required for the

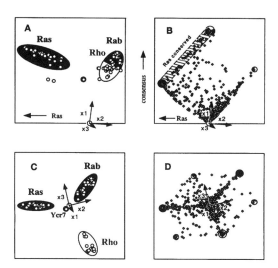

Figure 2: Sequence space analysis of the Ras Rab Rho superfamily; a family of GTP-binding regulatory proteins:

Two projections of sequence space of Ras Rab Rho superfamily onto the subspace defined by the 3 principal axes with largest eigenvalues, x_1, x_2, x_3. The 116 proteins contained in the multiple alignment that was analysed are represented as dots and shown on the left hand plots (A,C), positions of single sequence residues represented as diamonds projected onto the same plane are shown in corresponding plots right to it (B,D).

A and B) Projection of proteins (A) and residues (B) into a plane defined by the first two principal axes. The first and strongest pattern defines the direction of a consensus for the entire Ras, Rab, Rho-superfamily ($x1$), the second a Ras specific direction ($-x2$).

A) Ras proteins in $x1/x2$ plane: The more homologous to the complete family, the further up a protein is placed, the more typical representative of the Ras family, the further to the left.

B) Single residues in the $x1/x2$ plane: The more conserved in all Ras superfamily proteins the further up, the more Ras subfamily specific the more to the left residues are placed. Residues completely conserved in all three families occupy the extreme top corner in this plane, all of them are involved in GTP-binding or hydrolysis. Residues specific for Ras form a corner in the Ras specific direction (left). All residues conserved in the Ras family occupy the upper left edge in this representation.

C and D) Projection onto a plane containing the Ras specific direction ($-x2$) and a discriminating direction for Rho ($x3$).

C) Ras proteins in $x2/x3$ plane: In this representation three protein families form separate clusters that are easily identified. These three clusters contain the functionally distinct protein families of Ras proteins (in signal transduction pathway), Rab proteins (control of vesicle targeting) and Rho proteins (organisation of cytoskeleton). Ycr7, a yeast protein of unknown function (centre), is not member of any of these clusters and most likely the only representative of a new functional family. D) Single residues in the $x2/x3$ plane: Residues are located according to their specificity for any of the three subfamilies, residues occupying the remote corners in direction of Ras, Rab or Rho are uniquely specific for the corresponding family and predicted to participate in the specific function. (In case of Ras these residues perform recognition of and binding to components in the signalling cascade. These residues cluster in a confined molecular surface region of Ras known to transmit the GTP-hydrolysis signal to downstream partners. Specific residues shared by two families form corners in directions midway between those specific for the single families (at position of the vector sum).

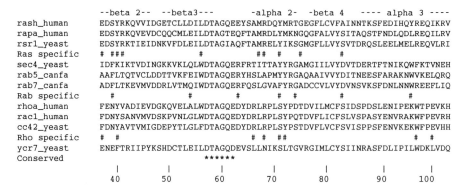

Figure 3: Example alignment illustrating patterns of conservation. This selected piece from the original alignment of Ras related sequences in the region known to forward the signal of GTP-hydrolysis downstream partners (switch II around alpha 2). Structural elements are labelled in the first line. This selected subset of sequences illustrates the essence of the method in a simple case. Conserved residues are indicated by an asterisk in line "conserved". All of them are involved in GTP binding and functionally important. Specific residues for the subgroups of Ras, Rab and Rho as obtained from this analysis are marked with asterisks in the corresponding lines. They cluster in regions important for signal readout like alpha 2.

individual functions of the subgroups (e.g. with proteins of the signalling pathway in the Ras family). The method has obvious limitations when sequence information is sparse and works best when ample sequences well dispersed in the subfamilies are available. In simple cases, the results of the method agree with intuitive analysis of conserved residues by mere inspection of multiple alignments, e.g., in the identification of completely conserved residues. However, identification of more subtle patterns by eye requires extensive experience and very tedious detailed inspection of both multiple sequence alignments and family trees. The real power of the method stems from the introduction of a conceptually novel view of sequence diversity, with complementary representation of both proteins and residues in the same mathematical space. The practical advantage of the method is brought out when a large sequence family is analysed or when conservation patterns are subtle.

We anticipate that the sequence space method will be a very useful tool for molecular biologists for predicting and classifying functional residues and planning residue-specific functional experiments.

References

[1] D. J. Lipman and W. R. Pearson, Rapid and sensitive protein similarity searches, *Science*, 227, 1435-1441, 1985.

[2] S. F. Altschul, W. Gish, W. Miller, E. W. Myers and D. J. Lipman, Basic local alignment search tool, *J. Mol. Biol.*, 215, 403-410, 1990.

[3] E. V. Koonin, P. Bork and C. Sander, Yeast Chromosome III: New Gene Functions, *EMBO J.*, 13, 493-503, 1994.

[4] G. Casari, C. Sander and A. Valencia, A method to predict functional residues in proteins, *Nature Struct. Biol.*, 2, 171-178, 1995.

[5] R. F. Doolittle and D-. F. Feng, Nearest neighbor procedure for relating progressively aligned amino acid sequences, *Meth. Enzymol.*, 183, 659-669, 1990.

[6] L. Lebart, A. Morineau and K. M. Warwick, *Multivariate Descriptive Statistical Analysis*, John Wiley & Sons, 1984.

Fitting 1-D Predictions
into 3-D Structures

Burkhard Rost

EMBL, Meyerhofstrasse 1, D-69012 Heidelberg, Germany, rost@embl-heidelberg.de

Abstract

The experimental determination of protein structure cannot keep track with the rapid generation of new sequence information. Can theory contribute? The most successful prediction method — and the only one for prediction of 3-D structure — is homology modelling. It is applicable for about one quarter of the proteins. For the rest, the prediction task has to be simplified. An extreme simplification is to project 3-D structure onto 1-D strings of secondary structure or solvent accessibility. For these 1-D aspects of 3-D structure, prediction accuracy has been improved significantly by using evolutionary information as input to neural network systems. The gain in accuracy is based on the conservation of secondary structure and relative solvent accessibility within sequence families. Secondary structure and accessibility are conserved, as well, between remote homologues. This fact can be used by fitting 1-D predictions into 3-D structures to detect such remote homologues. In comparison to other threading approaches, 1-D threading is rather flexible. However, two factors decrease detection accuracy. Firstly, the loss of information by projecting 3-D structure onto 1-D strings (in particular the loss of distances between secondary structure segments). And secondly, the inaccuracy of predicting 1-D structure. A preliminary result is that every fifth remote homologue is detected correctly.

1   Introduction

Sequence determines structure, determines function. It is generally assumed that three-dimensional (3-D[1]) protein structure is uniquely determined by sequence [1]. There are proteins assisting the folding *in vitro*, the chaperones. Are such assistants necessary for the majority of folding pathways? And do chaperones purely prevent unfolding, or are they actually necessary for folding? Answers remain open [2, 3, 4]. Anyway, the assumption that sequence determines structure constitutes a reasonable approximation. The function(s) of a protein are determined by its structure and environment (reagents). Thus, protein sequence

---

[1] Abbreviations used: 3-D, three-dimensional; 2-D, two-dimensional; 1-D, one-dimensional; PDB, Protein Data Bank of experimentally determined 3-D structures of proteins; SWISSPROT, data base of protein sequences; DSSP, data base containing the secondary structure and solvent accessibility for proteins of known 3-D structure; HSSP, data base containing for each PDB protein of known 3-D structure the alignments of all SWISSPROT sequences homologue to the known structure; FSSP, data base of remote homologues of known 3-D structure; PHD, Profile based neural network prediction of secondary structure (PHDsec) and solvent accessibility (PHDacc).

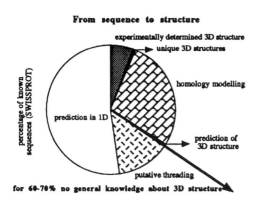 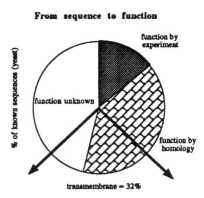

Figure 1: Prediction of protein structure and function — state of the art. *Prediction of structure:* For 70% of all known sequences, no knowledge about 3-D structure is available, in general. Threading methods may reduce this value to some 60% if they will become publicly available and sufficiently accurate for large scale sequence analysis. Today, for the majority of known protein sequences, the only successful sequence analyses are multiple alignments and predictions in 1-D. *Prediction of function:* For some 40-50% of the protein sequences obtained from sequencing whole genes (yeast III and VIII) some knowledge about function is either given by experiment or by homology modelling ([7]). Furthermore, for some 25-30% of the proteins transmembrane segments can be predicted (estimate derived from an analysis of 171 yeast VIII sequences, [68]).

determines function to a certain extent. Consequently, structure and function can, in principle, be induced from the sequence based on physico-chemical properties. In practice, this is prevented by the enormous complexity of the phase space. Can theory contribute to the advance of molecular biology, nevertheless?

The objective of theory is to reduce the sequence-structure and sequence-function gaps. Large scale gene-sequencing projects produce data of gene and consequently protein sequences at breathtaking pace [5, 6]. Knowledge about function and/or structure of the proteins plays a crucial role in designing experiments using such data. However, only for the minority of proteins with known sequence, the 3-D structure is also known. Experimental determination of protein function is easier than that of structure. Consequently, the sequence-function gap is less exposed than the sequence-structure gap [7]. In the near future, the gaps are unlikely to be reduced significantly by experiments. How does theory contribute today to reduce the gaps?

Homology modelling is the most powerful theoretical tool. The only reliable technique to predict both protein structure and protein function is homology modelling: for a search sequence its 3-D structure and function is predicted based on a sequence alignment to proteins of known 3-D structure and/or function [8, 9, 10, 11, 12]. This method increases the number of known 3-D structures by a factor of five [13], and the number of proteins with some knowledge about function by a factor of three [7, 14] (Fig. 1). What if there is no protein with significant sequence identity ($> 25\%$) in the data base of known structures?

Threading techniques may become a second comprehensive tool. Roughly, every fifth protein in PDB is remotely homologue to another PDB protein [15], i.e. has a homologous 3-D structures but no significant pairwise sequence similarity ($< 25\%$ [16]). Thus, theory could reduce the sequence-structure gap by another 10-20% of the known sequences if remote homology were detected based on sequence information (as homology is by sequence alignment). One way to predict remote homology is by threading sequences into structures [17, 18, 19, 20, 21, 22, 23, 24, 25, 26, 27]. The principle objective is to define a criterion that enables to evaluate whether or not the sequence fits into the structure. If both homology modelling and threading fail, can theory predict 3-D structure from sequence?

In general, prediction is limited to 1-D. Despite advances in detail, the ability to predict 3-D structure from sequence by theoretical means has not much improved. In general, 3-D structure cannot be predicted ab initio. The prediction problem has to be simplified. One extreme simplification is projecting 3-D structure onto 1-D strings of secondary structure assignments (e.g. helix, strand, rest). Improving the accuracy of secondary structure prediction has been protruded for the last three decades. Another 1-D feature of 3-D structure that had been subject to prediction methods is the position of a residue with respect to the surface of a protein, i.e. its solvent accessibility. Predictions of such 1-D features are of limited accuracy, but are applicable in general. Can predictions of simplified 1-D aspects of 3-D structure be used successfully as a starting point to predict structure or function?

In some cases, 1-D predictions can be used to infer aspects of function and 3-D structure. Supposed, the pattern of predicted secondary structure elements, e.g. "helix-strand-helix-strand", were similar to either the secondary structure pattern of a protein with known 3-D structure, or to the pattern of a protein for which secondary structure is predicted and not experimentally determined. Then, the hypothesis that the two proteins are remote homologues may be used to predict 3-D structure and/or function. For selected cases, remote homology modelling has been used to predict 3-D structure (e.g. [28]). Is such a procedure necessarily restricted to selected cases, or can it be done automatically?

Can 1-D predictions seed an automatic prediction of remote homologues? Here, some preliminary results will be given to answer this question. The goal is to recognise remote homologues based on alignments of a projection of 3-D structure onto 1-D strings of secondary structure and solvent accessibility assignments. First, the results of the underlying methods for predicting secondary structure and solvent accessibility will be sketched briefly. Second, the principles of the threading method will be described, and some strategies for the optimisation of free parameters will be given.

2   Combining evolutionary information and neural networks

2.1   Prediction of secondary structure

Prediction of secondary structure based on single sequences is limited to $< 65\%$ accuracy. The basic idea of most prediction methods is that stretches of adjacent residues from protein sequences are unique. E.g. given a pentapeptide of five consecutive residues, is the central residue of all equal pentapeptides always observed in the same secondary structure? For pentapeptides, this is indeed not the case [29]; peptides of e.g. 13 residues are unique. However, for prediction purposes it is not sufficient to just search for an identical peptide of 13 residues, as it may not be contained in the data base. Instead, the goal is to classify similar patterns in either of the three classes: helix, strand, or rest. Secondary structure prediction based on pattern classification has been pursued even before the first X-ray structure was determined [30, 31, 32]. A decade ago, prediction accuracy reached some 50-55% three-state accuracy [33] (percentage of residues predicted correctly in either of the three states). More advanced algorithms and increased data bases pushed the accuracy to 60-65%, a mark that was long taken as insurmountable [34, 35, 36, 37, 38, 39, 40, 41, 42, 43, 44]. The main

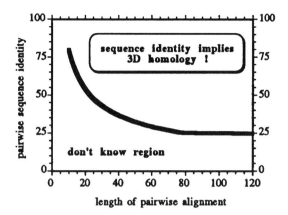

Figure 2: Information about 3-D structure contained in evolutionary records. All protein pairs in the current data base (PDB [69]) that have 30 out of 100 aligned residues in common have homologous 3-D structure [16]. Thus, any sequence pair above the line for which one sequence has a known 3-D structure, can be used for prediction of 3-D structure by homology modelling. All 3-D homologues that fall below the line are referred to as remote homologues; some 4,000 remote homologues are known today (FSSP, [15]). Remote homologues could be detected based on sequence information by successful threading techniques. To illustrate the problem of threading by numbers: more than one billion pairs fall under the line, of these only some thousands of pairs are remote homologues.

difficulty was that the input information contained in stretches of 13-21 consecutive residues is not sufficient. Do protein sequences contain any additionally information about 3-D structure that could be used for prediction?

Sequence families contain much more information than single sequences. Protein sequence determines protein structure. But, how unique is this relation? How many residues can be exchanged in a protein without changing the 3-D structure? Evolutionary pressure to maintain protein function has explored paths to exchange about 75% of all residues without changing the 3-D structure (Fig. 2, [16]). Can any three out of four amino acid be exchanged against any other? Not at all, instead a random exchange of some residues will often be sufficient to destabilize a structure. Thus, the detailed pattern of amino acid exchanges found in sequence families is highly informative about the structure of that family [45]. Are 1-D projections of 3-D structure, such as secondary structure and solvent accessibility, conserved between 3-D homologues?

Secondary structure was conserved to some 90% between 3-D homologues. Sequence alignments can be used to predict secondary structure for proteins for which there is a known structure with significant sequence identity (all above the line in Fig. 2). Within sequence families, the pairwise identity of secondary structure segments was some 90% (Fig. 3, [46, 47]). In other words, two proteins can adopt the same 3-D structure and yet differ in the secondary structure assignment by about 10% Conservation was higher in the core than at the surface [46]. Can evolutionary information be used to improve secondary structure predictions?

Evolutionary information improved prediction accuracy to $> 72\%$. The way to use evolutionary information for prediction was the following. First, the data base of known

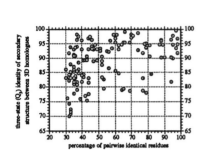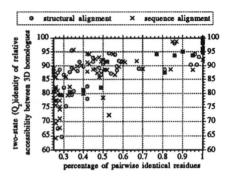

Figure 3: Conservation of 1-D structure between 3-D homologues. *(a)* Conservation of secondary structure (averaged over protein pairs) vs. the percentage of identical residues between the sequences of the pair. Homologues were aligned on sequence-based [16] comparisons. The identity is given as the overlap of secondary structure segments between the pairs [46]. *(b)* Conservation of relative solvent accessibility (averaged over protein pairs) vs. the percentage of identical residues between the sequences of the pair. Homologues were aligned both based on structure-based [15] and on sequence-based [16] comparisons. The identity is given as the percentage of residues in either of the two states for relative solvent accessibility (buried, exposed, [53]).

sequences was scanned by sequence alignment methods [16] for similar sequences. Second, the list of sequences found was filtered by the length-dependent threshold for significant sequence identity (Fig. 2). Third, for all probable 3-D homologues, a profile of amino acid exchanges was compiled. Fourth, this profile was used for prediction. The first method that has been proven in a cross-validation experiment based on 250 unique protein chains to predict secondary structure at a sustained level of $> 72\%$ three-state accuracy was a neural network [42, 48]. For this method the profiles, and additional information derived from the multiple sequence alignments, were fed as input into the neural network system. Various further details of the architectures of a network system composed of two layers of networks and a final compilation of an arithmetic average over independently trained networks, were important to yield a prediction with a high overall accuracy, a relative accurate prediction of strands, and succeeded to correctly predict secondary structure segments rather than single residues (Table 1, [42, 43]). For the 40% of all residues predicted with higher reliability, the method (dubbed PHDsec) reached a value of 90%, i.e. was as accurate as homology modelling would be if applicable. Almost ten percentage points of the improvement in overall accuracy stemmed from using evolutionary information. Does evolutionary information also improve the prediction of other aspects of 3-D structure?

2.2 Prediction of solvent accessibility

Solvent accessibility depends on residue type and structural environment. The solvent accessibility of a residue embedded in a protein can be measured by the number of water (solvent) molecules that can be placed around it [49]. Values typically vary between 0 and 200 Å^2. To compare residues of different sizes, a relative solvent accessibility has to be compiled

Table 1: Accuracy of secondary structure prediction.
Abbreviations of methods: HM, homology modelling; RAN, random sequence alignments; PHDsec, neural network prediction using multiple alignment information as input [42, 48]; SIMPA, similarity based statistical prediction method using single sequence information only [70](note: SIMPA has not the highest accuracy reported for classical methods, but it scored better than others on the particular data set used here [42]); LPAG, statistical prediction method using multiple alignment information [71].
Abbreviations of measures: Nprot, number of proteins used for testing (all prediction results hold for test proteins with less than 25% sequence identity to the proteins used to derive the prediction method); set, different test sets are numbered to indicate identical sets (1:[46], 2, 3, 4:[42], 5 and 6: proteins of recently determined 3-D structure); Q_3, three-state overall per-residue accuracy, i.e. number of residues predicted correctly in either of the three states helix, strand, rest; I, information, entropy measure for prediction accuracy [46, 48]; Sov_3, three-state overall per-segment accuracy, i.e. the overlap of predicted and observed secondary structure segments (rather than single residues) [46]; date, whenever new protein structures are added to the data base (PDB) the neural network prediction was re-evaluated.

method	set	Nprot	Q_3	I	Sov_3	date
HM	set 1	80	88.4	0.62	89.7	
RAN	set 1	80	35.2	0.01	30.6	
PHDsec	set 2	126	71.6	0.27	72.8	Jun, 93
PHDsec	set 3	124	72,5	0.28	75.6	Aug, 93
SIMPA	set 3	124	60.7	0.12	61.7	
PHDsec	set 4	60	74.8	0.34	76.8	
LPAG	set 4	60	68.5			
PHDsec	set 5	27	72.0	0.28	72.4	May, 94
PHDsec	set 6	59	73.0	0.30	75.7	Nov, 94

[51, 52, 53]. Conservation of solvent accessibility between 3-D homologous pairs is best analysed by computing the correlation between the relative solvent accessibility of the two [53]. Here, a simpler measure is used, a two-state description of solvent accessibility (buried < 16% solvent accessible; exposed ≥ 16% solvent accessible, [54, 55, 56]). If protein cores were conserved completely between 3-D homologues, the two-state identity should be 100%. Is solvent accessibility conserved that well within protein families?

Solvent accessibility was conserved to some 85% between 3-D homologues. Conservation of solvent accessibility in two states is found to be clearly less than 100% (Fig. 3, [53]). A possible reason may be that sequences were not correctly aligned at low levels of sequence identity (sharp decrease around 40%, Fig. 3). Indeed, the decrease in conservation was less significant for structural alignments of the same protein pairs (Fig. 3). However, even for structural alignments, solvent accessibility was conserved to only 85% in two states. Furthermore, conservation dropped for low levels of sequence identity (Fig. 3). This observation sheds a light on why the accuracy of automatic homology modelling decreases with decreasing sequence identity. When three states were distinguished for relative solvent accessibility (buried,

Table 2: Accuracy of solvent accessibility prediction.

<u>Abbreviations of methods:</u> HM: SeqAli, homology modelling, alignments based on sequence comparisons [53]; HM: StrAli, homology modelling, alignments based on structural comparisons [53]; PHDacc, neural network prediction based on multiple alignments [53]; Wako, statistical prediction method based on multiple sequence alignments[72].

<u>Abbreviations of measures:</u> The protein sets are as in Table 1 (set 3a is a subset of set 3); Q_3, three-state overall per-residue accuracy, i.e. percentage of residues correctly predicted in either of the three-states buried, intermediate, exposed [53]; Q_2, two-state overall accuracy (buried, exposed); Corr, correlation between predicted and observed relative solvent accessibility [53].

method	set	Nprot	Q_3	Q_2	Corr	date
HM: SeqAli	set 1	80	71.6	83.8	0.68	
HM: StrAli	set 1	80	73.6	84.8	0. 77	
RAN	set 1	80	33.9	52.0	0.01	
PHDacc	set 2	126	57.9	75.0	0.54	
PHDacc	set 3a	112	57.9	74.7	0.54	Mar, 94
PHDacc	set 7	13	60.8	79.2	0.61	
Wako	set 7		76.5			
PHDacc	set 5	27	57.6	73.4	0.55	May, 94
PHDacc	set 6	59	57.0	74.0	0.54	Nov, 94

intermediate, exposed), the identity for 3-D homologues was reduced to an average of $< 75\%$ [53]. As the distribution of these three states is comparable to that of the three secondary structure states, the conclusion is that solvent accessibility is less well conserved in evolution than is secondary structure. Does this imply that the prediction of solvent accessibility is less accurate than the prediction of secondary structure?

Solvent accessibility was predicted at 75% two-state accuracy. The profile based neural network system used (named PHDacc) was similar to PHDsec [53]). A cross-validation experiment on 238 unique protein chains yielded an expected two-state accuracy of 75% (residues correctly predicted as either buried or exposed), and an expected three-state accuracy (buried, intermediate, exposed) of <60% (Table 2). Thus, solvent accessibility was predicted less accurately than secondary structure. Does this imply that the network has intrinsically more difficulties with the accessibility prediction? To find out, the prediction accuracy was normalised such that on the normalised scale a prediction by homology yielded 100% and a random prediction 0%. On this normalised scale solvent accessibility prediction turned out to be more accurate than secondary structure prediction [53]. In other words, PHDacc came closer to the optimal prediction performance given by the conservation of solvent accessibility than PHDsec to the mark given by the conservation of secondary structure (Table 1, Table 2). Thus, the low level of accuracy for predicting solvent accessibility mainly stems from the fact that this aspect of 3-D structure is less conserved between 3-D homologues.

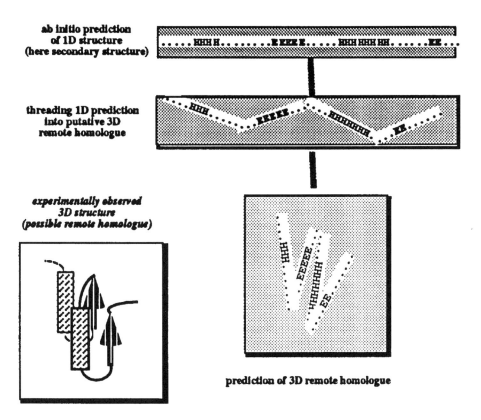

prediction of 3D remote homologue

Figure 4: Threading 1-D strings into 3-D structures. The principle idea of threading 1-D predictions into 3-D structures is the following. First, for a search sequence secondary structure and solvent accessibility are predicted. Second, the known 3-D structures are projected onto 1-D strings of secondary structure and solvent accessibility (DSSP, [50]). Third, the predicted 1-D strings are aligned to the 1-D strings of known structures. The best match of the dynamic programming algorithm constitutes the predicted remote homologue for the search sequence.

3 Aligning 1-D strings of secondary structure and solvent accessibility

3.1 Principle idea of 1-D threading

How can 1-D predictions be used to predict more aspects about 3-D structure? The simple idea is the following. Protein folds often are described by motifs of secondary structure (e.g. H-E-H-E) in combination with a table of inter segment distances (e.g. "H1 near to H2, E1 near to E2, strands on top of helices"). But even without the distance table, a prediction of "H-E-H-E" combined with a certain pattern of solvent accessibility states should suffice to, at least, formulate the hypothesis that the structure sketched in figure 4 is homologue to the search sequence.

Detection of motifs by alignment of 1-D strings. The mostly studied technique to detect similar motifs in 1-D strings is dynamic programming [57, 58, 59, 60]. The application to

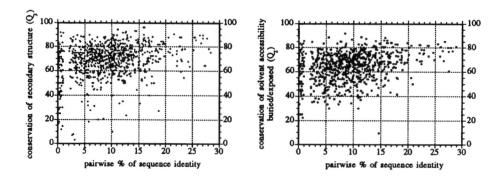

Figure 5: Conservation of secondary structure and solvent accessibility between remote homologues. The conservation of secondary structure is given as the percentage of identical residues in either of the three states helix, strand and rest; the conservation of solvent accessibility as the percentage of residues identical in either of the two states buried (relative accessibility < 16%) and exposed (relative accessibility 3 $\geq$ 16%). Each point reflects one of a total of 2211 protein pairs structurally aligned in the FSSP data base [15].

1-D threading worked as follows. First, for a list of proteins of known 3-D structure (typically unique set, [61]) projections of 3-D structure onto strings of secondary structure and relative solvent accessibility assignments were computed (DSSP, [50]). Second, a search sequence of unknown structure was aligned against the sequence data base (SWISSPROT [62]), and used as input to neural network systems that predicted secondary structure and solvent accessibility. Third, prediction and observation were extracted into strings composed of a six letter alphabet (3 × 2), for the three secondary structure states, and the two relative accessibility states. Fourth, the string predicted for the search sequence was aligned with the strings extracted from the data base of observed structures. (The program used for the alignment procedure was a modified version of the sequence alignment program *MaxHom* [13, 16]).

Secondary structure and solvent accessibility was conserved between remote homologues. 1-D threading is possible only if secondary structure and solvent accessibility are conserved, not only within sequence families (Fig. 3), but also between remote homologues. The average conservation of secondary structure was 69% (Fig. 5, overall three-state identity, one standard deviation 13%); the average conservation of relative solvent accessibility 65% (Fig. 5, overall two-state identity, one standard deviation 10%). Thus, both secondary structure and relative solvent accessibility were largely conserved between remote homologues. An interesting detail was that, although both 1-D aspects were less conserved for remote homologues than for homologues with significant pairwise sequence identity (Fig. 3), the conservation did not decrease significantly with sequence identity.

3.2   Adjusting free parameters for alignment

How can free alignment parameters be optimised? The success of alignment algorithms depends on two important groups of free parameters. First, the values for the comparison matrix: matches or mismatches between the six states of the strings aligned have not equal significance with respect to the structural motif searched for. Second, the penalty given for introducing a gap ("gap open penalty") and for continuing a gap ("gap elongation penalty"). Less important (in terms of less sensitive to the stability of the resulting alignment) are the minimal and maximal value for the scoring matrix (chosen as: maximal match score =1; minimal (mis-)match score = -1). Optimisation of the free parameters is a highly non-trivial task; the main obstacle being the lack of a clear-cut optimisation criterion. In the following some optimisation strategies and some particular choices for the free parameters will be discussed.

Distinguishing random alignments and true remote homologues. Some relations between the elements of the scoring matrix are evident from expert knowledge. For example, a mismatch between buried helix and exposed strand is much worse than a mismatch between buried helix and buried loop. But how should the values be chosen exactly? What is the optimisation criterion for the choice of the scoring matrix? The alignment goal is to detect true remote homologues. This implies not only that remote homologues are detected, but also that the alignment procedure distinguishes between remote homologues (termed "correct hits") and non-homologous proteins (termed "false positives" or "incorrect hits"). Thus, one idea for the optimisation of the scoring matrix is to choose the values such that scores for correct and incorrect hits become maximally separated.

Different concepts of maximal separation of distributions. For some thousand pairs, the scores were computed for random alignments (incorrect hits) and structurally aligned remote homologues (correct hits). The distributions do overlap (Fig. 6). Various matrices were generated by expert driven trial and error. No choice resulted in an overlap of zero. Thus, the next question is what 'maximal separation' means. Various concepts are feasible: (i) maximize the difference between the averages of the distributions, (ii) maximize the quotient between the differences of averages normalised with the product of the standard deviations, or (iii) minimize the area of overlap. The alternatives (i)-(iii) did not result in the same choice for the free variables of the scoring matrix. The separation shown in Fig. 6 was optimal with respect to criterion (ii) (and almost best for (i) and (iii)).

Secondary structure and solvent accessibility superior to either of the two. Would the separation between correct and incorrect hits be less distinct, if either only secondary structure or only accessibility were used, instead of both combined? Indeed, the separation was less for either of the two 1-D features alone than for a combination of the two. However, the degree of separation that was gained by adding relative solvent accessibility states to the description in terms of secondary structure assignments, was rather small (Fig. 6).

Optimisation of gap penalties with respect to remote homologues detected. There are three reasons to introduce gaps. First, loop regions can be inserted between regular secondary structure segments without influencing the basic fold [63]. Second, slightly elongated or shortened helices or strands can form similar motifs[46]. Third, predictions are generally more accurate for the core of predicted segments than at the ends, in other words it is less likely that a whole segment is predicted falsely than that some residues at the ends of segments are predicted wrongly [43]. The optimisation criterion for gap penalties is different than that for the scoring matrix in that gap penalties have to be optimised with respect to a given alignment list (3.3.). If the goal is to minimize the percentage of false positives (3.3.), then the optimal values for a search with PDB against PDB (3.4.) were: gap open penalty = 1.0; gap elongation penalty = 0.1. However, if the goal is to have one correct prediction at first rank, higher values (3/0.3, 5/0.5) are better.

3.3 Measuring prediction accuracy for threading

Sorting the alignment list by normalised alignment scores. For one sequence (search sequence), the predicted strings are aligned against a list of typically some 300 proteins of known structure.

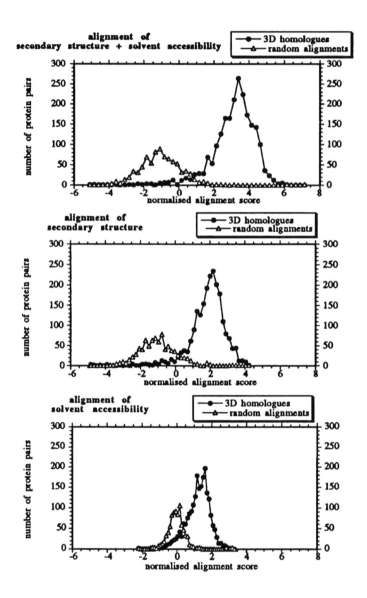

Figure 6: Separation of 3-D homologues and random alignments. For three different scenarios, the separation of random alignments (generated by sequence alignments of non-homologous PDB pairs with no significant pairwise sequence identity) and structural alignments of 3-D homologues (taken from FSSP, [15]) are compared. First, strings of secondary structure and relative solvent accessibility were aligned (six-letter alphabet: 3×2, for three secondary structure types helix, strand, rest and two states for relative solvent accessibility, buried and exposed). Second, strings of secondary structure were aligned (3 states). And third, strings of relative solvent accessibility were aligned (2 states).

Since alignments can involve different sub-regions of a protein, the result of one threading experiment is a list of several hundreds of alignments. Previously published threading methods uncovered that it is crucial for the success, to adequately sort the alignment hit list. Sorting by scores, comparable to the alignment score compiled here, is not sufficient [64, 65]. Instead, only if the score is normalised with respect to the background given by the data base, the distinction between correct and false positives becomes feasible [64]. The normalisation used here does not alter the simple sorting of the hit list by the alignment score, but enables a comparison of scores between different search sequences:

$$zE_i = \frac{E_i - \langle E \rangle}{\sigma} \tag{1}$$

where E_i is the alignment score for the i'th hit in the list of all alignments obtained for a search protein, $< E >$ is the average over all hits for that sequence and σ the standard deviation of the distribution of all hits. In other words, zE_i describes the significance of a given hit i, for a search sequence.

Lack of widely accepted standards to measure accuracy. Due to historical reasons, threading results in the past have put too much emphasis on "find-self" measures, i.e. the ability of a threading potential to correctly find the search sequence among a large number of decoys [22, 23, 64, 65, 66]. The measures defined here are restricted to analysing the detection of remote homologues. Another important issue is the correctness of the alignment (Holm, Ouzounis, Sander, Sippl, manuscript in preparation).

Definition of simple measures for accuracy in detecting remote homologues. Given a list of true remote homologues and another of predicted homologues, various measures for accuracy can be defined (Table 3). The most important is the simplest: how many of the first hits are correct (eq. (T3a))? Less strict is to cut the alignment list at a given threshold and to count the percentage of correct hits in the remaining list (eq. (T3c)). Such a number is of interest if an expert user could manage to reduce the list further, or if it were more important for the user to detect a remote homologue than to rely on the correctness of a given hit.

More than some "favourable cases" are necessary for evaluating threading. So far, most publications on the threading issue used a couple of "favourite remote homologues" to test the method. Such a procedure is rather arbitrary. A more reasonable approach would be to start with a list of unique proteins [61, 67], and to compile for each of these proteins all remote homologues. A first version of such an approach has been explored here. All results given are based on structural alignments of 46 protein chains. (A more comprehensive list is currently being collected.)

3.4 Preliminary results

Expert knowledge helps to separate correct hits from false positives. For some 40% of all proteins, one correct hit was found in the alignment list among the first four hits. As an explicit example for a 1-D threading the first 15 hits for the search sequence TU-elongation factor (1etu) are shown (Fig. 7). Due to the high number of inserted residues (*IDEL* in Fig. 7) an expert would have probably ignored all hits before the fourth (dihydropteridine reductase, 1dhr), or even before the sixth (ras-p21, 5p21). Both are correctly detected remote homologues. For the TU-elongation factor many of the first hits were correct and the only hits without exceptionally long insertions were correct. The optimistic conclusion is that 1-D threading is successful in detecting remote homologues. Does this hold in general? Is it always possible to distinguish between correct and incorrect hits based on some expert criteria?

Three scenarios: PDB vs. PDB; PHD vs. PDB; and PHD vs. PHD. Three different scenarios were compared to analyse threading performance. Firstly, the case of an error-

Table 3: Measures for accuracy in detecting remote homologues.

For each prediction of a remote homologue (each search sequences) there are two lists of alignments, one summarising the true remote homologues (as given in e.g. FSSP [15]), and the other the predicted homologues (sorted by any score). Q_{1st} estimates how often a correct answer will come out if only the first hit is used as prediction; $Q_{1stcorrect}$ gives the average position of a correct hit; $Q_{zE(n)}$, gives the percentage of correct hits if the alignment list is cut according to a given criterion (e.g. how many of the hits with a z-score (Eq. (1)) zE > n are correct?); $Cov_{zE(n)}$ coverage of true positives (i.e. how many of the true remote homologues are predicted at a given cut-off threshold). Note: all counts refer to lists, which a purged off from trivial hits (such as hits with significant pairwise sequence identity). In practice, this is accomplished by simply excluding all hits from the list, which are contained in HSSP files [13], i.e. could have been detected by simple sequence alignment.

$$Q_{1st} = 100 \times \frac{\text{number of correct first hits}}{\text{number of all proteins}} \qquad \text{(T3a)}$$

$$Q_{1stcorrect} = 100 \times \frac{1}{\text{position of first correct hit}} \qquad \text{(T3b)}$$

$$Q_{zE(n)} = 100 \times \frac{\text{number of correct first hits with zE > n}}{\text{number of hits with zE > n}} \qquad \text{(T3c)}$$

$$Cov_{zE(n)} = 100 \times \frac{\text{number of correct first hits with zE > n}}{\text{number of true remote homologues } (N_T)} \qquad \text{(T3d)}$$

free prediction of secondary structure and solvent accessibility represented by alignments of observed with observed strings (PDB-PDB). Secondly, predicted strings are aligned with observed ones (PHD-PDB). Thirdly, predicted strings for the search sequence are aligned with predicted strings for the putative homologues. The first case of an optimal prediction was tested to analyse the degree to which the reduction of the information by predicting 3-D structure onto 1-D strings (and by loosing distance information) results in ambiguities. The last case of aligning predictions with predictions was motivated by the hypothesis that prediction errors may to a certain degree be non-random, i.e. the prediction may e.g. always fail to predict a certain twisted strand in a fold. In that case the prediction for the search sequence and for the remote homologue may align better than the prediction for the search sequence and the observed structure for the remote homologue.

High accuracy in predicting the 1-D strings is crucial. The following four results can be summarised. First, a high accuracy in predicting secondary structure and solvent accessibility is very important for the 1-D threading to work out (Table 4): an alignment of PDB with PDB (i.e. observation with observation) is almost twice as accurate as an alignment of PHD with PDB (i.e. prediction with observation). Second, the projection of 3-D structure onto 1-D results in a detection accuracy of about 50%. Third, an alignment of PHD with PDB is slightly superior to an alignment of PHD with PHD, i.e. the errors in secondary structure and solvent accessibility prediction are to a certain extent not random. Fourth, the accuracy in detecting remote homologues was about 20%.

Refinement by filtering the alignment list. The single prediction example discussed (Fig. 7) suggested that there may be other criteria than the z-score (eq. (1)) to distinguish between correct and false positives. Preliminary results confirm what has been uncovered by others before (e.g. Braxenthaler and Eisenberg, these Proceedings): an adequate combination of

POS	E	LEN	IDEL	ZE	%IDE	STRH	OK	ID2	NAME2
1	80.5	141	135	2.23	0.11	0.96		2ctc	CARBOXYPEPTIDASE A
2	79.7	139	103	2.20	0.07	0.91	*	1dri	D-RIBOSE-BINDING PROTEIN
3	78.6	141	73	2.15	0.08	0.90	*	1dhr	DIHYDROPTERIDINE REDUCTASE
4	78.0	141	152	2.12	0.09	0.92		1gsc	HEAT-SHOCK PROTEIN
5	79.0	139	123	2.11	0.10	0.94		1bll	LEUCINE AMINOPEPTIDASE
6	77.9	122	49	2.11	0.09	0.91	*	5p21	RAS P21 PROTEIN
7	76.4	141	120	2.04	0.06	0.91		1gal	GLUCOSE OXIDASE
8	76.4	141	138	2.04	0.11	0.91	*	1gd1	GLYCERALDEHYDE-PHOSPHATE DEHYDROGENASE
9	76.0	141	65	2.02	0.07	0.82	*	1fnr	FERREDOXIN
10	75.6	141	111	2.00	0.08	0.87	*	1ipd	3-ISOPROPYLMALATE DEHYDROGENASE
11	75.3	141	118	1.98	0.10	0.90		1fba	FRUCTOSE-BISPHOSPHATE ALDOLASE
12	75.1	135	90	1.98	0.08	0.87	*	1pfk	PHOSPHOFRUCTOKINASE
13	74.8	141	107	1.96	0.09	0.88		1pda	PORPHOBILINOGEN DEAMINASE
14	74.7	140	134	1.96	0.08	0.93		1omp	D-MALTODEXTRIN-BINDING PROTEIN
15	74.7	141	134	1.96	0.06	0.90	*	8abp	ARABINOSE-BINDING PROTEIN

Figure 7: Example for a threading list. Search sequence was 1etu, the TU-elongation factor. Abbreviations: POS, position in list; E, alignment score; LEN, length of alignment; IDEL, number of residues inserted in either of the two aligned strings; ZE, z-score for alignment score (Eq. (1)); %IDE, ratio of pairwise sequence identity; STRH, structural homology (identical symbols in six-letter alphabet); OK = *, if the pair is a true 3-D homologue, i.e. is contained in the FSSP data base [15]; ID2, PDB identifier of aligned 3-D structure; NAME2, SWISSPROT name of aligned 3-D structure.

information from the alignment list (number of residues inserted, length of alignment, length of search sequence and of remote homologue) improves the accuracy in detecting remote homologues. In general, there as a trade-off between a high level of reliability of the prediction (eq. (T3c)) and the likelihood that an existing remote homologue is detected (eq. (T3d)). Different threshold criteria can shift the balance between higher coverage and higher accuracy (Fig. 8).

4   Conclusions

Evolutionary information is the key to accurate predictions in 1-D. Predictions of secondary structure and solvent accessibility were improved significantly by tailoring the neural network systems to the problem. However, the most significant improvement resulted from including evolutionary information (Fig. 4, Table 1, Table 2). The final predictions of secondary structure were very accurate: three thirds of all segments were predicted correctly, and for the 40% of the residues predicted at higher reliability the prediction accuracy was comparable to homology modelling [42]. Solvent accessibility was more difficult to predict than secondary structure. This was largely due to a lower degree in conservation of solvent accessibility (Fig. 3). This suggests that prediction methods should focus on features of protein structure that are

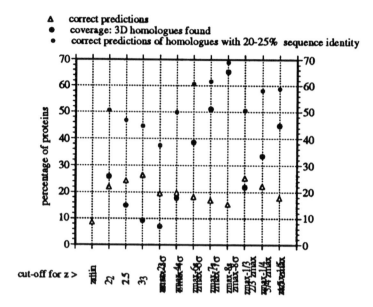

Figure 8: Preliminary results for detection of remote homologues. The alignment list is cut-off at various values for the alignment z-score (eq. (1)), i.e. only hits with a value larger than the threshold are taken as predicted remote homologues. The cut-off values given are: $zE > zmin$, i.e. all hits are taken; $zE > 2, 2.5, 3$, i.e. hits for which the z-score exceeds a value independent of the search sequence; $zE > (zmax - n \times \sigma)$, with $n = 2, 4, 6, 7, 8$, i.e. hits for which the z-score exceeds a value defined by the standard deviation and the maximal z-score for all alignments with a search sequence; and $zE > r \times zmax$, with $r = 0.66, 0.75, 0.8$, i.e. hits for which the z-score has a maximal difference to the maximal z-score for the search sequence. For all cut-off thresholds n the percentage of correct hits (Q_{zE}, eq. (T3c), open triangles) and the coverage, i.e. the percentage of true homologues detected at that threshold ($Cov_{zE}(n)$, eq. (T3d), filled circles) are plotted. Using additionally sequence information for the alignment improves the detection accuracy for pairs with a pairwise sequence identity above the average for remote homologues (20-25%, circles with point), but below the average of a significant detection of homology based on sequence information alone (> 25%, for more elaborate alignment procedures).

conserved in evolution. Are 1-D predictions useful in practice?

Conservative evaluations of accuracy are more productive than best-case expectations. A common fault in evaluating prediction methods is that free parameters are fitted on the data sets used for evaluation. However, the opposite is more useful: the performance on a set of new proteins should tend to be higher rather than lower than the published expected accuracy (Table 1, Table 2). The neural network based predictions of secondary structure and solvent accessibility are being used frequently (more than 80 requests per day to an automatic prediction service, for information, send the word *help* to the internet address *PredictProtein@EMBL-Heidelberg.DE*, or use the World Wide Web (WWW) site *http://www.embl-heidelberg.de/predictprotein/predictprotein.html*). Users find the 1-D pre-

Table 4: Accuracy of 1-D threading.
Values are given as percentages. Abbreviations of measures as in Table 3. Two cut-off thresholds are compared: zE > 3; and zE > 3/4 of the maximal value for zE for a given alignment list. Abbreviations of methods: PDB-PDB, the aligned strings of the search sequence and the putative homologue both originate from experimentally determined structures, i.e. these values describe the detection accuracy for ideal predictions of secondary structure and solvent accessibility; PHD-PDB, alignment of predicted (search sequence) and observed (to be detected homologues) strings (the predictions were done by cross-validation, i.e. no protein used to train the neural network systems did have more than 25% pairwise sequence identity to the search sequence of the threading); PHD-PHD, the aligned strings of the search sequence and the putative homologue both originate from predictions. E.g. if only those alignments between a 1-D prediction for a search sequence and 1-D strings extracted from a data base of experimentally determined 3-D structures with zE > 3 were taken, then 27% of these hits had been correct hits, and 8% of all true positives had been found above this threshold (21% of all first hits had been correct).

method	Q_{1st}	$Q_{zE(n)}$	$Cov_{zE(n)}$	$Q_{zE(n)}$	$Cov_{zE(n)}$
comment:		zE > 3	zE > 3	zE > $\frac{3}{4}$ × z_{max}	zE > $\frac{3}{4}$ × z_{max}
PDB-PDB	28	46	10	42	28
PHD-PDB	21	27	8	22	28
PHD-PHD	19	21	13	19	28

dictions useful. But, can 1-D predictions be used to predict more aspects of 3-D structure?

Standards for evaluating threading techniques are becoming required. How can threading experiments be evaluated? Appropriate evaluation consists of two parts, first, the choice of a representative data set, and second, the definition of adequate measures for prediction accuracy. The data set used here, was a first attempt to validate threading experiments on more than just a handful of proteins. The measures defined here, were restricted to analysing the detection of remote homologues. The most stringent measure is the percentage of proteins for which the first predicted 3-D homologue is correct (Table 3). Given these definitions, does 1-D threading work?

1-D threading possible, but so far very inaccurate. The positive message is "sometimes 1-D threading does work" (Fig. 7). How often? Three important results are. First, erasing the inter-segment distances reduces the 3-D information too drastically (PDB vs. PDB, Fig. 6, Table 4). Second, the inaccuracy of the neural network predictions reduces the accuracy in detecting 3-D homologues further, but is relatively less harmful than the loss of distance information (PHD vs. PDB, Table 4). Third, the accuracy in detecting remote homologues is about 20%. Does this imply that 1-D threading is a flop?

1-D threading is intrinsically more flexible than other threading techniques. The threading approach presented here differs from threading tools based on potentials of mean-force in that it is more coarse-grained. Although, a large scale comparison is not yet available, it appears to be very likely that mean-force based approaches, at least, the better ones (Braxenthaler, these Proceedings and [64]), are more accurate than 1-D threading. However, this still does not imply that 1-D threading is of academic interest, only. Fitting 1-D predictions into 3-D structures uses completely different information than mean-force based threading techniques. This raises the hope, that the two could be combined to more reliably filter out false positives from an alignment list.

Acknowledgements

First of all, thanks to Chris Sander(EMBL) for his intellectual, emotional, and financial support. Second, thanks to Reinhard Schneider(EMBL) for valuable ideas, important discussions, and for having tailored his alignment program *MaxHom* to the purpose of threading 1-D predictions into 3-D structures. Furthermore, thanks to Michael Braxenthaler(Washington) and Manfred Sippl(Salzburg) for fruitful discussions about threading details. Thanks also to Christos Ouzounis(EMBL); Henrik Bohr, Søren Brunak, Jacob Engelbrecht, and Jan Hansen(all four Copenhagen), and Tim Hubbard(Cambridge) for helpful discussions. Last not least, I should like to express my gratitude to all those who contributed by human or financial resources to organise a rather inspiring workshop embedded into an outstanding program for the discussions outside the halls of the Royal Danish Academy of sciences. To mention only three: thanks to Johanne Keiding, Henrik Bohr and Søren Brunak.

References

[1] C. J. Epstein, R. F. Goldberger and C. B. Anfinsen, The genetic control of tertiary protein structure: studies with model systems, *Cold Spring Harbour Symp. Quant. Biol.*, 28, 439-449, 1963.

[2] J. Martin and F. U. Hartl, Protein folding in the cell: molecular chaperones pave the way, *Structure*, 1, 161-164, 1993.

[3] T. J. P. Hubbard and C. Sander, The role of heat-shock and chaperone proteins in protein folding: possible molecular mechanisms, *Prot. Engin.*, 4, 711-717, 1991.

[4] F.-U. Hartl, R. Hlodan and T. Langer, Molecular chaperones in protein folding: the art of avoiding sticky situations, *TIBS*, 19, 20-25. 1994.

[5] S. Oliver, *et al.*, The complete DNA sequence of yeast chromosome III, *Nature*, 357, 38-46, 1992.

[6] M. Johnston, *et al.*, Complete Nucleotide Sequence of Saccaromyces cerevisiae Chromosome VIII, *Science*, 265, 2077-2082, 1994.

[7] P. Bork, C. Ouzounis and C. Sander, From genome sequences to protein function, *Curr. Opin. Str. Biol.*, 4, 393-403, 1994.

[8] J. Greer, Comparative Modeling of Homologous Proteins, *Meth. Enzymol.*, 202, 239-252, 1991.

[9] M. S. Johnson, J. P. Overington and T. L. Blundell, Alignment and Searching for Common Protein Folds Using a Data Bank of Structural Templates, *J. Mol. Biol.*, 231, 735-752, 1993.

[10] A. C. W. May and T. L. Blundell, Automated comparative modelling of protein structures, *Curr. Opin. Biotech.*, 5, 355-360, 1994.

[11] A. Sali and T. Blundell, Comparative Protein Modelling by Satisfaction of Spatial Restraints, in: H. Bohr and S. Brunak eds., *Protein Structure by Distance Analysis*, Amsterdam, Oxford, Washington: IOS Press, 64-87, 1994.

[12] G. Vriend and C. Sander, Detection of Common Three-Dimensional Substructures in Proteins, *Proteins*, 11, 52-58, 1991.

[13] C. Sander and R. Schneider, The HSSP database of protein structure-sequence alignments, *Nucl. Acids Res.*, 22, 3597-3599, 1994.

[14] A. Bairoch, The PROSITE Dictionary of Sites and Patterns in Proteins, its Current Status, *Nucl. Acids Res.*, 21, 3097-3103, 1993.

[15] L. Holm and C. Sander, The FSSP database of structurally aligned protein fold families, *Nucl. Acids Res.*, 22, 3600-3609, 1994.

[16] C. Sander and R. Schneider, Database of Homology-Derived Structures and the Structurally Meaning of Sequence Alignment, *Proteins*, 9, 56-68, 1991.

[17] R. Abagyan, D. Frishman and P. Argos, Recognition of distantly related proteins through energy calculations, *Proteins*, 19, 132-140, 1994.

[18] T. L. Blundell and M. S. Johnson, Catching a common fold, *Prot. Sci.*, 2, 877-883, 1993.

[19] J. U. Bowie, N. D. Clarke, C. O. Pabo and R. T. Sauer, Identification of Protein Folds: Matching Hydrophobicity Patterns of Sequence Sets With Solvent Accessibility Patterns of Known Structures, *Proteins*, 7, 257-264, 1990.

[20] G. M. Crippen and V. N. Maiorov, A Potential Function that Identifies Correct Protein Folds, in: H. Bohr and S. Brunak eds., *Protein Structure by Distance Analysis*, Amsterdam, Oxford, Washington: IOS Press, 158-174, 1994.

[21] K. Nishikawa and Y. Matsuo, Development of pseudoenergy potentials for assessing protein 3-D-1-D compatibility and detecting weak homologies, *Prot. Engin.*, 6, 811-820, 1993.

[22] C. Ouzounis, C. Sander, M. Scharf and R. Schneider, Prediction of protein structure by evaluation of sequence-structure fitness: Aligning sequences to contact profiles derived from 3-D structures, *J. Mol. Biol.*, 232, 805-825, 1993.

[23] M. J. Sippl and S. Weitckus, Detection of Native-Like Models for Amino Acid Sequences of Unknown Three-Dimensional Structure in a Data Base of Known Protein Conformations, *Proteins*, 13, 258-271, 1992.

[24] M. Wilmanns and D. Eisenberg, Three-dimensional profiles from residue-pair preferences: Identification of sequences with b/a-barrel fold, *Proc. Natl. Acad. Sc. U.S.A.*, 90, 1379-1383, 1993.

[25] D. Eisenberg, R. Lüthy and A. D. McLachland, Secondary structure-based profiles: Use of structure-conserving scoring tables in searching protein sequence databases for structural similarities, *Proteins*, 10, 229-239, 1991.

[26] J. U. Bowie, R. Lüthy and D. Eisenberg, A Method to Identify Protein Sequences That Fold into a Known Three-Dimensional Structure, *Science*, 253, 164-169, 1991.

[27] D. T. Jones, W. R. Taylor and J. M. Thornton, A New Approach to Protein Fold Recognition, *Nature*, 358, 86-89, 1992.

[28] T. Meitinger, A. Meindl, P. Bork, B. Rost, C. Sander, M. Haasemann and J. Murken, Molecular modelling of the Norrie disease protein predicts a cysteine knot growth factor tertiary structure, *Nature Gen.*, 5, 376-380, 1993.

[29] W. Kabsch and C. Sander, On the use of sequence homologies to predict protein structure: Identical pentapeptides can have completely different conformations, *Proc. Natl. Acad. Sc. U.S.A.*, 81, 1075-1078, 1984.

[30] A. G. Szent-Gysrgyi and C. Cohen, Role of Proline in Polypeptide Chain Configuration of Proteins, *Science*, 126, 697, 1957.

[31] J. C. Kendrew, R. E. Dickerson, B. E. Strandberg, R. J. Hart, D. R. Davies and D. C. Phillips, Structure of myoglobin: a three-dimensional Fourier synthesis at 2 Åresolution, *Nature*, 185, 422-427, 1960.

[32] M. F. Perutz, M. G. Rossmann, A. F. Cullis, G. Muirhead, G. Will and A. T. North, Structure of haemoglobin: a three-dimensional Fourier synthesis at 5.5 Åresolution, obtained by X-ray analysis, *Nature*, 185, 416-422, 1960.

[33] W. Kabsch and C. Sander, How good are predictions of protein secondary structure?, *FEBS Lett.*, 155, 179-182, 1983.

[34] J. Garnier and J. M. Levin, The protein structure code: what is its present status?, *CABIOS*, 7, 133-142, 1991.

[35] J. M. Levin and J. Garnier, Improvements in a secondary structure prediction method based on a search for local sequence homologies and its use as a model building tool, *Biochim. Biophys. Ac.*, 955, 283-295, 1988.

[36] V. Biou, J. F. Gibrat, J. M. Levin, B. Robson and J. Garnier, Secondary structure prediction: combination of three different methods, *Prot. Engin.*, 2, 185-91, 1988.

[37] O. Gascuel and J. L. Golmard, A simple method for predicting the secondary structure of globular proteins: implications and accuracy, *CABIOS*, 4, 357-365, 1988.

[38] N. Qian and T. J. Sejnowski, Predicting the Secondary Structure of Globular Proteins Using Neural Network Models, *J. Mol. Biol.*, 202, 865-884, 1988.

[39] H. Bohr, J. Bohr, S. Brunak, R. M. J. Cotterill, B. Lautrup, L. Nørskov, O. H. Olsen and S. B. Petersen, Protein secondary structure and homology by neural networks, *FEBS Lett.*, 241, 223-228, 1988.

[40] X. Zhang, J. P. Mesirov and D. L. Waltz, Hybrid System for Protein Secondary Structure Prediction, *J. Mol. Biol.*, 225, 1049-63, 1992.

[41] B. Rost, C. Sander and R. Schneider, Progress in protein structure prediction?, *TIBS*, 18, 120-123, 1993.

[42] B. Rost and C. Sander, Combining evolutionary information and neural networks to predict protein secondary structure, *Proteins*, 19, 55-72, 1994.

[43] B. Rost and C. Sander, 1-D secondary structure prediction through evolutionary profiles, in: H. Bohr and S. Brunak eds., *Protein Structure by Distance Analysis*, Amsterdam, Oxford, Washington: IOS Press, 257-276, 1994.

[44] R. M. Sweet, Evolutionary similarity among peptide segments is a basis for prediction of protein folding, *Biopolymers*, 25, 1565-1577, 1986.

[45] B. Rost and C. Sander, Improved prediction of protein secondary structure by use of sequence profiles and neural networks, *Proc. Natl. Acad. Sc. U.S.A.*, 90, 7558-7562, 1993.

[46] B. Rost, C. Sander and R. Schneider, Redefining the goals of protein secondary structure prediction, *J. Mol. Biol.*, 235, 13-26, 1994.

[47] R. B. Russell and G. J. Barton, The limits of protein secondary structure prediction accuracy from multiple sequence alignment, *J. Mol. Biol.*, 234, 951-957, 1993.

[48] B. Rost and C. Sander, Prediction of protein secondary structure at better than 70% accuracy, *J. Mol. Biol.*, 232, 584-599, 1993.

[49] B. K. Lee and F. M. Richards, The interpretation of protein structures: Estimation of static accessibility, *J. Mol. Biol.*, 55, 379-400, 1971.

[50] W. Kabsch and C. Sander, Dictionary of Protein secondary structure: Pattern recognition of hydrogen bonded and geometrical features, *Biopolymers*, 22, 2577-2637, 1983.

[51] C. Sander, M. Scharf and R. Schneider, Design of protein structures, in: A. R. Rees, M. J. E. Sternberg and R. Wetzel eds., *Protein Engineering*, Oxford: IRL Press, 89-115, 1992.

[52] G. D. Rose, A. R. Geselowitz, G. J. Lesser, R. H. Lee and M. H. Zehfus, Hydrophobicity of Amino Acid Residues in Globular Proteins, *Science*, 229, 834-838, 1985.

[53] B. Rost and C. Sander, Conservation and prediction of solvent accessibility in protein

families, *Proteins*, 20, 216-226 1994.

[54] T. J. P. Hubbard and T. L. Blundell, Comparison of solvent-inaccessible cores of homologous proteins: definitions useful for protein modelling, *Prot. Engin.*, 1, 159-171, 1987.

[55] J. Janin, Surface and inside volumes in globular proteins, *Nature*, 277, 491-492, 1979.

[56] S. Miller, J. Janin, A. M. Lesk and C. Chothia, Interior and Surface of Monomeric Proteins, *J. Mol. Biol.*, 196, 641-656, 1987.

[57] T. F. Smith and M. S. Waterman, Identification of common molecular subsequences, *J. Mol. Biol.*, 147, 195-197, 1981.

[58] S. F. Altschul, Amino Acid Substitution Matrices from an Information Theoretic Perspective, *J. Mol. Biol.*, 219, 555-565, 1991.

[59] A. D. McLachlan, Tests for comparing related amino acid sequences, *J. Mol. Biol.*, 61, 409-424, 1971.

[60] S. B. Needlman and C. D. Wunsch, A General Method Applicable to the Search for Similarities in the Amino Acid Sequence of Two Proteins, *J. Mol. Biol.*, 48, 443-53, 1970.

[61] U. Hobohm and C. Sander, Enlarged representative set of protein structures, *Prot. Sci.*, 3, 522-524, 1994.

[62] A. Bairoch and B. Boeckmann, The SWISS-PROT protein sequence data bank: current status, *Nucl. Acids Res.*, 22, 3578-3580, 1994.

[63] A. M. Lesk, *Protein Architecture — A Practical Approach*, Oxford, New York, Tokyo: Oxford University Press, 1991.

[64] M. J. Sippl and M. Jaritz, Predictive Power of Mean Force Pair Potentials, in: H. Bohr and S. Brunak eds., *Protein Structure by Distance Analysis*, Amsterdam, Oxford, Washington DC: IOS Press, 113-134, 1994.

[65] M. J. Sippl, Boltzmann's Principle, Knowledge Based Mean Fields and Protein Folding. An Approach to the Computational Determination of Protein Structures, *J. Comput. Aided Mol. Design*, 7, 473-501, 1993.

[66] M. J. Sippl, Recognition of Errors in Three-Dimensional Structures of Proteins, Proteins, 17, 355-362, 1993.

[67] L. Holm and C. Sander, Parser for Protein Folding Units, *Proteins*, 19, 256-268, 1994.

[68] B. Rost, R. Casadio, P. Fariselli and C. Sander, Prediction of helical transmembrane segments at 95% accuracy, *Prot. Sci.*, in press 1995.

[69] F. C. Bernstein, T. F. Koetzle, G. J. B. Williams, E. F. Meyer, M. D. Brice, J. R. Rodgers, O. Kennard, T. Shimanouchi and M. Tasumi, The Protein Data Bank: a computer based archival file for macromolecular structures, *J. Mol. Biol.*, 112, 535-542, 1977.

[70] J. M. Levin, B. Robson and J. Garnier, An algorithm for secondary structure determination in proteins based on sequence similarity, *FEBS Lett.*, 205, 303-308, 1986.

[71] J. M. Levin, S. Pascarella, P. Argos and J. Garnier, Quantification of Secondary Structure Prediction Improvement Using Multiple Alignments, *Prot. Engin.*, 6, 849-854, 1993.

[72] H. Wako and T. L. Blundell, Use of Amino Acid Environment-dependent Substitutioin Tables and Conformational Propensities in Structure Prediction from Aligned Sequences of Homologous Proteins I. Solvent Accessibility Classes, *J. Mol. Biol.*, 238, 682-692, 1994.

Determination of Membrane Bound Protein Structure and Function

Modelling α-helical Integral Membrane Proteins

Dan Donnelly and John B. C. Findlay

Department of Biochemistry and Molecular Biology, The University of Leeds, Leeds LS2 9JT, U.K.

Abstract

This chapter reviews an approach towards obtaining structural information from sequence alignments of transmembrane segments. The approach has facilitated the construction of models of the G protein-coupled receptors. Amino acid substitution tables have been calculated using two reaction centre structures for those residues where the sidechain is accessible to the lipid. The patterns of residue substitutions show that the lipid accessible residues have distinctly different substitution patterns from residues buried in the core of proteins and also from residues exposed to an aqueous environment. The observed substitution patterns obtained from sequence alignments of putative transmembrane regions can be compared with the patterns derived from the substitution tables in order to predict the accessibility of some residues to the lipid. A Fourier transform method, similar to that used for the calculation of a hydrophobic moment, is used to detect periodicity in the predicted accessibility. If this periodicity is compatible with that of an α-helix, then the putative transmembrane region is designated as helical and the buried and lipid-exposed faces can be discriminated. Once these faces have been identified, the presence of charged residues on the lipid exposed face can help to identify the regions that are in contact with the polar environment on the borders of the bilayer. This is also possible by comparing the direction of the internal/conserved face with the hydrophobic face. These faces should be equivalent for a helical region outside the bilayer but opposite for a membrane buried region. Taken together, this information provides valuable data for the construction of 3-D models and for the planning of new experiments.

1 Predicting membrane protein structure

Integral membrane proteins play a crucial role in cellular communication and transport. However, the scarcity of available structures means that homologous protein modelling is not generally useful for building 3-dimensional (3D) models and hence other more crude approaches have to be used (although this is not always the case e.g. [1]). This may seem to be unrealistic but since membranes are essentially 2-dimensional (2D), they provide a powerful constraint upon the arrangement of the elements that cross them. In many cases, these transmembrane segments are likely to be α-helices arranged approximately perpendicular to the plane of the membrane so that they pack together in a parallel or anti-parallel fashion. Therefore, the task of constructing a 3D model of the transmembrane region of an α-helical membrane protein can be viewed as a 2D problem for which four pieces of information are required.

- The regions of sequence that form the transmembrane helices.
- The side of each helix that faces the interior of the helical bundle.
- The relative depth that each helix is inserted into the membrane.
- The manner in which the individual transmembrane domains pack together.

The transmembrane regions can be identified from the amino acid sequence by hydrophobicity and hydropathy analysis, by proteolytic cleavage and by reporter enzyme or chemical probe methods (e.g. [2] for a review). This chapter describes an approach that attempts to address the second and third requirements. The prediction of the arrangement of the transmembrane domains is less straight-forward. However, since the helices are likely to pack in an approximately parallel or an anti-parallel manner, their possible arrangement is limited once the number and the relative directions of the helices are known (e.g. [3, 4]).

Comparisons between the reaction centre structures and those of water soluble proteins have shown the expected difference in surface polarity [5]. However, a feature common to both membrane and water soluble proteins is that the surface residues are less conserved than those in the interior [6, 7, 8]. In order to identify amphipathic helices from sequences and sequence alignments, Fourier transform methods have been used to identify the periodic differences of hydrophobic and hydrophilic residues [9, 10]. Likewise, the periodicity of conserved/variable residues can also be used to predict the presence of helices [6]. This provides a method that is not only independent of the hydrophobicity procedure but one that is likely to be more reliable in many cases since the difference between the polarity of buried and lipid-facing residues can be small [5].

The differences between the substitution patterns of surface and buried residues have been described for water-soluble proteins [11, 12] and also for membrane proteins [13]. These environment-specific substitution tables can be used to assign a value at each position in a sequence alignment that quantifies the extent to which that particular position is buried in the protein core. The periodicity in these values can be used to predict the presence of α-helices and the buried face of each helix can be identified. Once this information is available, it can then be used to predict the point at which the helix makes contact with the aqueous environment at the boundaries of the bilayer.

2   Computational Methods

2.1   Construction of Substitution Tables

The two L and two M subunits from the reaction centres from *Rhodopseudomonas viridis* [14] and *Rhodobacter sphaeroides* [5] were aligned using the alignment program COMPARER [15] which takes into account features of the 3D structures of the proteins being compared. The structurally aligned proteins showed between 28-58% pairwise sequence identity. The regions of the transmembrane helices that are within the lipid portion of the bilayer [5] were aligned with the equivalent sequences of five bacterial and cyanobacterial reaction centre sequences, and also with 28 sequences from the D1 and D2 subunits from photosystem II in green plants and algi (sequences extracted from the OWL database [16]). Identical sequences within each of the five alignments were removed. The single lipid spanning regions of the H subunits from the two structures were aligned to give a sixth alignment.

The percentage sidechain accessibility (a, [17]) was calculated for all of the residues in both structures from the intact L, M and H complex, including the cofactors. Those residues

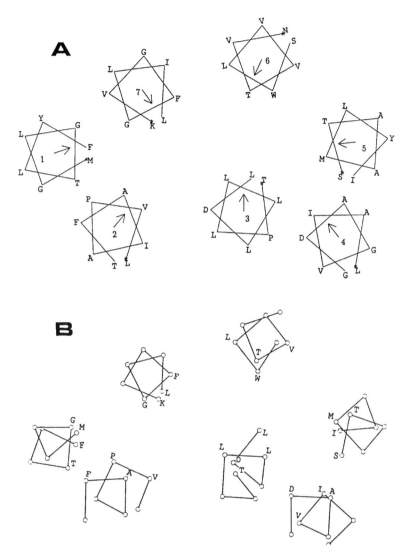

Figure 1: A The predicted orientation of the seven helices of bacteriorhodopsin individually arranged in an anti-parallel fashion. The predicted internal face of each helix is orientated towards the interior of the bundle. The internal faces are compatible with those in the structure shown in B. Only 8 residues in each helix are shown for clarity. (This figure originally appeared in Donnelly *et al.*, 1993).

within the lipid region of the bilayer with a greater than 7% [18] were considered as lipid accessible. The sequence of each one of the four subunit structures was compared, in a pair-wise fashion, with each other structure and sequence in the alignment. The residue substitutions observed for the lipid accessible residues were scored in a 20 x 20 matrix F^l composed of elements f^l_{ik} that represent the frequency of substitutions of the lipid accessible residue type k to residue type i. 3853 residue substitutions were observed.

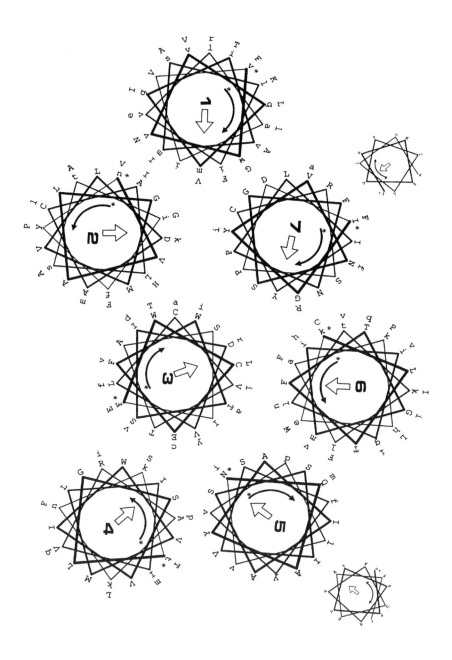

Figure 2: The predicted helical wheels calculated from an alignment of 59 aminergic G protein-coupled receptors (sequence shown is that of the human β2-adrenergic receptor). The helical wheels are arranged according to Schertler *et al.* (1993) and Baldwin (1993). The cytoplasmic protrusion of helix 5 and the extracellular protrusion of helix 7 are shown by the smaller wheels. The residues in the regions connecting the transmembrane helices to the protruding helices are not in a helical conformation. The view is from the extracellular side of the bilayer and the large arrows indicate the internal face of the helices. (This figure originally appeared in Donnelly *et al.*, 1994a)

This frequency matrix was converted to a probability matrix by dividing the frequency of each substitution by the total number of substitutions observed for that particular residue type. The resultant probability matrix P^l is composed of elements p^l_{ik} representing the probability of the substitution of residue type k to i.

The difference between the substitution patterns of lipid accessible residues and those residues buried in the cores of water soluble proteins (P^b, from [12] can be readily observed by calculating the difference matrix D^{bl})

$$d^{bl}_{ik} = p^b_{ik} - p^l_{ik}. \tag{1}$$

A difference probability greater than 0 indicates that the substitution (from a residue k to residue i) is more likely if residue type k is buried, whereas a value less than 0 indicates that the substitution is more likely at a position exposed to lipid.

The substitution tables show distinct patterns depending on the environment. For example, buried isoleucine residues are usually conserved, but when they are substituted, it is usually by valine or leucine. Solvent accessible isoleucine residues are less conserved and although valine and leucine are still the most probable substitutions, there is a general increase in the probability of substitutions to nearly all the other amino acid types. In the case of lipid accessible isoleucine residues, there is still a reduction in the conservation but there is not a general increase in substitutions to other amino acids. Rather an increase only in substitutions by uncharged residues. This reduction in the conservation and the absence of substitutions by charged residues is typical of the substitution patterns for lipid facing residues.

2.2 Application of the Fourier Transform Method

We use the substitution tables to predict whether a position in a sequence alignment is buried or exposed. Using the difference matrix D^{bl} described above, the difference probability profile S (composed of elements S_j) is calculated. S_j is the average value of the difference probabilities for all pairwise substitutions at each position j in the alignment. Therefore, for an alignment of y sequences, there are $y(y-1)$ pairwise substitutions possible. However, sequences that are identical over the window being used are included only once.

For a window of length N over the sequence alignment, the periodicity in the values of S_j can be calculated using the Fourier transform procedures described in [13]. A property profile U is calculated so that a property U_j is assigned at each position j in a sequence or sequence alignment over a window size N. The moment M can be calculated as

$$M = \left\{ [\sum_{j=1}^{N} U_j \sin(j\omega)]^2 + [\sum_{j=1}^{N} U_j \cos(j\omega)]^2 \right\}^{1/2} \tag{2}$$

where ω is the angle between adjacent side chains when the sequence is considered as a regular structure and viewed down an axis defined by the Cα atoms. If the values of U_j represent the hydrophobicities (H_j) of the residues then M is the hydrophobic moment (μ, [9]).

When calculating the periodicity in the values of U_j, the Fourier transform power spectrum is calculated by

$$P(\omega) = [x]^2 + [y]^2 \tag{3}$$

where

$$x = \sum_{j=1}^{N} U^n_j \sin(j\omega) \tag{4}$$

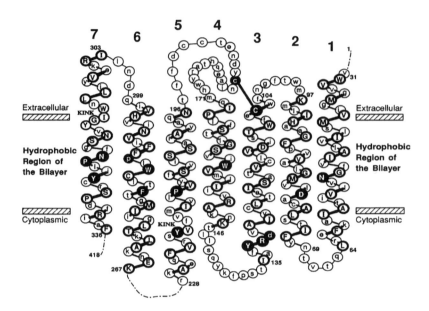

Figure 3: The GPCR model based on the Fourier transform analysis (the sequence shown is that of the human β2-AR). The figure is constructed as if the helical bundle was cut between helices 1 and 7 and opened up. Therefore, the residues on the inside of the bundle are projected out of the plane of the page and are in uppercase. Residues on the outside face of the helices or in the loop regions are shown in lowercase. Residues which are highly conserved across the GPCR superfamily are shown in black. (This figure originally appeared in Donnelly *et al.*, 1994a).

$$y = \sum_{j=1}^{N} U_j^n \cos(j\omega) \tag{5}$$

and where

$$U_j^n = U_j - \bar{U} \quad (j = 1,2,...N) \tag{6}$$

$\bar{U}$ is the average value of U_j over the window. U^n is therefore a normalised version of the profile U adjusted so that $\sum_{j=1}^{N} U_j^n = 0$ and hence $\bar{U}^n = 0$. The new profile U^n consists of elements U_j^n in which the periodicity in internal/external residues is predicted by the periodicity in positive/negative values (or negative/positive values) of U_j^n. This results in cleaner power spectra (since $P(\omega) = 0$ when $\omega = 0$) so that the alpha periodicity index AP can be calculated as

$$\text{AP} = [(1/30) \int_{90°}^{120°} P(\omega)d\omega]/[(1/180) \int_{0°}^{180°} P(\omega)d\omega] \tag{7}$$

AP is analogous to ψ used in [6] and to the amphipathic index AI used in [10] (although the precise boundaries of the helical regions of the power spectrum differ in the latter). AP is a ratio of the extent of the periodicity in the helical region of the spectrum compared with that over the whole spectrum. Komiya *et al.* [6] suggest that a value of AP greater than 2 indicates that the helical periodicity is significant. This suggests the presence of a helix within

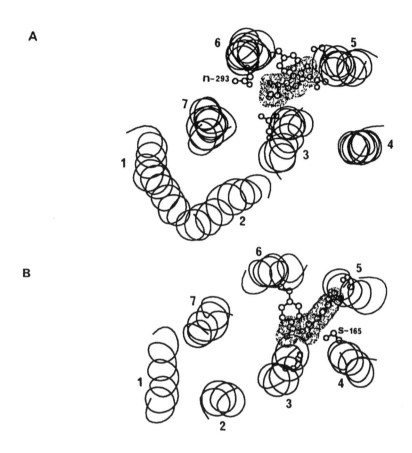

Figure 4: Two models of the human β2-adrenergic receptor, each with a docked ligand (dot surface). (A) is the model of Donnelly *et al.* (1994), while (B) shows the model described in Findlay and Donnelly (1993). The latest model suggests that Asn-293 (helix 6) interacts with the β-hydroxyl group of adrenaline rather than Ser-165 (helix 4). Other ligand binding residues are shown with a ball and stick representation (Asp-113, helix 3; Ser-204 and Ser-207, helix 5; Phe-290, helix 6).

the window of sequence used, but it is difficult to predict the precise start and finish of the helix. More recently, we have used a slightly altered definition of AP for the prediction of transmembrane α-helices [19].

$$AP^n = [(1/11) \int_{95°}^{106°} P(\omega)d\omega]/[(1/180) \int_{0°}^{180°} P(\omega)d\omega] \qquad (8)$$

This definition results in a greater value of AP for power spectra with sharper, more narrow peaks above 100°. Narrow maxima are more typical of longer regions of periodic sequence which should be the case for transmembrane helices.

The direction of the internal face of a predicted helix can be estimated from the direction of the moment $\sqrt{P(\omega)}$ when $\omega = 100°$. This is the moment produced by the profile U^n when the sequences form an ideal alpha helix. θ is the angle describing the direction of the moment relative to the first residue ($j = 1$). θ can be calculated by

$$\gamma = \arccos[y/\sqrt{P(\omega)}] \tag{9}$$

where γ is greater than $0°$ and less than $180°$.

$$\theta = \begin{cases} \gamma & \text{if } x > 0 \\ 360 - \gamma & \text{if } x < 0 \end{cases} \tag{10}$$

The point at which the lipid-accessible face contacts the more polar environment of the phosphate head groups and surrounding aqueous environment can be estimated by the point at which charged residues appear on this side of the helix. Charged residues should not be present on the lipid facing side of a transmembrane helix.

The analogous calculations can be carried out to calculate the direction of the hydrophobic and conserved face of the helix so that the results of the three approaches can be compared. This allows us to predict whether the helix is in an aqueous or lipid environment since the conserved and hydrophobic faces should be equivalent for the former but opposite for the latter. This can be useful for predicting the point at which a transmembrane helix protrudes from the lipid region of the bilayer into the more polar regions at the bilayer boundaries since the direction of the hydrophobic face should change by approximately $180°$ relative to the direction of the conserved/internal face [19, 20].

2.3   Testing the Methodology

The Fourier transform analysis of the amino acid substitution patterns observed in sequence alignments may provide a means of predicting and orientating α-helices. In order to test this, the method was applied to a sequence alignment of three members of the bacteriorhodopsin family [13].

Figure 1 shows a comparison of the prediction with the determined structure of bacteriorhodopsin [21]. The estimated orientation of each of the helices correlates well with the structure and suggests that the method can be used for prediction. The method has also been applied to the prediction of α-helices in water-soluble proteins [22].

3   Modelling G Protein-Coupled Receptors

G Protein-coupled receptors (GPCRs) are a large and extremely diverse super-family of integral membrane proteins. The prediction methods described above have been applied to a sequence alignment of 59 GPCRs that bind amine ligands [19]. A region of helical periodicity can be detected in each of the putative transmembrane segments and the orientation of each helix relative to the core of the bundle can be determined (Fig. 2).

The point at which the fifth transmembrane helix protrudes into the cytoplasm and the point at which the seventh transmembrane helix protrudes on the extracellular side of the bilayer are detected by the relative direction of the hydrophobic and buried faces as described above. There appears to be a small non-helical region dividing the main transmembrane helices from the shorter protruding helical regions. For helix 7, the non-helical region includes residues Asn-312 and Trp-313 (residues and numbers correspond to the human β2-adrenergic receptor: hβ2-AR). One consequence of this prediction is that the position equivalent to the retinal binding lysine residue in rhodopsin (Lys-296; equivalent to Tyr-316 in hβ2-AR) is very close to the extracellular side of the bilayer (Fig. 3).

This is in contrast to the retinal binding lysine in bacteriorhodopsin (Lys-216) which is buried in the centre of the bilayer.

Detailed 3D models of various GPCRs have been constructed using these data [19, 23]. These models are *not* based upon the arrangement of helices found in bacteriorhodopsin but rather upon the arrangement observed in the projection map of bovine rhodopsin [24] using the connectivity suggested by Baldwin [4]. The close proximity of helices 3 and 7 in bovine rhodopsin (relative to that observed in bacteriorhodopsin) results in the ligand-binding site for adrenaline in the hβ2-AR lying between helices 3, 5, 6 and 7. In bacteriorhodopsin-based models, the binding site tends to involve only helices 3, 4, 5 and 6 (Figure 4). Although both types of model allow the ligand to interact with Asp-113, Ser-204, Ser-207 and Phe-290, the interactions with helices 4 and 7 differ. Moreover, the more recent model suggests Asn-293 as the principle interaction site for the β-hydroxyl group of adrenaline rather than Ser-165 (see Fig. 4).

4 Summary

The number of known amino acid sequences of integral membrane proteins is increasing rapidly. However, very few of these proteins either occur or can be expressed in sufficiently large quantities for structural studies. The methods described here attempt to derive structural information from the available protein sequences. The methods do not attempt to replace the need for experimentally determined structures but rather they provide a means of conceiving experiments that explore the ways in which particular proteins may function.

Acknowledgements

The authors are grateful to Prof. T. L. Blundell and Dr. J. P. Overington for their valuable contributions to the work described in this chapter.

References

[1] S. V. Ruffle, D. Donnelly, T. L. Blundell and J. H. A. Nugent, A three-dimensional model of the photosystem II reaction centre of *Pisum asvtivum*, *Photosynthesis Research*, 34, p. 287-300, 1992.

[2] M. J. Jennings, Topography of membrane proteins, *Ann. Rev. Biochem.*, 58, p. 999-1027, 1989.

[3] D. M. Engelman, R. Henderson, A. D. McLachlan and B. A. Wallace, Path of the polypeptide chain in bacteriorhodopsin, *Proc. Nat. Acad. Sci. USA*, 77, p. 2023-2027, 1980.

[4] J. M. Baldwin, The probable arrangement of the helices in G protein-coupled receptors, *EMBO J.*, 12, p. 1693-1703, 1993.

[5] D. C. Rees, H. Komiya, T. O. Yeates, J. P. Allen and G. Feher, The bacterial photosynthetic reaction center as a model for membrane-proteins, *Ann. Rev. Biochem.*, 58, p. 607-633, 1989a.

[6] H. Komiya, T. O. Yeates, D. C. Rees, J. P. Allen and G. Feher, Structure of the reaction center from Rhodobacter sphaeroides R-26: Symmetry relations and sequence

comparisons between different species, *Proc. Natl. Acad. Sci., USA*, 85, p. 9012-9016, 1988.

[7] E. L. Smith, The evolution of proteins, *Harvey Lect.*, 62, p. 231-256, 1968.

[8] C. Chothia and A. M. Lesk, The relationship between the divergence of sequence and structure in proteins, *EMBO J.*, 5, p. 823-826, 1986.

[9] D. Eisenberg, R. M. Weiss and T. C. Terwilliger, The hydrophobic moment detects periodicity in protein hydrophobicity, *Proc. Natl. Acad. Sci., USA*, 81, p. 140-144, 1984.

[10] J. L. Cornette, K. B. Cease, H. Margalit, J. L. Spouge, J. A. Berzofsky and C. DeLisi, Hydrophobicity scales and computational techniques for detecting amphipathic structures in proteins, *J. Mol. Biol.*, 195, p. 659-685, 1987.

[11] J. P. Overington, M. S. Johnson, A. Šali and T. L. Blundell, Tertiary structural constraints on evolutionary diversity: templates, key residues and structure prediction, *Proc. R. Soc. Lond.*, B 241, p. 132-145, 1990.

[12] J. Overington, D. Donnelly, M. J. Johnson, A. Šali and T. L. Blundell, Environment–specific amino acid substitution tables: Tertiary templates and prediction of protein folds, *Protein Sci.* 1, p. 216-226, 1992.

[13] D. Donnelly, J. P. Overington, S. V. Ruffle, J. H. A. Nugent and T. L. Blundell, Modeling α-helical transmembrane domains: the calculation and use of substitution tables for lipid-facing residues, *Protein Sci.*, 2, p. 55-70, 1993.

[14] J. Deisenhofer, O. Epp, K. Miki, R. Huber and H. Michel, Structure of the protein subunits in the photosynthetic reaction centre of Rhodopseudomonas viridis at 3Å resolution, *J. Mol. Biol.*, 180, p. 385-398, 1984.

[15] A. Šali and T. L. Blundell, Definition of general topological equivalence in protein structures: a procedure involving comparison of properties and relationships through simulated annealing and dynamic programming, *J. Mol. Biol.*, 212, p. 403-428, 1990.

[16] A. J. Bleasby and J. C. Wootton, Construction of validated, nonredundant composite protein sequence databases, *Prot. Engng.*, 3, p. 153-159, 1990.

[17] B. Lee and F. M. Richards, The interpretation of protein structures: Estimation of static accessibility, *J. Mol. Biol.*, 55, p. 379-400, 1971.

[18] T. J. P. Hubbard and T. L. Blundell, Comparison of solvent-inaccessible cores of homologous proteins — definitions useful for protein modelling, *Prot. Engng.*, 1, p. 159-171, 1987.

[19] D. Donnelly, J. B. C. Findlay and T. L. Blundell, The evolution and structure of aminergic G protein-coupled receptors, *Receptors and Channels*, 2, p. 61-78, 1994.

[20] D. Donnelly and R. J. Cogdell, Predicting the point at which transmembrane helices protrude from the bilayer: a model of the antenna complexes from photosynthetic bacteria, *Prot. Engng.*, 6, p. 629-635, 1993.

[21] R. Henderson, J. M. Baldwin, T. A. Ceska, F. Zemlin, E. Beckmann, and K. H. Downing, Model for the structure of bacteriorhodopsin based on high-resolution electron cryomicroscopy, *J. Mol. Biol.*, 213, p. 899-929, 1990.

[22] D. Donnelly, J. P. Overington and T. L. Blundell, The prediction and orientation of α-helices from sequence alignments: the combined use of environment-dependent substitution tables, Fourier transform methods and helix capping rules, *Prot. Engng.*, 7, p. 645-653, 1994.

[23] N. Bhogal, D. Donnelly and J. B. C. Findlay, The ligand binding site of the neurokinin 2 receptor, *J. Biol. Chem.*, 269, p. 27269-27274, 1994.

[24] G. F. X. Schertler, C. Villa and R. Henderson, Projection structure of rhodopsin, *Nature*, 362, p. 770-772, 1993.

Use of Small Organic Compounds and Metal-ions as structural and functional probes in 7TM receptors

Thue W. Schwartz, Christian E. Elling, Søren Møller Nielsen, Kenneth Thirstrup, Sannah Zoffmann, Mette Rosenkilde, Danielle Marchal, Roos den Hollander, Ulrik Gether and Siv A. Hjorth

Laboratory for Molecular Pharmacology 6321, University Department for Clinical Pharmacology, Rigshospitalet, Blegdamsvej 9, DK-2100 Copenhagen, Denmark

1   Background

Structures of both intracellular and extracellular proteins are today characterized in great number by x-ray crystallography and NMR. However it has as yet only been possible to solve the structure of very few membrane proteins to a resolution where amino acid sidechains and small ligands could be identified. Most chemical messengers, both polar and lipid ones, act through membrane receptors, which convey the signal to the inside of the cell. Thus, knowledge concerning the structure and function of these important membrane proteins is greatly needed.

1.1   7TM G-protein coupled receptors

7TM G-protein Coupled Receptors — GTP-binding proteins, G-proteins, act as transducers between a large superfamily of membrane receptors and a relatively small number of intracellular effector systems [1, 2, 3, 4]. In fact the number of G-protein coupled receptors are counted in hundreds just in a given mammalian organism. In vertebrates there are three main families of G-protein coupled receptors for which the only common structural feature is a group of seven hydrophobic segments that are believed to represent transmembrane helices. G-protein coupled receptors thus are seven helical bundle proteins embedded in the cell membrane (Fig. 1) [5, 6]. The family of rhodopsin-like receptors is the quantitatively dominating group of receptors through which a true multitude of chemical messengers of great chemical variance act: from calcium ions, over amino acids, monoamines, lipid messengers, and purines to peptide hormones, neuropeptides, glycoprotein hormones, and some proteases. Within the rhodopsin-like family of receptors, a pattern of loops — well-conserved in absolute length but not in amino acid sequence — appear to define a two-domain structure, in which transmembrane segments I (TM-I) through TM-V and connecting loops constitute an A-domain, and TM-VI and -VII constitute a B-domain. An important, highly conserved disulfide bridge from the top of TM-III forms two extra loops between this central "column" of the receptor and the top of TM-IV and -V. This disulfide bridge appear to be important for stabilizing mainly the structure of the A-domain. Three conserved proline residues placed in the middle portion of

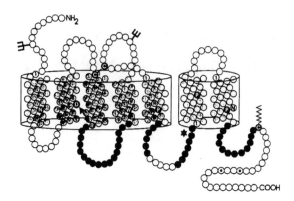

Figure 1: Serpentine model of a prototype G-protein coupled receptor of the rhodopsin-like type. The key residues conserved found in the transmembrane segments among members of this family are indicated in white on black. Residues in the dark grey shaded area are involved in G-protein binding.

TM-V, TM-VI, and TM-VII may be of importance in the dynamic function of these receptors as "weak points" in the transmembrane helices involved in the conformational interchange which are believed to be part of the intra-molecular signal transduction process.

1.2   Non-peptide ligands for peptide 7TM receptors

Around 45 to 50 peptide messengers, neuropeptides and peptide hormones act through 7TM receptors. In recent years a series of non-peptide compounds have furthermore been developed for many of these peptide receptors as drug candidates [7]. Most of these compounds act as receptor blockers, *antagonists*. However, the first non-peptide *antagonists* are currently being discovered in several receptor systems [8]. Chemically these non-peptide ligands are significantly different from the peptides. In general the non-peptide ligands are composed of three to four heterocyclic, often aromatic ring systems linked through conformationally constrained bonds. Despite the lack of chemical similarity the non-peptide compounds function as high-affinity competitive ligands on the peptide receptors. In figure 2 are shown examples of a few non-peptide ligands for the tachykinin NK-1 (substance P) receptor of which the quinuclidine compound, CP96,345, is the prototype antagonist.

2   Localization of binding sites by receptor mutagenesis

Ligand binding sites have been characterized in many 7TM receptor systems mainly through receptor mutagenesis. Initially most of our knowledge was derived from studies on a series of very similar monoamine receptors, especially the adrenergic receptors [1, 2, 3]. However, in recent year this initial, rather uniform picture has been supplemented extensively by data from studies of, for example, peptide and protease receptors [9]. These studies have demonstrated that ligands may activate 7TM receptors in many different ways. The classical picture of, for example noradrenalin binding, would be that the amine group interact with an aspartate

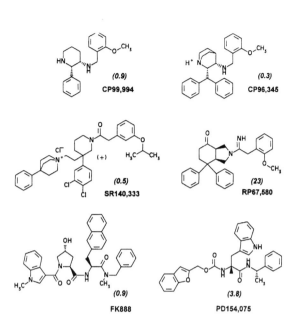

Figure 2: A selection of non-peptide antagonists for the tachykinin NK-1 (substance P) receptor. The affinity of the various compounds for the human NK-1 receptor is indicated in brackets. The quinuclidine compound, CP96,345, is the prototype NK-1 antagonists for which the binding site has been characterized in greatest detail.

residue in TM-III (AspIII:08), the two hydroxyl groups on the catechol-ring form hydrogen-bonds with two serines in TM-V (SerV:09 and Ser V:12), and the catecholring itself makes an aromatic-aromatic interaction with a phenylalanine in TM-VI (PheVI:17) [3, 10]. This binding pocket is located relatively deep between TM-III, IV, -V, and -VI. It was initially envisioned that all other agonists would interact with residues located at similar positions in their respective target receptors[11]. However, studies mainly on peptide receptors have now demonstrated that this may not be the case [9].

2.1 Peptide agonists bind to residues scattered in the exterior segments

In almost all systematic studies of binding sites for peptides larger than 3-4 residues, the main interaction point have been found in the more exterior part of the receptors [12, 13, 14, 15, 16, 17, 18, 19, 20, 21, 22, 23, 24, 25, 26]. Frequently, a series of crucial residues for a given peptide agonist are located in the N-terminal segment and/or in extracellular loop-3. In some cases, additional interaction points have been found in the upper part of the transmembrane segments, for example often in TM-III, -V, and -VI, and in the other loops. In the folded structure of the receptor these presumed contact points could be envisioned to cluster in a central and rather wide "pocket" around the outer "opening" of the seven-helical bundle of the receptor.

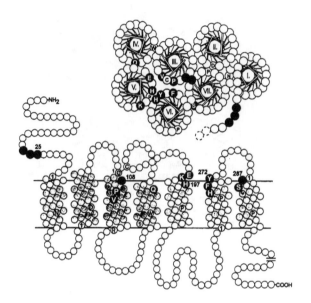

Figure 3: Complementary binding site for the agonist substance P and the antagonists CP96,345 on the tachykinin NK-1 receptor. Mutational hits which exclusively affect the binding of the agonist substance P are indicated in black on grey symbols. Mutational hits which exclusively affect the binding of the non-peptide antagonist CP96,345 are indicated in white on black symbols. Both a helical wheel and a serpentine model are shown.

2.2 Non-peptide antagonists bind between the transmembrane segments

In contrast to the contact points for the peptide ligands, the mutational "hits" for non-peptide antagonists have been found more deeply in the seven-helical bundle of the receptor structure, i.e. between the transmembrane segments [27, 28, 29, 30, 31, 32, 33, 34, 35, 36, 37]. In several cases, the mutations which seriously impair the binding of the non-peptide antagonists do not affect the binding of the peptide ligands, just as the mutations which eliminate the binding of the peptide do not affect the binding of the non-peptide antagonists. This picture is, however, not all that clear in every peptide receptor system. Thus, some non-peptide antagonists may bind in a rather similar fashion as their corresponding peptide agonist. However, in the tachykinin NK-1 receptor system a very clear picture of an entirely complementary binding mode for two competitive ligands is observed. Here, the mutational hits for the prototype antagonist, CP96,345, cluster on opposing faces of TM-III, -V, and -VI, whereas the presumed interaction points for the peptide agonists are found in the N- terminal segment and at the top of TM-III (higher up) and TM-VII, as shown in figure 3. In fact, as yet, no major, common interaction point for these competitive ligands has been identified.

2.3 Agonists and antagonists stabilize respectively "active" and "inactive" conformations of the receptor

Since some ligands in 7TM receptors could function as *competitive* ligands and still bind to different sites (*allo-sterically*) it has been suggested that they act as "allosteric competitive

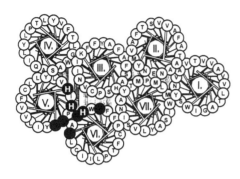
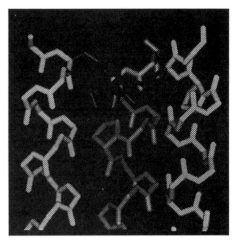

Figure 4: A high affinity zinc-binding site introduced into the tachykinin NK-1 receptor by systematically substituting residues in the presumed binding site for the non-peptide antagonist CP96,345 with His residues. Residues which were probed individually or in combinations with His substitutions are shown in black. The three His residues which are believed to coordinate the zinc-ion are indicated both on the helical wheel model and on the molecular model to the right. The two blue His residues to the left are located at the top of TM-V and the single His residue to the right are located at the top of TM-VI. In the back TM-III is seen.

ligands". That is, they associate with residues that are presented by the dynamic membrane protein in two different conformations, and bind in a mutually exclusive fashion as they prevent the interchange between these conformations [38]. In the monoamine systems, it has become more and more clear over the last couple of years that most antagonists — whether or not they are classical competitive ligands — act as so-called *inverse agonists*. The antagonists inhibits not only the agonist stimulated function of the receptors, but even the constitutive function, i.e. the activity of these receptors observed in the total absence of agonist [39]. Thus, antagonists have a property of their own right, and are not just compounds that prevent the binding and function of agonists. Thus, monoamine antagonists act in an agonist independent manner; which fits well with the observations in the peptide receptors, where antagonists can bind in an agonist independent fashion. In fact, agonists and antagonists simply act by stabilizing respectively active or inactive conformations of the receptor.

3 Binding sites can be moved between 7TM receptors by genetic transfer

Among homologous receptors the binding sites or rather essential parts of the binding sites for non-peptide antagonists have been moved from one to the other. Thus, for example, the genetic transfer from the NK-1 to the previously unresponsive NK-3 receptor of two relatively small segments around the top of TM-V and -VI increased the affinity for CP96,345 from being around mmol/l (on the NK-3) to only one order of magnitude from the nanomolar affinity it has on the wild-type NK-1 receptor [27]. An even more striking result is found in the transfer of the high affinity binding of the non-peptide antagonist SR48,968 (30) from the NK-2 receptor to the previously unresponsive NK-1 receptor by exchanging only three non-conserved residues around the top of TM-VI and -VII (unpublished results).

4 Binding sites for non-peptide antagonist can be structurally and functionally exchanged with metal-ion sites

The close spatial proximity of the mutational "hits" for the non-peptide antagonist CP96,345 on opposing faces of especially TM-V and -VI tempted us to try to exchange the binding site for this 6 x 9 x 12 Å compound with a binding site for the much smaller (1.4 Å) zinc-ion — hoping that the possible flexibility of the transmembrane segments would allow the formation of the metal-ion site. Much knowledge is available concerning metal-ion sites both in natural proteins and in *de novo* designed proteins [40, 41, 42, 43, 44, 45]. Systematic substitutions of the presumed contact points for CP96,345 with His residues gradually decreased the binding affinity for this compound, while an 800-fold increase in the binding affinity of zinc-ions step-wise was introduced into the receptor [46].   More than sub-micromolar affinity was found in a mutant receptor in which two His residues (one of which was found in the wild-type receptor) located around the top of TM-V and one introduced at the top of TM-VI are presumed to coordinate a single zinc-ion, possibly with a water molecule as the fourth ligand in a tetrahedral coordination-system. The introduction of the two new His residues had no effect on the high affinity binding and function of the agonist, substance P. Importantly, however, when the mutant receptor was treated with zinc-ions the binding of the agonist peptide was inhibited. And, the zinc-ions also functioned as blockers of the stimulatory effect of the natural agonist, substance P. Thus, the metal-ions substituted both structurally and functionally for the non-peptide antagonists [46]. This obviously have significance in respect of trying to understand the molecular pharmacological properties of agonist and antagonists in these 7TM receptors (as discussed above). However, the mere fact that artificial metal-ion sites can be introduced into 7TM receptors open up for an entirely new type of structural analysis of these membrane proteins.

5 Metal-ion sites may be used to study helix-helix and other interactions in membrane proteins

The well known distance and geometry constraints in the coordination of imidazole side chains by zinc-ions, imposes some important constraints on the possible distances between the three His residues in the receptor structure. Thus, a distance constraint or triangular "NOE" has in this way been introduced into the molecular models of the NK-1 receptor. Importantly, the high affinity zinc-site can also be transferred to, for example the opiate kappa-receptor, by introducing His residues at the corresponding three positions of that receptor. Apparently many if not all rhodopsin-like receptors have or can have a similar arrangement of at least TM-V and VI. Metal-ion sites may be used in general in studies of the relative interaction of transmembrane segments and, in fact, possibly also loops. Obviously, this is just one of the first small steps towards obtaining experimental data to elucidate helix-helix interaction in 7TM receptors. Many such metal-ion sites and, for example artificially introduced disulfide bridges, will have to be built before we have probed the overall structure of 7TM receptors well enough to build models of a reasonable resolution. Our current knowledge about 7TM receptor structure is in fact surprisingly limited — we do not even know for sure whether the seven helical bundle is arranged in a clock-wise or an counter-clock-wise fashion. In addition, introduction of metal-ion sites also opens for other kinds of biophysical studies of the receptor structures.

References

[1] H. G. Dohlman, J. Thorner, M. G. Caron and R. J. Lefkowitz, Model systems for the study of seven-transmembrane segment receptors, *Ann. Rev. Biochem.*, 60, p. 653-688, 1991.

[2] B. Kobilka, Adrenergic receptors as models for G protein-coupled receptors, *Ann. Rev. Neurosci.*, 15, p. 87-114, 1992.

[3] C. D. Strader, I. S. Sigal, R. A. F. Dixon, Structural basis of β-adrenergic receptor function, *FASEB J.* 3, p. 1825-1832, 1989.

[4] P. A. Hargrave, Seven-helix receptors, *Curr. Op. Struct. Biol.*, 1, p. 575-581, 1991.

[5] R. Henderson, J. M. Baldwin, T. A. Ceska, F. Zemlin, E. Bekckmann and K. H. Downing, Model for the structure of bacteriorhodopsin based on high-resolution electron crymicroscopy, *J. Mol. Biol.*, 213, p. 899-929, 1990.

[6] G. F. Schertler, C. Villa and R. Henderson, Projection structure of rhodopsin, *Nature*, 362, p. 770-772, 1993.

[7] R. M. Freidinger, Towards peptide receptor ligand drugs: Progress on nonpeptides, *Progr. Drug. Res.*, 40, p. 33-98, 1993.

[8] S. Perlman, H. T. Schambye, R. A. Rivero, W. Greenlee and T. W. Schwartz, Non-peptide Angiotensin Agonist — Functional and Molecular Interaction with the AT1 Receptor, *J. Biol. Chem.*, 270, p. 1493-1496, 1995.

[9] T. W. Schwartz, Locating Ligand Binding Sites in 7TM Receptors by Protein Engineering, *Curr. Opin. Biotech.*, 5, p. 434-444, 1994.

[10] C. D. Strader, T. Gaffney, E. E. Sugg, M. R. Candelore, R. Keys, A. A. Patchett and R. A. F. Dixon, Allele-specific activation of genetically engineered receptors, *J. Biol. Chem.*, 266, p. 5-8, 1991.

[11] S. Trumpp-Kallmeyer, J. Hoflack, A. Bruinvels and M. Hibert, Modeling of G-Protein-Coupled Receptors, p. Application to Dopamine, Adrenaline, Serotonin, Acetylcholine, and Mammalian Opsin Receptors, *J. Med. Chem.*, 35, p. 3448-3462, 1992.

[12] T. M. Fong, H. Yu, R. C. Huang and C. D. Stader, The extracellular domain of the neurokinin-1 receptor is required for high-affinity binding of peptides, *Biochemistry*, 31, p. 11806-11811, 1992.

[13] C. Mauzy, L. Wu, A. Egloff, T. Mirzadegan and F. Chung, Substitution of Lysine-181 to aspartic acid in the third transmembrane region of the endothelin (ET) Type B receptor selectively reduces its high-affinity binding with ET-3 peptide, *J. Cardiovasc. Pharmacol.*, 20, p. S5-S7, 1992.

[14] T. M. Fong, R. C. Huang and C. D. Stader, Localization of agonist and antagonist binding domains of the human neurokinin-1 receptor, *J. Biol. Chem.*, 267, p. 25664-25667, 1992.

[15] S. Zoffmann, U. Gether and T. W. Schwartz, Conserved His VI-17 of the NK-1 receptor is involved in binding of non-peptide antagonists but not substance P, *FEBS Lett.*, 336, p. 506-510, 1993.

[16] U. Gether, T. E. Johansen and T. W. Schwartz, Chimeric NK1 (Substance P) NK3 (Neurokinin B) Receptors, *J. Biol. Chem.*, 268, p. 7893-7898, 1993.

[17] C. A. Hébert, A. Chuntharapai, M. Smith, T. Colby, J. Kim and R. Horuk, Partial Functional Mapping of the Human Interleukin-8 type A Receptor, *J. Biol. Chem.*, 268, p. 18549-18553, 1993.

[18] T. Takasuka, T. Sakurai, K. Goto, Y. Furuichi and T. Watanabe, Human endothelin receptor ETB, *J. Biol. Chem.*, 269, p. 7509-7513, 1994.

[19] Z. Fathi, R. V. Benya, H. Shapira, R. T. Jensen and J. F. Battey, The fifth transmembrane segment of the neuromedin B receptor is critical for high affinity neuromedin B binding, *J. Biol. Chem.*, 268, p. 14622-14626, 1993.

[20] S. A. Hjorth, H. T. Schambye, W. J. Greenlee and T. W. Schwartz, Identification of peptide binding residues in the extracellular domains of the AT1 receptor, *J. Biol. Chem.*, 269, p. 30953-30959, 1994.

[21] J. A. Lee, J. A. Sutiphong, C. E. Peishoff, J. M. Stadel, C. Kumar, R. E. Naughton, F. A. Watson, E. H. Ohlstein, J. D. Elliott and J. Gleason, Lysine 182 of the human endothelin B receptor modulates peptide agonist selectivity and non-peptide antagonist affinity, *Proc. Natl. Acad. Sci. USA*, (in press) 1994.

[22] J. H. Perlman, C. N. Thaw, L. Laakkonen, C. Y. Bowers and R. Osman, Hydrogen bonding interaction of thyrotropin-releasing hormone (TRH) with transmembrane tyrosine 106 of the TRH receptor, *J. Biol. Chem.*, 269, p. 1610-1613, 1994.

[23] H. Ji, M. Leung, Y. Zhang, K. J. Catt and K. Sandberg, Differential structural requirements for specific binding of nonpeptide and peptide antagonists to the AT1 angiotensin receptor: Identification of amino acid residues that determine binding of the antihypertensive drug, losartan, *J. Biol. Chem.*, (in press) 1994.

[24] S. R. Krystek, P. S. Patel, P. M. Rose, S. M. Fisher, B. K. Kienzle, D. A. Lach, E. C. K. Liu, J. S. Lyneb, J. Novotny and M. L. Webb, Mutation of peptide binding site in transmembrane region of a G protein-coupled receptor accounts for endothelin receptor subtype selectivity, *J. Biol. Chem.*, 269, p. 12383-12386, 1994.

[25] L. Mery and F. Boulay, The NH2-terminal region of C5aR but not that of FPR is critical for both protein transport and ligand binding, *J. Biol. Chem.*, 269, p. 3457-3463, 1994.

[26] P. Walker, M. Munoz, R. Martinez and M. C. Peitsch, Acidic residues in extracellular loops of the human Y1 neuropeptide Y receptor are essential for ligand binding, *J. Biol. Chem.*, 269, p. 2863-2869, 1994.

[27] U. Gether, T. E. Johansen, R. M. Snider, J. A. Lowe III, S. Nakanishi and T. W. Schwartz, Different binding epitopes on the NK1 receptor for substance P and a non-peptide antagonist, *Nature*, 362, p. 345-348, 1993.

[28] M. Beinborn, Y. M. Lee, E. M. McBride, S. M. Quinn and A. S. Kopin, A single amino acid of the cholecystokinin-B/gastrin receptor determines specificity for non-peptide antagonists, *Nature*, 362, p. 348-350, 1993.

[29] T. M. Fong, M. A. Cascieri, H. Yu, A. Bansal, C. Swain and C. D. Strader, Amino-aromatic interaction between histidine 197 of the neurokinin-1 receptor and CP 96345, *Nature*, 362, p. 350-353, 1993.

[30] U. gether, Y. Yokota, X. Emonds-Alt, J. Breliere, J. A. Lowe III, R. M. Snider, S. Nakanishi and T. W. Schwartz, Two nonpeptide tachykinin antagonists act through epitopes on corresponding segments of the NK1 and NK2 receptors, *Proc. Natl. Acad. Sci. USA*, 90, p. 6194-6198, 1993.

[31] U. Gether, L. Nilsson, J. A. Lowe and T. W. Schwartz, Specific residues at the top of transmembrane segment V and VI of the NK-1 receptor involved in binding of the non-peptide antagonist CP96,345, *J. Biol. Chem.*, 269, p. 23959-23964, 1994.

[32] T. M. Fong, H. Yu, M. A. Cascieri, D. Underwood, C. J. Swain and C. D. Strader, The role of Histidine 265 in antagonist binding to the neurokinin-1 receptor, *J. Biol. Chem.*, 269, p. 2728-2732, 1994.

[33] U. Gether, X. Emonds-Alt, J. Breliere, T. Fujii, D. Hagiwara, L. Pradier, C. Garret, T. E. Johansen and T. W. Schwartz, Evidence for a common molecular mode of action for

chemically distinct nonpeptide antagonists at the neurokinin-1 (substance P) receptor, *Mol. Pharm.*, 45, p. 500-508, 1994.

[34] M. A. Cascieri, A. M. Macleod, D. Underwood, L. Shiao, E. Ber, S. Sadowski, H. Yu, K. J. Merchant, C. J. Swain, C. D. Strader and T. M. Fong, Characterization of the interaction of N-Acyl-L-Tryptophan Benzyl Ester Neurokinin Antagonists with the Human Neurokinin-1 receptor, *J. Biol. Chem.*, 269, p. 6587-6591, 1994.

[35] H. T. Schambye, S. A. Hjorth, D. J. Bergsma, G. Sathe and T. W. Schwartz, Differentiation between binding sites for angiotensin II and non-peptide antagonists on the AT1 receptors, *Proc. Natl. Acad. Sci. USA*, 91, p. 7046-7050, 1994.

[36] H. T. Schambye, S. A. Hjorth, J. Weinstock and T. W. Schwartz, Specific interaction between the non-peptide angiotensin antagonist SK&F108,566 and His^{256} in the AT-1 Receptor, *Mol. Pharm.*, in press 1995.

[37] S. A. Hjorth, K. Thirstrup, K. L. Grandy and T. W. Schwartz, Analysis of a selective binding epitope for the $_K$-opiate receptor antagonist norbinaltorphimine, *Mol. Pharm.*, in press 1995.

[38] M. M. Rosenkilde, M. Cahir, U. Gether, S. A. Hjorth and T. W. Schwartz, Mutations along TM-II of the NK-1 receptor affect substance P competition with non-peptide antagonists — but not substance P binding, *J. Biol. Chem.*, 269, p. 28160-28164, 1994.

[39] R. J. Lefkowitz, S. Cotecchia, P. Samama and T. Costa, Constitutive activity of receptors coupled to guanine nucleotides regulatory proteins, *Trend Pharmacol. Sci.*, 14, p. 303-307, 1993.

[40] J. P. Glusker, Structural aspects of metal liganding to functional groups in proteins, *Adv. Prot. Chem.*, 42, p. 3-76, 1991.

[41] P. Chakrabarti, Geometry of interaction of metal ions with histidine residues in protein structures, *Prot. Engineer.*, 4, p. 57-63, 1990.

[42] R. Jerigan, G. Raghunanthan, I. Bahar, Characterization of interactions and metal ion binding sites in proteins, *Curr. Opin. Struct. Biol.*, 4, p. 256-263, 1994.

[43] L. Regan, The design of metal-binding sites in proteins, *Ann. Rev. Biophys. Biomol. Struct.*, 22, p. 257-281, 1993.

[44] T. M. Handel, S. A. Williams and W. F. DeGrado, Metal ion-dependent modulation of the dynamics of a designed protein, *Science*, 261, p. 879-885, 1993.

[45] S. F. Betz, D. P. Raleigh and W. F. DeGrado, *Curr. Opin. Struct. Biol.* 3, p. 601-610, 1993.

[46] C. Elling, S. M. Nielsen and T. W. Schwartz, Conversion of Antagonist Binding Site to Metal Ion Site in the Tachykinin NK-1 Receptor, *Nature*, 374, p. 74-77, 1995.

Using Sequence Information and Model Building to explore Subtype Specificity in GPCRs

Robert Bywater[*], Gert Vriend[†], Laerte Oliveira[‡] and [§] Daan van Aalten

[*] Biostructure Department, Novo Nordisk A/S, DK-2880 Bagsværd, Denmark
[†] BIOcomputing, EMBL, D-6990 Heidelberg, Germany
[‡] Escola Paolista de Medicina, São Paolo, Brazil
[§] Biochemistry Department, University of Leeds, Leeds, England

Abstract

The amino acid sequences of more than 650 G-protein coupled receptors (GPCRs), together with their mutual alignments, are currently available [1]. Making use of this data, and using the published electron crystallographic structure of bacteriorhodopsin [2] as a template, molecular models of many different GPCRs have been published by several groups [3, 4]. In this work models of human dopamine receptor subtypes 1 and 2 have been constructed based on this template.

However, it is uncertain whether bacteriorhodopsin, which is not a GPCR, is suitable as a template for building such models. A low-resolution electron crystallography image of bovine rhodopsin, which is a true GPCR, has been published [5] and based on this data, a model has been constructed [6]. Using distance constraints derived from this model, molecular dynamics simulations were performed on one of the above models of the dopamine receptor and the resulting structure compared qualitatively with the published model of bovine rhodopsin and with the model based on bacteriorhodopsin.

Subtype specificities for ligands can be investigated at the sequence level. Correlations between patterns of known subtype preferences and sequence reveal the residues in the sequence that are likely to be decisive for determining subtype specificity.

1   Introduction

In the quest for new, more specific and potent drugs, knowledge of the structure of the protein target is of inestimable value. Having access to a model of the target protein allows the drug designer to ask much more pertinent questions about how ligands bind to the receptor, and even to answer many of them. Furthermore, it becomes possible to make use of some recently developed *de novo* ligand design tools [7].

The requirements of increased specificity and absence of side effects put extra constraints on the design of suitable ligands. Therefore, access to a structure not only of the target

```
TM1
                    D1    VRILTACFLSLLILSTLLGNTLVCAAVIR
                    D5    ..VVTACLLTLLIIWTLLGNVLVCAAIVR
                    D2    HYNYYATLLTLLIAVIVFGNVLVCMAIVR
                    D3    PHAYYALSYCALILAIVFGNGLVCMAVLK
                    D4    QGAAALVGGVLLIGAVLAGNSLVCVSVAT
      bovine rhodopsin    QFSMLAAYMFLLIMLGFPINFLTLY....
    bacteriorhodopsin     PEWIWLALGTALMGLGTLYFLVKGM....
TM2
                    D1    TNFFVISLAVSDLLVAVLVMPWKAVAEI
                    D5    TNVFIVSLAVSDLFVALLVMPWKAVAEV
                    D2    TNYLIVSLAVADLLVATLVMPWVVYLEV
                    D3    TNYLVVSLAVADLLVATLVMPWVVYLEV
                    D4    TNSFIVSLAAADLLLALLVLPLFVYSEV
      bovine rhodopsin    LNYILLNLAVADLFMVFGGFTTTLYTST
    bacteriorhodopsin     ...DAKKFYAITTLVPAIAFTMYLSMLL
TM3
                    D1    FCNIWVAFDIMCSTASILNLCVISVdry
                    D5    FCDVWVAFDIMCSTASILNLCVISVdry
                    D2    HCDIFVTLDVMMCTASILNLCAISIdry
                    D3    CCDVFVTLDVMMCTASILNLCAISIdry
                    D4    LCDALMAMDVMLCTASIFNLCAISVdry
      bovine rhodopsin    GCNLEGFFATLGGEIALWSLVVLAIery
    bacteriorhodopsin     EQNPIYWARYADWLFTTPLLLLDLALL
TM4
                    D1    AAFILISVAWTLSVLISFIPVQLSW
                    D5    MALVMVGLAWTLSILISFIPVQLNW
                    D2    RVTVMISIVWVLSFTISCPLLFGLN
                    D3    RVALMITAVWVLAFAVSCPLLFGFN
                    D4    RQLLLIGATWLLSAAVAAPVLCGLN
      bovine rhodopsin    HAIMGVAFTWVMALACAAPPLVGWS
    bacteriorhodopsin     GTILALVGADGIMIGTGLVGAL...
TM5
                    D1    YAISSSVISFYIPVAIMIVTYTRIY
                    D5    YAISSSLISFYIPVAIMIVTYTRIY
                    D2    FVVYSSIVSFYVPFIVTLLVYIKIY
                    D3    FVIYSSVVSFYLPFGVTVLVYARIY
                    D4    YVVYSSVCSFFLPCPLMLLLYWATF
      bovine rhodopsin    FVIYMFVVHFIIPLIVIFFCYGQLV
    bacteriorhodopsin     WWAISTAAMLYILYVLFFGFT....
TM6
                    D1    KVLKTLSVIMGVFVCCWLPFFILNCI
                    D5    KVLKTLSVIMGVFVCCWLPFFILNCM
                    D2    KATQMLAIVLGVFIICWLPFFITHIL
                    D3    KATQMVAIVLGAFIVCWLPFFLTHVL
                    D4    KAMRVLPVVVGAFLLCWTPFFVVHIT
      bovine rhodopsin    EVTRMVIIMVIAFLICWLPYAGVAFY
    bacteriorhodopsin     EVASTFKVLRNVTVVLWSAYPVVWLI
TM7
                    D1    FCIDSNTFDVFVWFGWANSSLNPIIYV
                    D5    PCVSETTFDVFVWFGWANSSLNPVIYV
                    D2    CNIPPVLYSAFTWLGYVNSAVNPIIYG
                    D3    CHVSPELYSATTWLGYVNSALNPVIYT
                    D4    CSVPPRLVSAVTWLGYVNSALNPVIYT
      bovine rhodopsin    .DFGPIFMTIPAFFAKTSAVYNPVIYI
    bacteriorhodopsin     .NIETLLFMVLDVSAKVGFGLILLR..
```

Figure 1: Alignment of dopamine receptor subtype transmembrane regions with bovine rhodopsin and bacteriorhodopsin

molecule, but also that of other receptors to which it is wished that the drugs do not bind, would be of great value. In particular, it is important to be able to design a drug specific for only one member of a family of closely related receptors, and which does not to any appreciable extent bind to the other members of the family. Nature has solved this problem in the case of CNS receptors by ensuring that different subtypes get expressed only locally within an anatomically confined region of the brain [8]. By doing that, one and the same ligand can be used to activate all members of the family, but since the ligand will only be elicited locally, in response to a particular stimulus, only those receptor molecules located close to the site of ligand secretion will bind the ligand and convey the appropriate signal further down the signal transduction pathway. Pharmacologists do not have access to such sophisticated technology for drug administration; a drug administered to a patient either orally or intravenously or in almost any other way will, once it has crossed the blood-brain barrier, be distributed throughout the brain in a way that we can not control, so there is no way that we can prevent a non-specific drug from hitting the "wrong" target.

For the purposes of illustrating this problem, and attempting to find a solution, an example is taken from the dopamine family of G-protein coupled receptors. Many GPCRs, including those of the dopamine receptor family, are expressed in several structurally related subtypes, so the conclusions reached here could equally well be applied to any other family of GPCRs.

Like all other members of the GPCR superfamily, the dopamine receptors are characterized by a fold which consists of seven transmembrane helices[1] connected by three intracellular and three extracellular loops[2], and the entire molecule is oriented such that the N-terminal chain is extracellular, and the C-terminal chain is located inside the cell. In many members of the superfamily, this chain is anchored onto the inside of the membrane by a fatty acid chain covalently attached to a conserved cysteine residue within the C-terminal chain.

These receptors have been targets for a large number of drugs over the last 20 years or more, which have been designed without knowledge of the structures of these receptors. Instead, the techniques of classical medicinal chemistry and of "small molecule" modelling have been employed. Although some progress towards developing drugs with selectivity for different subtypes has been made, it is not easy to derive general rules which enable synthetic chemists to design yet more selective compounds by these methods.

In the case of the dopamine family, where a variety of behavioural and psychotic states can arise from an imbalance in the activity of the different receptor subtypes of which five (referred to as D1,......D5) have so far been identified, treatment has often been associated with certain unpleasant side-effects, typically affecting the motor system, which are directly caused by the activity of other dopamine subtypes than the one of interest. In the pursuit of more specific drugs, a large number of analogues has been tested, but the elimination of side-effects remains a problem. Despite this, there has been some success in separating D1 activity from D2. The question now is, to what extent can we make reliable models of the subtypes of the dopamine receptor, and to what extent will the differences we observe allow us to design subtype-specific ligands?

2 Methods and Results

2.1 Strategies for building receptor models

The only really reliable strategy for model building of proteins is that of homology modelling [9]. Comparisons of the tertiary structures of homologous proteins have shown that 3D structures have been better conserved in evolution than primary sequences [10, 11].

A necessary prerequisite to modelling by homology is the existence of a good alignment between the protein to be modelled and that of a protein with known structure. The sequences of the entire GPCR superfamily have been aligned [1] — the present count is over 650 such sequences. These are maintained on a database file server at EMBL, Heidelberg (tm7@embl-heidelberg.de), and the alignments are updated at regular intervals. Based on these alignments a large number of GPCR models has been constructed in many laboratories (see references [3] and [4] for a discussion).

The most widely-used approach has been to use as a template the only 7-transmembrane protein for which an experimental structure exists, the bacteriorhodopsin of *Halobacterium halobium* [2], and then build the desired structure by some standard homology modelling

---

[1]referred to as "TM1",.........,"TM7".
[2]referred to as "i1","i2","i3" and "o1","o2","o3" respectively.

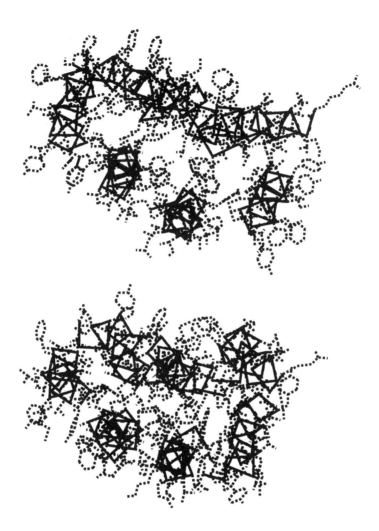

Figure 2: a. Dopamine D1 receptor model based on the bacteriorhodopsin[2] template.
b. Dopamine D1 receptor model based on the bovine rhodopsin [5] template.

technique. There are several objections to that approach. Although bacteriorhodopsin is constructed along similar lines to the GPCR family, being a 7-transmembrane protein with its N-terminal end on the extracellular side of the membrane, the bacterial protein has entirely different loop structures, especially on the cytosolic side, without any of the sequence motifs known to be essential for G-protein binding. It lacks the cys-cys disulfide bridge linking the top of TM3 and the middle of loop "o2", that is commonly found in GPCRs, and it lacks any immediately apparent sequence homology to the GPCRs. In addition to that, there is now preliminary structural data on a true GPCR, bovine rhodopsin [5], that suggests that there are considerable differences in the mutual packing and the tilt angles of the helices, between the structures of bacteriorhodopsin and bovine rhodopsin. If anyone is going to attempt to design ligands that bind to GPCRs, let alone try to go even further and design subtype-specific ligands, it is essential to resolve the issue of which template to use for homology building of GPCR models.

The published images [5] of bovine rhodopsin reveal the general packing scheme for the 7 TM helices, and *inter alia* show that TM3 is more "buried" in bovine rhodopsin than in bacteriorhodopsin, but nothing is revealed about the sequential arrangement of the helices i.e. whether they are ordered in the same sense (clockwise as seen from the cytosol). Indeed, some authors [12, 13] have proposed entirely different topologies. These will not be discussed here since the consensus of opinion within the GPCR community now favours the bacteriorhodopsin topology for a convincingly large number of reasons [14]. In this work, it is assumed that the topologies of the two proteins are the same, the question being which packing arrangement of the helices to use-that of bacteriorhodopsin [2] or bovine rhodopsin [6]. This different packing arrangement is also reflected in the tilt angles of the helices being different in the two molecules. An attempt has been made [15] to "explain away" this difference (with the aim maybe of trying to preserve some credence for bacteriorhodopsin as a suitable template) by proposing that the same structure can be obtained if one of them is tilted globally through 15° relative to the other. This suggestion has been refuted as being irreconcilable with the experimental techniques employed by the original authors of the bovine rhodopsin work [16], and it is shown later in this work, that the two structures can be modelled as two quite distinct, thermodynamically stable species without the need for a "fix" of this sort.

2.2 Construction of models of dopamine receptor with the bacteriorhodopsin template

To begin with, models of the human dopamine receptor subtypes were constructed in the most widely-used way, using bacteriorhodopsin as the template. The alignments for the subtypes were taken from the 7TM alignment available from the "TM7" ftp server referred to above, except for D3 for which the sequence was obtained by translation from the DNA sequence (with two frameshifts) and then aligned manually. The resulting alignment of all five known human dopamine receptor subtypes, alongside bovine rhodopsin and bacteriorhodopsin, is shown in fig. 1. Note that these sequences encompass the TM sequences but include the first few flanking sequences at each end. This is because there is no absolute criterion which can be used for deciding the exact start and end of the TM sequences, and because, later, when making mutations, it is important to include flanking sequences that are outside the helix since it has been shown [17] that side-chain rotamer angles are determined largely by the nature of the flanking residues. Furthermore, to the extent that there may be some unwinding of the helix from the ends during molecular dynamics (MD) simulations, it is preferable that the sequence abutting the ends of the helix is the natural sequence as far as possible, rather than some more arbitrary piece of chain such as $(gly)_n$. Otherwise, no special effort was made to model the loops, beyond the two features listed below, because the loops almost certainly interact with the lipid bilayer in some way (and we have not so far included the membrane in our models) and furthermore the loops "i2" and "i3", as well as the C-terminal chain are involved in binding the G-protein[3].

- On the cytosolic side, within the flanking regions and beyond into the loops, there is quite a large number of positively-charge residues. This is in accordance with the "positive inside" rule [22]. So long as the loop is not thereby made unduly long, these were incorporated into the loops. No attempt was made at this stage to compensate in any way for these charges, as the MD simulations in the absence of lipid are all carried

---

[3] Loops "i2" and "i3" is known from earlier work [18, 19, 20] to bind G-protein. Correlated mutation studies [21] show that loop "i2" and the first 18-20 residues of the C-terminal tail are also important for G-protein binding in a way that is *specific for G-protein type (G_s or G_i respectively).*

Table 1: RMS differences between backbones of original and mutated receptor molecules

	D1	D2	D2⇒D1
D1		0.918	0.826
D2			0.323

out *"in vacuo"*, where net charges on residues are neutral. Furthermore, although it is easy to establish from secondary structure assignments that loop "i2" consists probably of a beta-turn, loop "i3" starts and ends in a helix, and the C-terminal chain, which contains the conserved cys residue that is "anchored" into the membrane by a long alkyl chain, very likely starts with a helix, these features were not incorporated into the loops at this stage. Another feature, peculiar to D2, is a very long loop (157 residues) inserted between the helixes in "i3". This sequence was submitted to PredictProtein@embl-heidelberg.de [23] for secondary structure assignment and sequence homology determination. No hits were found from the sequence database apart from a similar loop in α-adrenoceptor. The structure of this loop and its function remain obscure at this stage, so it would be pointless to try and model it further.

• The loop "o2" was modelled in its entirety (13 residues) because it contains the important cysteine residue that is linked via a disulfide bond to the cysteine at the top of TM3.

Models of D1 (Fig. 2a shows the arrangement of helices as seen from the cytosolic side of the membrane) and D2 receptors were constructed on the bacteriorhodopsin template, using the homology modelling routine in WHAT IF, and subsequently energy minimized followed by 100 ps of MD using the program GROMOS. Despite the fact that they were built on the same template, the structures drifted away from one another. Since the treatment has been identical in both cases, this can only be due to the differences in sequence between the two subtypes. In order to check the significance of this observation, D1 was mutated back to D2 and re-run through energy minimization and MD. The structure reconverged towards the D2 structure and at the end of the MD run was closer to that structure than to the parent D1 structure as shown by the RMS values listed in table 1.

2.3   Construction of models of dopamine receptor with the bovine rhodopsin template

There are no published coordinates for the bovine rhodopsin structure. However, a model has been proposed for this protein [6] and differences between the proposed model and that of bacteriorhodopsin illustrated in the form of diagrams showing "slices" across the molecules at three levels, from the cytosolic end of the molecule down to a depth of 11 Å, the middle 11 Å, and from the extracellular face down to 11 Å, for both molecules. From the diagram for bovine rhodopsin, a set of approximate "distance constraints" (listed in table 2) were extracted from the figure using the bond lengths in the figure for calibration. These "distance constraints" were applied to a model of the D2 receptor built according to the bacteriorhodopsin template in a GROMOS simulation run for 100 ps. The resulting structure (fig. 2b) resembles, at least by visual inspection, the electron microscope images [5] and the proposed model structure [6]. This is perhaps not surprising, although the method of extracting the constraints is prone to all sorts of errors. What is of greater interest, however, is to see what happens when the

Table 2: List of CA-CA distance constraints (all set at 0.8 nm with constraint force set at 1000 kJ/mol/nm^2) applied in formation of the receptor structure according to the bovine rhodopsin model. (NB. New numbering scheme[1]).

V	I103	T	I106
V	133	T	CO2
I	338	T	413
S	337	V	527
V	412	Y	528
I	160	T	604
A	127	D	224
A	223	A	328
T	327	S	423
L	220	S	726
S	329	A	727
S	423	S	516
F	521	I	615
F	614	N	725
T	120	V	231
V	231	S	716
A	119	S	716
T	123	T	719
W	234	F	318
D	322	V	509
F	318	L	431
L	431	V	509
A	717	Y	528

constraints are relaxed. Constraints such as these are valid only for the purposes of forcing a rapid displacement through phase space such as when setting up a starting structure.

When the constraints were relaxed, and a new minimization carried out, followed by a 100 ps MD trajectory, the resulting structure was stable, maintaining essentially the same structure as the original constrained molecule (RMS difference of 0.159 nm). This indicates that the structure obtained is at least stable, and is qualitatively similar to the published structure of bovine rhodopsin.

In all protein model building, validation is a key issue. If predictions can not be checked against experimentally determined structures, they should at least be subjected to a rigorous analysis in which structural features such as packing, torsion angles, absence of bumps and buried polar groups etc. are examined. A procedure for doing this is present in WHAT IF. The report of this protein analysis stated that there were no bad bondlengths, and otherwise, no more bumps and other deficiencies than are normally found in proteins built by homology. Of the few "buried' polars, virtually all were in fact polar residues that line the binding cavity and are required for activity. An important *caveat* with any of the current checking procedures is that they use databases containing data derived only from the structures of water-soluble globular proteins. Consequently, certain features that may turn out to be quite normal in the context of membrane proteins may be interpreted as incorrect, while some serious errors may pass unnoticed. We do not yet have any database of accurately determined membrane protein structures. Having said that, it is worth recalling that when backbones of e.g. water-soluble globular proteins having a four helix bundle topology are superimposed on any four of the seven TMs in protein models similar to this, the packing arrangements appear to be quite conventional [3].

2.4 Correlating Subtype Sequence and Subtype Specificity for Ligands

Binding constants for a panel of ligands binding to all five known subtypes[4] were made available [24] for this work. These were used as input for a method [25] of determining statistical correlations between differential ligand binding and sequence differences between subtypes. The actual correlations were carried out using the implementation of this method in the protein modelling program WHAT IF [26].

The results are shown in Color plate 12 (page xxvi), in which the sites at which different combinations of subtypes differ can be observed. It will be apparent that the sequences fall into two major subgroups, referred to as the D1 and D2 subfamily. That there are so many differences is reflected in the fact that is has been much easier to find compounds that are selective between these subfamilies than to find compounds selective for subtypes within the subfamilies, using conventional medicinal chemistry procedures. What one really needs to know, however, is which of the sites in the protein that are identified as being significant for subtype specificity are *adjacent to the bound ligand*. For it is only those that are likely to have any direct influence on the way in which the ligand docks, and hence on the selectivity. Other sites in the protein that the correlation analysis points to which do not line the binding pocket, or are not close to it, may exert their influence in other ways, e.g. by influencing some details of the overall conformation of the molecule in such a way as to change the shape of the binding pocket, but we can not use this information in order to design new drugs or modify existing ones. It is therefore of more interest to examine where in the molecule these key residues are located.

2.5 Docking of ligands onto receptor models

It is easy to dock a variety of ligands into the binding cavity of models of D1 and D2 receptor, built on both templates without needing to twist the ligands away from the conformation they would be likely to adopt in solution, or more commonly, in gas-phase (determined by e.g. the SYBYL force field [27]). However, in the case of flexible ligands, such as dopamine itself, it is by no means certain that this solution structure is the one which would be observed when bound to the receptor[5]. In this work, an extended conformation was used for dopamine, which superimposed well onto a rigid agonist (Fig. 3).

The ligands typically sit in a cage of aromatic side chains, positioned in an edge-on positioned relative to the planes on the phenyl rings in the ligands, although no special "tweaking" of the sidechain rotamer angles was necessary to achieve this. The rotamer angles were assigned using the rotamer database in WHAT IF. One residue that does need "tweaking" is the conserved (throughout all amine-binding GPCRs) asp residue on TM3, D322 (the now standard [1] numbering system for GPCRs is used throughout here). Although the ligands dock naturally with their amino-nitrogen atoms aligned close to this residue, the only way to obtain a contact distance of approximately 3 Å, typical of an ionic interaction of this type, is to change the dihedral angle χ_1 of the sidechain hydroxyl from -72 to 64 °. Given that the former figure is the one favoured by the rotamer database, and is retained during the GROMOS runs in the absence of ligand, it suggests that this switch in χ_1-angle for the asp sidechain might

---

[4]NB. for this panel of compounds, data related to agonist or antagonist activity was not complete, but accurate binding constants were available for the whole set. Full details of this will be published separately.

[5]There is a precedent for the occurrence of conformational changes on binding of ligands which lack a rigid, polycyclic structure - acetylcholine, for example, which according to solution NMR data normally adopts an extended conformation but which changes to a bent structure on binding to the nicotinic acetylcholine receptor as shown by transferred NOE data [28].

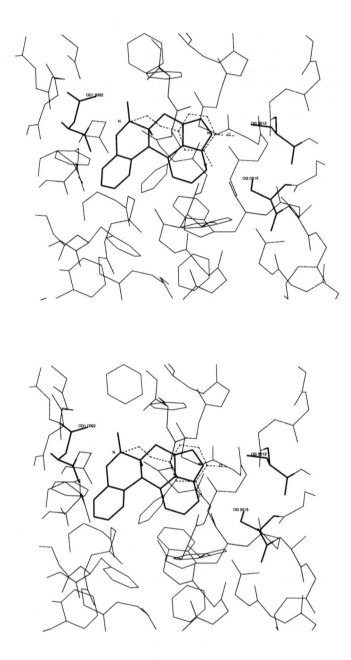

Figure 3: Dopamine (—-) and the D1 agonist benzergoline docked between D322, S512 and S516.

well be important for triggering a signal transduction event. However, most antagonists also contain an (often alicyclic) amino nitrogen of this kind, and although it is a bit premature to propose how antagonists bind at this stage, there does not seem to be any simple way to account for how, if at all, this switch in χ_1-angle may trigger the signal transduction mechanism[6].

Another important question is the role of the serine hydroxyls on S512 and S516 and their significance in binding to the catechol hydroxyls in a pairwise hydrogen-bonding arrangement [30]. In figure 3, in which dopamine has been docked into the D1 model, the two hydroxyls of the dopamine are shown docked onto these serines. The same figure shows benzergoline, a potent D1-selective agonist [31] docked into the binding site, with the amino function located within 3 Å of the conserved asp residue (D322), as in the case of dopamine, and the aromatic moieties docked comfortably into the aromatic pocket. This time, however, the ligand possesses only a single hydrogen bond donor, and the docking has been carried out so as to bring this into juxtaposition with the hydroxyl oxygen of S512, but this choice is quite arbitrary.

Since we know that a) agonists do not always possess two hydroxyls (a single hydrogen-bond donor is a requirement as in the above case) and b) in many amine receptors, at least one of the serines can be mutated to residues not capable of forming hydrogen bonds, without affecting binding or agonist activity, we should perhaps consider finding another hydrogen bond acceptor. A possible candidate for this is a naked backbone carbonyl group situated on TM4, four residues downstream from a conserved proline (*but conserved only within the subfamily - position 430 in the D1 subfamily and 429 in the D2 group*). The fact that the carbonyl group is displaced by one residue in the two subfamilies (residue I426 in D1 and residue T425 in D2, respectively) suggests that this could be a key determinant of selectivity between these subfamilies. Of course, this can not be considered as conclusive, until confirmed by experiment, but the carbonyl group presents an alternative mode of binding to the conventionally accepted one, and one which has the merit of at least offering an explanation for the observed difference in suptype specificity between ligands selective for the D1 and D2 subfamilies.

On this question of selectivity for individual members of the subfamilies, it is proposed that use may be made of the correlation studies mentioned earlier. Although the models are not accurate enough for *de novo* ligand design, they will be useful for qualitative ligand design studies. If a ligand is docked e.g. as described above, then there are certain constraints as to which residues may or may not be in close proximity to the docked ligand. Whenever a residue that is close to the docked ligand, and can be identified as significant for subtype-specific binding as discussed in section 2.4. (See also Fig. 1 and Color plate 12, page xxvi) then there are clearly possibilities for either building up the ligand, or reducing the bulk of the ligand at that site, or changing polar character, whatever the case may be. This question is being penetrated more deeply and will be reported on in future publications. Likewise, the model based on bovine rhodopsin rather than bacteriorhodopsin (Fig. 2b) will feature in these studies also.

3   Conclusions

1) The sequence-function correlation method [10] identifies sites in the receptor molecules which are determinants of function and of differences in functional properties between the subtypes. These include subtype-specific ligand binding, in which the residues

---

[6]Before we search for mechanism based on some kind of "charge relay" system we should consider other possible mechanisms such as the proposal [29] that agonist activity merely reflects the stabilization by the agonist of the "active" form of the receptor, while antagonists stabilize the "inactive" form.

responsible for binding of ligands in a manner which discriminates between different subtypes, and additionally, those residues in the loops which act as a "switch" between different G-protein types (G_s or G_i) [24].

2) Model building of the various receptor subtypes enables these sites to be located within the context of a three dimensional structure. However, validation of these structures is still a problem. Attempts to resolve these problems has led to the proposal that two versions of each subtype be used in all ligand docking and design studies. These two versions are the structures which resemble the bacteriorhodopsin template and bovine rhodopsin template respectively. Further modelling work on the receptors should pay attention to the packing of lipid around the receptor molecule, the proper construction of the cytosolic loops, tethering of the C-terminal tail into the membrane, and the docking of models of G-proteins onto these loop structures. These are a necessary prerequisite before conclusions as to the mechanism of activation of GPCRs can be drawn.

3) The mode of docking has not been unequivocally settled. Until experimental data is available that resolves this issue, alternative modes of binding should be considered.

Acknowledgments

The authors wish to record their thanks to several experts in the GPCR field. In particular, to Professor John Findlay, a pioneer of GPCR research, for valuable discussions and for providing resources for doing this work. (D. v. A. is a PhD student with Professor Findlay at the present time). Dr. A. C. M. Paiva for providing facilities and support for this work. Dr. Chris Sander for hospitality and stimulating discussions. The members of the European 7TM Club for encouragement and helpful discussions. The ligand binding data were kindly supplied by Marit Kristiansen, Novo Nordisk A/S.

References

[1] L. Oliveira, A. C. M. Paiva and G. Vriend, *J. Comp. Aided. Mol. Des.*, 7, p. 649-658, 1993.
[2] R. Henderson, J. M. Baldwin, T. A. Ceska, F. Zemlin, E. Beckmann and K. H. Downing, Model for the structure of bacteriorhodopsin based on high-resolution electron cryo-microscopy, *J. Mol. Biol.*, 213, p. 899-929, 1990.
[3] P. Cronet, C. Sander and G. Vriend, *Prot. Eng.*, 6, p. 59-64, 1993.
[4] L. Oliveira, A. C. M. Paiva, C. Sander and G. Vriend, *TIPS*, 15, p. 170-172, 1994.
[5] G. F. X. Schertler, C. Villa and R. Henderson, Projection structure of rhodopsin, *Nature*, 362, p. 770-772, 1993.
[6] J. M. Baldwin, The probable arrangement of the helices in G-protein coupled receptors, *EMBO J.*, 12, p. 1693-1703, 1993.
[7] I. D. Kuntz, *Science*, Structure-based strategies for Drug Design and Discovery, 257, p. 1078-1082, 1992.
[8] U. Ungerstedt, Stereotaxic mapping of the monoamine pathway in the rat brain, *Acta Physiol. Scan.*, S367, p. 1-48, 1971.
[9] M. B. Swindells and J. M. Thornton, *Curr. Opin. Struct. Biol.*, 1, p. 219, 1991.
[10] M. Bajaj and T. L. Blundell, Evolution and the tertiary structure of proteins, *Ann. Rev. Biophys. Bioeng.*, 13, p. 453-492, 1984.

[11] D. Bashford, C. Chothia and A. M. Lesk, Determinants of a protein fold: Unique features of the globin amino acid sequences, *J. Mol. Biol.*, 196, p. 199-216, 1987.

[12] D. Zhang and H. Weinstein, Signal transduction by a 5-HT2 receptor: a mechanistic hypothesis from molecular dynamics simulations of the three-dimensional model of the receptor complexed to ligands, *J. Med. Chem.*, 36, p. 934-938, 1993.

[13] K. MaloneyHuss and T. Lybrand, Three dimensional structure for the β_2 adrenergic receptor protein based on computer modeling studies *J. Mol. Biol.*, 225, p. 859-871, 1992.

[14] G. Vriend, *7TM*, 4, p. 4-11, 1994.

[15] J. Hoflack, S. Trumpp-Kallmeyer and M. Hibert, *TIPS*, 15, p. 7-9, 1994.

[16] R. Henderson, *personal communication*.

[17] V. De Filippis, C. Sander and G. Vriend, *Prot. Eng.*, 7, p. 1203-1208, 1994.

[18] R. A. F. Dixon, I. S. Sigal and C. D. Strader, *Cold Spring Harbor Symp. Quant. Biol.*, 53, p. 487-498, 1988.

[19] B. F. O'Dowd, M. Hnatowich, J. W. Regan, W. M. Leader, M. G. Caron and R. J. Lefkowitz, *J. Biol. Chem.*, 263, p. 15985-15992, 1988.

[20] R. R. Franke, T. P. Sakmar, D. A. Oprian and Khorana, *J. Biol. Chem.*, 263, p. 2119-2122, 1988.

[21] L. Oliveira, G. Vriend *et al.*, to be published 1995.

[22] G. Von Heijne, The Distribution of Positively Charged Residues in Bacterial Inner Membrane Proteins Correlates with the Trans-Membrane Topology, *EMBO J.*, 5, p. 3021-3027, 1986.

[23] B. Rost and C. Sander, *Proteins: Struc. Funct. Gen.*, 19, p. 55-72, 1994.

[24] Dopamine project group, Novo Nordisk A/S

[25] W. Kuipers, L. Oliveira, A. C. M. Paiva, F. Rippmann, C. Sander, G. Vriend and A. P. IJzerman, *Proceedings of Molecular Graphics and Modelling Society Meeting on Membrane Proteins*, Leeds, 28-30 March, 1994.

[26] G. Vriend, *J. Mol. Graph.*, 8, p. 52-56, 1990.

[27] Tripos Associates, St. Louis, Missouri, USA.

[28] R. W. Behling, T. Yamane, G. Navon and L. Jelinski, Conformation of acetylcholine bound to the nicotinic acetylcholine receptor, *PNAS*, 85, p. 6721-6725, 1988.

[29] T. W. Schwartz, *this volume*, 1995.

[30] C. D. Strader, I. S. Sigal and R. A. F. Dixon, *FASEB J.*, 3, p. 1825-1832, 1989.

[31] M. Seiler, P. Floersheim, R. Markstein and A. Widmer, *J. Med. Chem.*, 36, p. 977-984, 1993.

Statistical Mechanics and Kinetics of Protein Folding Processes

Proposed Rules of the Protein Folding Game

M. Crippen and Vladimir N. Maiorov

College of Pharmacy, University of Michigan, Ann Arbor, Michigan 48109, U.S.A.

Abstract

In an attempt to reduce confusion in the field of protein folding calculations, we propose simple definitions for the protein folding problem (FP) and the inverse folding problem (IFP). As more tractable subsets of these very general problems, we define the structure identification problem (3DID) and the sequence identification problem (SEQID), for which there exist effective algorithms. In 3DID, the inputs are an amino acid sequence and a large set of three-dimensional structures that sequence might adopt, including the native one; the desired output is the unambiguous identification of the native structure. In SEQID, the inputs are a sequence and its native structure, along with a large set of other sequences; the output should be a selection of those sequences that prefer to fold to the given template structure, even when the homology with the given sequence is minimal. We then debunk a number of popular misconceptions, particularly the notion that algorithms for 3DID must necessarily solve SEQID and vice versa, and the idea that since gapped alignment is a necessary feature of SEQID, it must be used also in 3DID.

Associated with all these definitions, algorithms, and misconceptions is the customary comparison of protein structures by their root-mean-square deviation (RMSD) in atomic coordinates after optimal rigid body superposition. What is not so clear is the significance of different RMSD values, particularly above the customary arbitrary cutoff for obvious similarity of 2–3 Å. Our earlier work argued for an intrinsic cutoff for protein similarity that varied with the number of residues in the polypeptide chains being compared. Here we introduce a new measure, ρ, of structural similarity based on RMSD that is independent of the sizes of the molecules involved, or of any other special properties of molecules. When $\rho < 0.3$, protein structures are visually recognized to be obviously similar, but the mathematically pleasing intrinsic cutoff of $\rho < 1.0$ corresponds to overall similarity in folding motif at a level not usually recognized until smoothing of the polypeptide chain path makes it striking.

1 Problem definition

There has been a lot of excitement in the recent literature about computer calculations that "fold up proteins", particularly methods that employ specially designed potential functions that are not general purpose molecular mechanics force fields, yet somehow incorporate information about protein folding. Along with all the excitement and optimistic claims of success has come a great deal of confusion over who has really done what, and what does it mean in other contexts. Our purpose here is not to give an authoritative review of the field, but rather to clear up some of the misconceptions and define some terms precisely enough to explain what we have been doing.

The long term goal of many investigators has been the protein folding problem (FP): given only the amino acid sequence, calculate the detailed three-dimensional (3D) structure of the protein. However, this statement of FP is insufficient. We must add the target accuracy of the prediction and a requirement of generality. The experimental answer the calculation is trying to match is almost always taken to be a high-resolution X-ray crystal or NMR structure. There is also consensus that the appropriate measure of protein conformational similarity is the root-mean-square deviation in C^α coordinates after optimal superposition by rigid body translation and rotation (denoted here by RMSD). (We believe that the test of "topological similarity" is so ill-defined as to be a meaningless measure.) Unfortunately, there is no consensus about how small the RMSD between the calculated and crystal structure must be to count as success. We have recently proposed an objective RMSD cutoff between similar and dissimilar protein structures that depends on chain length, but is free of arbitrary decisions [1]. Using this criterion we find several cases where various authors have calculated the tertiary structure of small proteins nearly well enough, and one or two cases where they have barely succeeded. Yet no one has succeeded on more than one protein, to our knowledge. This brings up the requirement of generality. A particular folding algorithm may inadvertently or intentionally incorporate information about the protein being predicted, or it may be subtly biased toward producing structures of that type. Success in FP must include the ability to function on a variety of different protein structural types, as well as extension beyond the set of proteins that may have been used to develop the method. Just how broad the range of proteins must be is up for debate, but we would propose that a successful method should work at least for α, β, and α/β types of globular, water soluble proteins.

There is a second major goal that is of more recent interest than FP and opposite to it, namely the inverse folding problem (IFP). Here the intent is to calculate a sequence or sequences that will uniquely fold to a given 3D structure. In IFP the solution is not unique, as we know from the great similarity of the many mutant T4 lysozyme crystal structures, but otherwise the accuracy and generality issues are the same. The experimentally determined 3D structure of the designed amino acid sequence must be unique enough to crystallize, and must lie within the proposed RMSD limit compared to the given target structure. Furthermore, this must be generally true for some wide variety of proteins, particularly those that are significantly different from structures used to develop the method.

FP and IFP so formulated are probably distant goals, and we need easier problems for now, such that their solution will lead the way to success on the more difficult ones. Certainly if we can't even distinguish between correctly and incorrectly folded structures of the same sequence, we have little hope of solving FP. Our research has therefore centered around what we will call the structure identification problem (3DID): given a particular amino acid sequence and a large collection of 3D protein structures of the correct chain length, one of which is the correct native structure, select that native structure. Once again, the problem statement needs to be refined as to accuracy and generality.

Most investigators of 3DID have used a statistical treatment of accuracy by developing a scalar function of structure that can be used to rank all the structures given, and then noting that the native lies far out on the favorable end of the distribution [2, 3, 4]. We have adopted the much more stringent, nonstatistical requirement that the native must always be ranked first, just as the real protein folds to its one native structure and no other. As for generality, there is the range of applicability concerning sizes and types of native proteins, as well as the range of nonnative structural types. We consider only native proteins that are compact, globular, and water soluble, consisting of one or more polypeptide chains of naturally occurring amino

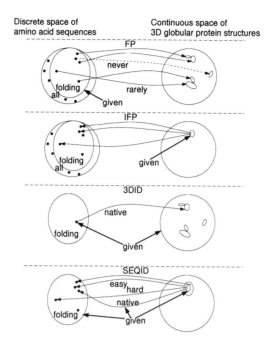

Figure 1: Schematic representation of different folding problems as mappings.

acids. They may be of any folding motif and have associated ions, small ligands and prosthetic groups, but otherwise the set of polypeptide chains comprising the native structure must be able to fold up independently of other macromolecules. For example, if the experimentally stable state of a protein is the dimer, we must consider both chains at once, not just the monomer. As far as the diversity of the alternative structures goes, we assume that the obviously bad ones have already been rejected by some structure quality assessment program that looks for left-handed α-helices, van der Waals contacts, unusual ϕ/ψ values, etc. Otherwise, they may be compact or noncompact, similar to the native or very dissimilar. As does the Sippl group, we generate our alternatives by cutting out contiguous segments of polypeptide chain the length of the native from larger PDB entries.

The opposite of 3DID and a restriction of IFP is what we will call the sequence identification problem (SEQID): given a particular native sequence and its high-resolution 3D structure, select from a large set of sequences the one or more that will fold to the target structure. As in IFP, the answer is clearly not unique, given a large assortment of sequences, although the native sequence should certainly be one of the hits. A successful algorithm should be applicable to a broad class of native protein 3D types. The accuracy issue is not so straightforward. Suppose the algorithm ranks sequences according to their suitability for the target structure, which is a globin, for instance. If the target is globin A, and it differs only a little in RMSD from globin B, then is ranking sequence B ahead of sequence A a mistake? Perhaps sequence B is more strongly biased toward the globin folding motif than sequence A is.

One further question of problem definition common to both 3DID and SEQID is the treatment of insertions and deletions. In the same way that permitting indels is essential to the success of sequence alignment algorithms, this is a reasonable feature of SEQID. Without it, one can well expect to identify only the native sequence, even when clearly homologous

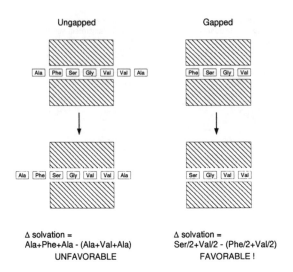

Figure 2: Shifting a strand by one residue as it forms a buried core segment and parts of the adjacent solvated loop regions.

sequences are available for selection. Similarly, it has often been argued that 3DID must select the native structure on the basis of the conserved interior strands (the "core" residues) alone, so that if the assortment of structures to choose from does not happen to include the native, the algorithm will at least recognize some homologous structure. We present the argument in the next section that such a goal for a 3DID algorithm is incompatible with experiment and with the previously stated objectives of the problem. In any case, we have strictly considered 3DID without gaps of any sort.

2   Misconceptions

There are some persistent myths in the protein folding field shared by many. The first is that 3DID is easy to solve, and that several different approaches have already solved it. The fact is that the problem is rather hard if the criteria for success are high, but it can always be trivialized by relaxing the standards. One should keep in mind the numbers and structural diversity of the alternative conformations compared to the native. It is quite easy to discriminate against a few tens of alternatives, or even hundreds, particularly if they are all clustered near the native in conformation or all are near each other but far away from the native. When there are 10^4 or even 10^6 alternatives taken from all over the structures in the Protein Data Bank, the problem is qualitatively different. When the native must be recognized as the single best structure for many natives, the problem is much more demanding than asking that it be statistically outstanding.

The second myth is that a method adapted from statistical mechanics is essential for success in 3DID. Both the Boltzmann distribution approach of Sippl et al. [5] and the spin glass approach of Wolynes et al. [4] view a collection of alternative conformations derived from PDB as an ensemble of conformational states resulting from the energy function that will be subsequently used as the ranking potential in 3DID. As a heuristic, these approaches

Table 1: Residue-residue contact contributions for some protein crystal structures, broken down according to core and loop interactions.

Protein	% of Total Potential Value		
(PDB code)	Core-Core	Core-Loop	Loop-Loop
1sn3	42.1	44.1	13.7
351c	72.0	10.5	17.5
1ubq	65.5	30.9	3.7
1hoe	86.8	18.5	−5.4
5cyt.R	40.1	36.5	23.4
5cpv	35.7	42.4	21.9

have been empirically validated by producing reasonably successful potentials. However, since PDB structures or fragments of them neither sample all polypeptide conformational possibilities nor are in equilibrium with each other, one cannot take the underlying physical theory too seriously. In particular, the fact that the associated physical theory may produce a potential with units of energy, does not necessarily lend it more validity. In 3DID, the distribution of energies of the alternatives is irrelevant; the only thing that counts is that the native is more favored than any alternative. If that is not true, the method doesn't solve the problem. If it is true, the method does solve the problem regardless of the shape of the distribution of the alternatives.

The third myth reasons that since 3DID and SEQID both deal with the compatibility of sequence and structure, an algorithm that solves one must necessarily solve the other. To paraphrase Sippl's argument [5] against this common error, think of the potential function $f(x, y)$, where x is sequence and y is structure, expressed in some sort of parameterization. If f solves 3DID, then $f(x_i, y)$ always has its *global* minimum at $y = y_i$, where x_i and y_i are the native sequence and native structure for protein i=1,2,...,1000. Alternatively if f solves SEQID, then $f(x, y_i)$ always has its global minimum at x_i for all i. There is absolutely no mathematical reason in the world that the first property of f implies the second, or vice versa. For example, $f(x_i, y)$ might have its global minimum at y_i for a particular protein i, but the global minimum of $f(x, y_i)$ can easily be $x = x_j$. Now this does leave open the possibility that one could devise some $f(x, y)$ that handles both problems, although success so far has been limited [2]. We view this as a dubious undertaking because while we do know the native structure for a few sequences and that these sequences do not fold to other structures, we don't know what sequence most prefers a given structure. Empirical as these potentials may be, at least they are trying to mimic a property of the real free energy in 3DID, and there are experimental data to compare with. In SEQID, there is no corresponding physical energy, nor corresponding experimental process like protein refolding.

The fourth myth has it that gapped alignment is an essential feature of any 3DID method. As we have recently summarized elsewhere [6], our potential solves the ungapped 3DID for practically all proteins in PDB compared with literally millions of alternatives. Furthermore, it correctly disfavors a fragment taken out of context, such as one chain of a multimeric complex or a postprocessed protein locked into the conformation favored by its pro-protein by disulfide

Table 2: For compact globular proteins having n residues, the minimal radius of gyration is R. If two such structures have $D = 3$ Å, then the corresponding values of ρ are shown; if instead they have $\rho = 0.26$, then the corresponding D values are shown.

n	R (Å)	ρ	D (Å)
25	6.90	0.45	1.77
50	9.02	0.34	2.31
100	11.69	0.26	3.00
200	15.06	0.20	3.86
400	19.30	0.16	4.95

bonds. In particular it treats proteins having more than one polypeptide chain as well as those having only one. Having thus reached a high level of confidence with our potential, consider what gapped structure identification looks like to it. The isolated core segments are supposed to prefer their relative positions taken from the native structure over any other arrangement, even more compact ones. Breaking the chain in a few places within a domain and removing many residues, even those on the surface, would almost certainly prevent the remaining fragments from folding up as they did before. Why should anyone expect a potential to correctly agree with so many experimental facts and then give a bogus result that violates common experience in protein chemistry? These potentials are indeed empirical, but in some sense they have assimilated a lot of knowledge about protein folding.

A second way to look at this last myth is that introducing gaps adds degrees of freedom to the calculation that a real protein doesn't have. When different members of a homologous series of proteins fold to similar core structures except for the positioning of their different surface loops, alternative placements for all the residues must be taken into consideration, and the native fold is the most favorable structure each sequence can choose. In the corresponding calculations, when we introduce gaps into the native sequence and/or gaps into the structures we are comparing, some residues and their interactions with the rest of the protein effectively disappear. This can lead to the curious result of a nonnative gapped alignment of the native sequence onto the native structure being preferred over the native alignment.

3   Gapped 3DID

Lathrop, Smith, and coworkers have been examining the gapped 3DID problem using pairwise interaction potentials [7]. Assuming the native structure must be recognizable from the interactions between residues in the structural core (as opposed to core-loop or loop-loop interactions), they represent each native globular protein by only a set of core strands, determined by an examination of the crystal structure. For example, for sea snake neurotoxin (1sn3) these are chosen to be residues 1–4 (extended), 23–32 (helix), 37–41 (extended), and 46–50 (extended) [8]. Then the given native sequence is presented with the native structure's core strands and the cores of any other known protein structures such that the sum of the residues in the core does not exceed the length of the given sequence. A threading of the sequence onto some core amounts to assigning a contiguous sequence segment of the correct length to each

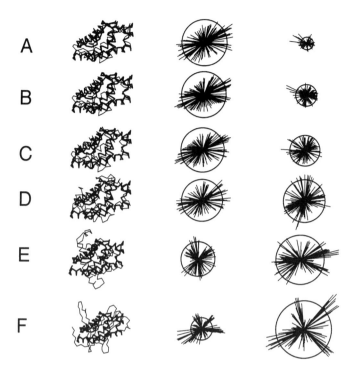

Figure 3: Spatial similarity, sum, and difference structures. The left column shows examples of optimally superimposed polypeptide chains (heavy vs. light lines) which have increasing dissimilarity going from case A to F. The center column shows the corresponding sum structure vectors, s_i and a circle proportional to its radius of gyration, R_s. The right column shows the corresponding difference structure vectors and its radius of gyration.

core structure segment. Each core residue position is used exactly once, each sequence residue is used at most once, and the order of core segments matches the order of used sequence segments. In other words, all the core residue positions are assigned residues, but there will be unassigned sequence residues that effectively vanish.

This formulation of gapped 3DID then amounts to finding the optimal (lowest) potential threading of the given sequence onto all the cores and seeing whether this one is the native alignment of the native sequence onto the native core. Since loop segments have been removed from the structures, there are many ways to thread even the native sequence onto the native core. Using our standard 112 parameter potential, the native threading of the 1sn3 sequence onto its core corresponds to a value of −229.7 arbitrary units [8]. However, a nonnative threading of this sequence onto the same core yields the markedly better score of −395.7 units (sequence segments 5–8, 14–23, 37–41, and 44–48 onto core structure segments 1–4, 23–32, 37–41 and 46–50, respectively). Furthermore, the same sequence prefers some threadings onto the cores of other proteins even more.

We have two explanations for why our potential does so well with ungapped threading and so poorly at gapped threading. The first is the idea that gapped threading allows the calculation of some freedom that the real protein does not have, and our potential has been trained in more realistic comparisons. Suppose the native threading of the native sequence onto the native structure has some residues ...Phe-Ser-X-X-Val-Ala... where the first four residues are in an

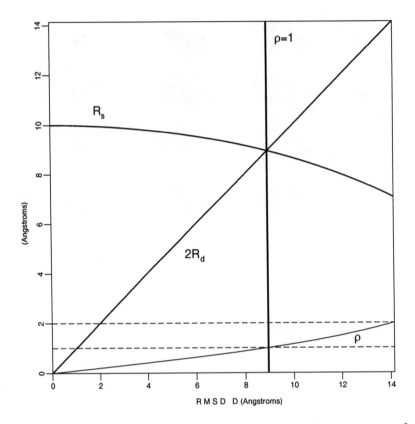

Figure 4: A plot of $2R_d$, R_s, and ρ as a function of D for $R_A = R_B = 9.94\,\text{Å}$.

interior core strand, so that Phe and Ser are buried, but Val and Ala are exposed. Shifting the alignment one residue to the left would expose Phe in exchange for burying Val, which would probably be a net loss in stability for the real protein and for our potential in an ungapped calculation. On the other hand, considering only core strands means that the Phe would be pushed off the end of the strand so that it disappears and no longer interacts with anything, Ser becomes more exposed to solvent, and Val enters the buried core strand, a net favorable move.

Our second explanation questions the assumption that only core-core interactions are important in determining protein folding. Given reasonable assignments of core strands for several proteins [8], we calculated for several native proteins the fractions of the total contact potential values arising from core-core, core-loop, and loop-loop interactions (Table 1). Depending on the protein, core-core interactions accounted for anywhere between 30% and 90% of the stabilization of the native structure. (For 1hoe, the calculated loop-loop interactions are a net destabilization.) Of course, our potential is only an empirical construct that does not necessarily quantitatively translate into free energy, but it is so successful at 3DID that these observations cannot be dismissed out of hand.

4   Conformational Similarity vs. Size

Consider two arbitrary configurations, A and B, each consisting of n points in three-dimensional space. Assume we have numbered the points so that the given correspondence

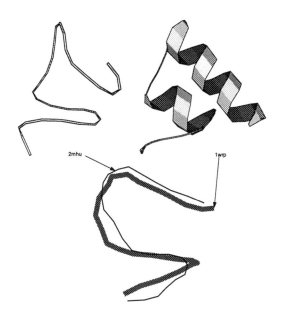

Figure 5: Molscript [13] diagrams for 2mhu and 1wrp in relative orientations corresponding to their optimal superposition. Smoothed C^α tracings show their superposition.

matches point i in A with point i in B for $i = 1, ..., n$. Denote the Cartesian coordinates of the points by $\mathbf{a}_i$ and $\mathbf{b}_i$. Our concern here is the optimal superposition of these matching pairs of points by rigid body translation and rotation of A and B. It is well known that such a superposition requires that the centroids of A and B must coincide [9], so we will assume in all that follows that the centroids of both have already been translated to the origin, i.e. $\sum_i \mathbf{a}_i = \sum_i \mathbf{b}_i = 0$. Then there are many algorithms (see references in [1]) for finding the proper rotation matrix, $\mathbf{R}$, where $\det (\mathbf{R}) = 1$, that minimizes

$$D^2 (A, B) = n^{-1} \sum_i (\mathbf{R}\mathbf{a}_i - \mathbf{b}_i)^2 \tag{1}$$

so that D is the desired RMSD between the two configurations. Now the value of D reflects not only the similarity in relative placement of the points, but also the sizes of A and B and the disparity in their sizes. Let us take as our measure of size the radius of gyration, which can be calculated from either the magnitudes of the center-of-mass coordinate vectors $\mathbf{r}_i$ or the interpoint distances [10] d_{ij}

$$R^2 = n^{-1} \sum_i r_i^2 = n^{-2} \sum_{i<j} d_{ij}^2 \tag{2}$$

Suppose for a moment that A and B are completely similar figures up to a scaling factor f, so that $\mathbf{b}_i = f\mathbf{a}_i$. Then in Eq. (1) the optimal rotation matrix $\mathbf{R} = \mathbf{I}$, the identity matrix, because the steepest descents rotation axis is $\sum_i \mathbf{a}_i \times \mathbf{b}_i = f \sum_i \mathbf{a}_i \times \mathbf{a}_i = 0$. Using this and Eq. (2), Eq. (1) simplifies to $D^2 = (1 - f)^2 R_A^2$. Of course $D = 0$ when $f = 1$, and in the limit of B being much smaller than A, $f \to 0$ and $D \to R_A$. For some fixed value of $f \neq 1$, the magnitude of D is just proportional to R_A, so that judging similarity by a single cutoff in D

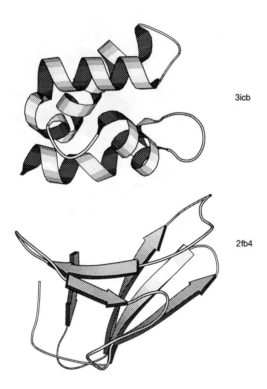

Figure 6: Molscript diagrams for 3icb and 2fb4 in relative orientations corresponding to their optimal superposition.

for all sizes of configurations is clearly inappropriate. At the other extreme of very dissimilar configurations [11],

$$\max_B D^2(A, B) = R_A^2 + R_B^2 \tag{3}$$

It would be preferable to have some measure of dissimilarity that compensated for these simple size effects. Let us start with center of mass coordinates of A and B where A has already been optimally rotated onto B so that Eq. (1) simplifies to

$$D^2 = n^{-1} \sum_i (\mathbf{a}_i - \mathbf{b}_i)^2 \tag{4}$$

which can be expanded and simplified by Eq. (2) to

$$D^2 = R_A^2 + R_B^2 - \frac{2}{n} \sum_i \mathbf{a}_i \cdot \mathbf{b}_i \quad . \tag{5}$$

It is helpful to introduce two artificial configurations: the "sum" or mean structure

$$\mathbf{s}_i = (\mathbf{a}_i + \mathbf{b}_i)/2, \quad i = 1, \ldots, n \tag{6}$$

and the "difference" structure

$$\mathbf{d}_i = (\mathbf{a}_i - \mathbf{b}_i)/2, \quad i = 1, \ldots, n \quad . \tag{7}$$

Since $\mathbf{a}_i = \mathbf{s}_i + \mathbf{d}_i$ and $\mathbf{b}_i = \mathbf{s}_i - \mathbf{d}_i$, we can express $\mathbf{a}_i \cdot \mathbf{b}_i = s_i^2 - d_i^2$, which simplifies Eq. (5) to

$$D^2 = R_A^2 + R_B^2 - 2R_s^2 + 2R_d^2 \qquad (8)$$

where R_s and R_d are the respective radii of gyration of the sum and difference configurations. Since Eq. (4) expresses D in terms of the difference structure, Eq. (7), the definition of the radius of gyration, Eq. (2), results in

$$R_d^2 = D^2/4 \qquad (9)$$

so that Eq. (8) can be rearranged to give

$$2R_s^2 = R_A^2 + R_B^2 - D^2/2 \quad . \qquad (10)$$

As shown in Figures 3 and 4, as one progresses from similar to dissimilar configurations, the sum structure shrinks while the difference structure expands, and the radius of gyration of the difference structure is just proportional to D. As a measure of dissimilarity, we propose a ratio of the radii of gyration of the difference and sum structures, namely

$$\rho = \frac{2R_d}{R_s} = \frac{2D}{(2R_A^2 + 2R_B^2 - D^2)^{1/2}} \quad . \qquad (11)$$

Remembering that D can range from 0 to Eq. (3), we see that $0 \le \rho \le 2$, independent of R_A and R_B (Figure 2). In the case of configurations differing only by a scaling factor f, Eq. (11) reduces to $\rho = 2\,|1 - f|\,/\,|1 + f|$, which is minimal $\rho = 0$ at $f = 1$ and maximal $\rho = 2$ at $f = 0$ or $f \to \infty$. As a matter of mathematical esthetics, we suggest $\rho < 1$ for a size-independent criterion of similarity.

5   Large Scale Similarity in Protein Structures

So far, the configurations A and B have been completely arbitrary arrangements of n points in three-dimensional space, and the comparison assumes the ith point of A is supposed to match the ith point of B. In order to relate ρ to protein conformational studies, we will now identify the ith point with the C^α atom of residue i in an n-residue contiguous polypeptide chain. We will not consider the more complicated matching problem with insertions and deletions.

Traditionally, $D < 2$ to 3 Å has been used as a criterion for spatial similarity of proteins. It turns out to be a substantial error to use such a fixed cutoff in D over the range of protein sizes commonly studied. Earlier we empirically observed [12] that the most compact globular proteins have

$$R = -1.26 + 2.79n^{1/3} \qquad (12)$$

in Å. Then Table 2 shows that if we compare two such compact 100-residue structures and find $D = 3$ Å, this corresponds to $\rho = 0.26$ according to Eq. 11. However, this same 3 Å cutoff in D when applied to all chain lengths amounts to requiring as loose a similarity as $\rho = 0.45$ for short chains or as stringent a similarity as $\rho = 0.16$ for long ones. To put it the other way around, adopting $\rho < 0.26$ as a criterion for obvious spatial similarity implies $D < 1.77$ Å for short chains but only $D < 4.95$ Å for long ones.

If $\rho < 0.2$ to 0.3 corresponds to the subjective consensus in the field for clear conformational similarity of globular proteins, then our proposed $\rho < 1$ test must imply only the most general level of similarity. Consider for example $n = 30$ and residues 1–30 of metallothionine (Brookhaven Protein Data Bank (PDB) entry 2mhu) compared to residues 54–83 of Trp repressor (1wrp, chain "R"). These segments have very similar radii of gyration (8.18 and 7.89

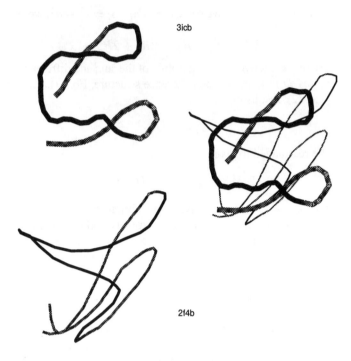

Figure 7: Smoothed C^{α} tracings of 3icb and 2fb4 in one view of the optimal superposition.

Å, respectively), and the optimal superposition gives $\rho = 0.54$, but the superposition matches α-helical segments with coil segments (see Figure 5). The similarity between the two becomes obvious, however, when the C^{α} coordinates are averaged over a 7–residue window sliding up each chain, because this at least straightens out the helical segments.

As a more striking example, residues 1–75 of bovine calcium-binding protein (3icb) form a helical bundle, while residues 9–83 of the FAB immunoglobulin KOL (2fb4, light chain) are β-sheet strands (Fig. 6). Their respective radii of gyration happen to be similar (11.15 and 12.68 Å), and $\rho = 0.76$. Figure 4 shows how their smoothed chain traces are obviously similar to the eye. We have found dozens of similar examples in PDB with such long chain segments, great differences in secondary structure, and yet $\rho < 1$. Clearly helical bundles and sheets are different folding motifs in the usually accepted sense, but from the broader perspective of $\rho < 1$, there may be a very limited number of different ways to pack a polypeptide chain up into an approximately spherical globule. Whether this is just a geometric restriction on curved lines in three-dimensional space or whether this says something special about protein folding, remains to be seen.

Acknowledgements

This work was supported by a grant from the Office of the Vice President for Research of the University of Michigan. We are indebted to all those who deposited their structural data into the Protein Data Bank.

References

[1] Maiorov, V. N. and Crippen, G. M. (1994) Significance of root-mean-square deviation in comparing three-dimensional structures of globular proteins, J. Mol. Biol. 235, 625-634.

[2] Bryant, S. H. and Lawrence, C. E. (1993) An empirical energy function for threading protein sequence, Proteins Struct. Func. Genetics 16, 92-112.

[3] Covell, D. G. and Jernigan, R. L. (1990) Conformations of folded proteins in restricted spaces, Biochemistry 29, 3287-3294.

[4] Goldstein, R. A., Luthey-Schulten, Z. A., and Wolynes, P. G. (1992) Protein tertiary structure recognition using optimized hamiltonians with local interactions, Proc. Natl. Acad. Sci. U. S. A. 89, 9029-33.

[5] Sippl, M. J. (1993) Boltzmann's principle, knowledge-based mean fields and protein folding. An approach to the computational determination of protein structures, J. Comp.-Aided Mol. Design 7, 473-501.

[6] Maiorov, V. N. and Crippen, G. M. (1994) Learning about protein folding via potential functions, Proteins: Struct. Func. Genetics, in press.

[7] Lathrop, R. and Smith, T.F. (1994) A branch and bound algorithm for optimal protein threading with pairwise (contact potential) amino acid interactions, In L. Hunter, (ed.), Proceedings of the 27th Annual Hawaii International Conference on Systems Sciences, Los Alamitos, CA: IEEE Computer Society Press, pp. 365-374.

[8] Buturovic, L. (1994) Personal communication.

[9] Zucker, M. and Somorjai, R.L. (1989) The alignment of protein structures in three dimensions, Bull. math. Biol. 51, 55-78.

[10] Crippen, G.M. and Havel, T.F. (1988) Distance geometry and molecular conformation, In D. Bawden, (ed.), Chemometrics Research Studies Series, Research Studies Press, Ltd. (Wiley) New York.

[11] MaLachlan, A.D. (1979) Gene dublications in the structural evolution of chymotrypsin, J. Mol. Biol. 128, 48-79.

[12] Maiorov, V. N. and Crippen, G. M. (1992) Contact potential that recognizes the correct fold of globular proteins, J. Mol. Biol. 227, 876-888.

[13] Kraulis, P. (1991) MOLSCRIPT: A program to produce both detailed and schematic plots of protein structures, J. Appl. Crystallogr. 24, 946-950.

Protein Folding Studied by Monte Carlo Simulations

Andrej Sali*, Eugene Shakhnovich and Martin Karplus [1]

Dept. of Chemistry, 12 Oxford St, Harvard University, Cambridge, MA 02138, U.S.A.
* Present address: The Rockefeller University, 1230 York Avenue, New York, NY 10021, U.S.A.

Abstract

The number of all possible conformations of a polypeptide chain is too large to be sampled exhaustively. Nevertheless, protein sequences do fold into unique native states in seconds (Levinthal paradox). To determine how the Levinthal paradox is resolved, we use a lattice Monte Carlo model in which the global minimum (native state) is known. The necessary and sufficient condition for folding in this model is that the native state be a pronounced global minimum on the potential surface. This guarantees thermodynamic stability of the native state at a temperature where the chain does not get trapped in local minima. Folding starts by a rapid collapse from a random-coil state to a random semi-compact globule. It then proceeds by a slow, rate-determining search through the semi-compact states to find a transition state close to the native state from which the chain folds rapidly to the native state. The elements of the folding mechanism that lead to the resolution of the Levinthal paradox are the reduced number of conformations that need to be searched in the semi-compact globule ($\approx 10^{10}$ *versus* $\approx 10^{16}$ for the random coil) and the existence of many ($\approx 10^3$) transition states. The results have evolutionary implications and suggest principles for the folding of real proteins.

[1] to whom correspondence should be addressed. Phone: +1 (617) 495 4018, Fax: +1 (617) 496 3204, E-mail: marci@tammy.harvard.edu

1 Introduction

The mechanism of protein folding is not understood, despite many studies devoted to this subject [1, 2, 3, 4]. The essential question is how a polypeptide chain is able to fold rapidly, in ms to s, to the stable native state in spite of the very large number of possible conformations that exist for the chain (Levinthal paradox) [5]. The mechanisms of protein folding are proposed on the basis of conceptual discussions [6, 7, 8, 9], simulations [10, 11, 12, 13, 14], and theory [15, 16, 17]. Theories of protein folding were recently reviewed in references [1, 2, 3, 4, 18, 19, 20, 21, 22, 23, 24, 25, 26, 27, 28].

While the dynamics of the native state can be characterized relatively well by molecular dynamics simulations [29], much less is known about the potential surface governing the non-native portion of conformation space that is involved in protein folding. It includes a wide range of structures which may differ by tens of angstroms. Concomitantly, instead of the time scale of picoseconds to nanoseconds that is required for exploring the neighborhood of the native state, the characteristic times corresponding to the motions in the full conformation space are in the nanosecond to second range. The existence of such a separation of time and length scales with fast local motions and slow large-scale motions makes it possible to introduce two simplifying concepts, which can serve as a basis for theoretical work on protein folding. The first simplification is an effective potential or potential of mean force and the second is a discretized description of the polypeptide chain. Both of these concepts are based on the idea of "preaveraging" the small-scale motions to obtain a "coarse grained" model, which can treat a molecule on the time and length scales at which protein folding occurs. This leads to simplified models of proteins that include only a subset of atoms [30] and to discretized conformational space of various lattice models [31, 32, 33] that employ Monte Carlo (MC) dynamics to simulate the kinetics.

Recently, lattice models have been used to address a variety of aspects of the protein folding problem [9, 10, 12, 34, 35, 36, 37, 38, 39, 40, 41, 42, 43, 44, 45]. In one particularly simple class of lattice models, the protein chain is represented as a string of beads on the 2D square lattice [33, 46] or 3D cubic lattice [16]. These models are generally not meant to simulate folding of any particular real amino acid sequence. However, the lattice models do capture the most essential features of proteins, including their heteropolymeric nature and the interactions between sequentially local and distant amino acid residues. Thus, the simple lattice models may be suitable for elucidating overall features of the folding process such as the main stages of folding. The advantages of simple lattice models are that simulations of many sequences are possible and that frequently the global energy minimum can be determined by enumeration.

As the model does not include side chains, the "native" state in the lattice model corresponds to a compact globule with the native fold of a real protein. Such structured globules may correspond to the experimentally observed molten globules, which (although expanded relative to the native state) preserve much of the backbone structure, and whose side chains are free to undergo dihedral angle transitions [47, 48, 49, 50]. Molten globules appear to be a late stage in the folding of some proteins and their formation involves resolution of the Levinthal paradox [48, 50, 51]. For further discussion of the suitability of lattice models to describe real proteins and of MC to represent molecular dynamics, see refs. [4, 38, 52, 53].

In this review, we summarize our results obtained by the use of MC simulations of 27-mer heteropolymers on a cubic lattice. We identified the features of the folding sequences that allow them to fold rapidly into a unique and stable native state [52] and the mechanism by which they achieve this state [12, 54].

---

[1] Abbreviations used: MC, Monte Carlo; 3SRS-mechanism, three-stage random search mechanism.

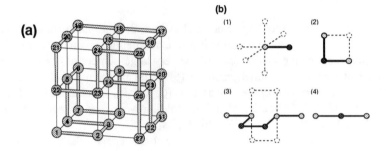

Figure 1: Lattice model of protein folding. *a*, An example of a compact self-avoiding structure of a chain of 27 monomers (filled numbered circles) with 28 contacts (thin lines). The structure shown is the native state of the folding random sequence 43 used as an example in this paper. The total energy of a conformation is the sum of contact energies: $E = \sum_{i<j} \Delta(r_i, r_j) B_{ij}$, where r_i are the positions of monomers i, B_{ij} are the contact energies for pairs of monomers i, j, and $\Delta(r_i, r_j)$ is 1 if monomers i and j are in contact and is 0 otherwise; two monomers are in contact if they are not successive in sequence and are at unit distance from each other. The values of the B_{ij} are obtained from a Gaussian distribution with a mean B_o and standard deviation σ_B. This particular model for B_{ij} corresponds to a heteropolymer with a random sequence of monomers of many different types whose heterogeneity is measured by σ_B [15]. The parameter B_o is an overall attractive term that emulates the hydrophobic effect observed in globular proteins. A particular *sequence* is defined by the matrix of contact energies B_{ij}. In terms of their magnitude and standard deviation, the B_{ij}'s correspond to the contact energies in real proteins [52], such as those described by Miyazawa and Jernigan[72]. The *native* conformation is the compact self-avoiding chain with the lowest energy. *b*, The three types of possible MC moves (1–3). Situation 4 shows a conformation where no move of the central monomer is possible. The current conformation is shown in thick lines. Possible new conformations are shown in dashed lines. A move is possible if all new positions are unoccupied. The monomers that are being moved are shown in dark gray.

2   Methods

We use a simplified model that consists of a 27-bead self-avoiding chain on a cubic lattice [10] (Figs. 1 and 2). The native (lowest-energy) state can be determined exactly [10] and a survey of the folding behavior of many sequences is possible [52]. In addition, the full phase space density of the system (Fig. 6) [12, 54] can be obtained and the thermodynamic properties can be calculated as a function of the folding "reaction coordinate" (Fig. 7) [12, 54]. The model is sufficiently complex that the Levinthal paradox exists: *i.e.*, some sequences find the native state in only $\approx 10^7$ MC (MC) steps even though there are $\approx 10^{16}$ possible conformations (Fig. 6b).

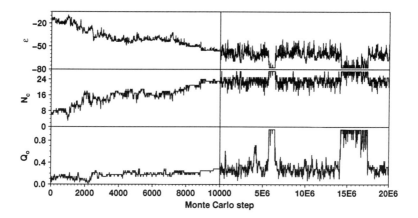

Figure 2: Typical trajectory for a folding random sequence ($T = 1.3$). Energy, ϵ (in units of k_BT); the number of contacts, N_c; fraction of the number of contacts in common with the native state, Q_o. The instantaneous values of these quantities are plotted every 10 MC steps in the first part of the trajectory (≤ 10000 MC steps) and every 20000 steps in the subsequent part. The folding trajectory starts with a random-coil conformation and consists of local MC moves described in Fig. 1b[52]; one MC step corresponds to a move and a test of its acceptance with the Metropolis criterion[73]. In the first part of the trajectory, $\approx 50\%$ of the MC moves are accepted, while only 5–10% of the moves are successful in the subsequent part of the simulation.

3 Results and Discussion

3.1 A pronounced energy minimum is necessary and sufficient for rapid folding to a stable native state

In the first part of the analysis, 200 sequences with random interactions were generated and subjected to MC folding simulations (Fig. 3) [52]. Of these, 30 chains found the known native state in a short time. These chains correspond to actual protein sequences in the present model; the remaining sequences, which do not fold, do not correspond to protein sequences and serve as controls. The 30 folding sequences were analyzed and compared with the non-folding sequences. Several suggested mechanisms for resolving the Levinthal paradox do not apply to the present model; *i.e.*, the features assumed to be responsible for rapid folding in these mechanisms are found to be the same for the folding and non-folding sequences. These include a high number of short *versus* long range contacts in the native state [8], a high content of secondary structure in the native state [7], a strong correlation between the native contact map and the interaction parameters [31], and the existence of a high number of low energy states with near-native conformations [10]. Moreover, there is no repetitive trapping of the non-folding sequences in the same local minimum, so that the native state cannot be a metastable state [55]. The only significant difference between the folding and non-folding sequences is that the native state is at a pronounced energy minimum (Fig. 3). This is the necessary and sufficient condition for a sequence to fold rapidly in the present model (Fig. 4). It is necessary because no sequences without a pronounced energy minimum fold to the native state and it is sufficient because all sequences with such a minimum do fold.

An essential element of the study was to examine a large number of sequences and separate

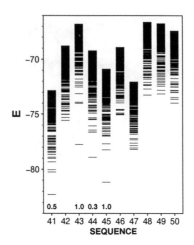

Figure 3: Energy spectra for 10 folding and non-folding random sequences. The energies of the 400 lowest compact self-avoiding conformations are shown. The native state corresponds to the bottom bar. The numbers below the spectra show the foldicities of the corresponding sequences; if no number is given, foldicity is 0. A sequence *folds* in a given MC simulation if it finds the native conformation within $50 \cdot 10^6$ MC steps. *Foldicity* of a given sequence is defined as the fraction of 10 MC runs that started with a random conformation and reached the native conformation under a given set of conditions. A sequence is a *folding sequence* if the native conformation is structurally unique and foldicity is high (≥ 0.4) under conditions where the native structure is thermodynamically stable. A sequence is a *non-folding sequence* if the foldicity is 0.0. There are 24 intermediate sequences that we do not consider here. Optimal values for parameters B_o (-2) and σ_B (1) were determined by exhaustive sampling of foldicity as a function of these two parameters[52]. Each sequence is studied at a temperature, T_x, slightly above the midpoint of the folding transition[52]. An order parameter that describes a transition of a chain from a degenerate state with many backbone conformations to a state with few, possibly only one, backbone conformation is $X(T) = 1 - \sum_i^M p_i^2$, where $p_i = \exp(-\frac{\epsilon_i}{k_B T})/Z$ and $Z = \sum_i^M \exp(-\frac{\epsilon_i}{k_B T})$. k_B is the Boltzmann constant set to 1 in this study, p_i is the Boltzmann probability for a system to be in state i, M is the number of all compact self-avoiding states, and Z is the configuration partition function of the chain. T_x is defined such that $X(T_x) = 0.8$ where the native state has a weight almost invariably larger than 0.2 relative to other compact-self avoiding conformations.

those that fold from those that do not. Consequently, a temperature at the neighbourhood of T_m, the mid-point of the folding transition, was used to speed up the reaction and save computer time (Fig. 3). Optimization of the folding rate was important to verify that certain sequences did not fold. If folding to the native state were always possible under the simulation conditions, there would not have been any nonfolding sequences and our computer experiment would have failed. Figure 5 shows the temperature dependence of the folding rate over a range where 0 to 50% of the polymers are in the native state at equilibrium. Linear folding kinetics is observed throughout the temperature range; this justifies the use of a relatively high temperature for the folding experiments (Fig. 3).

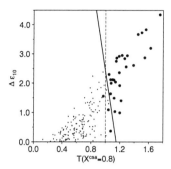

Figure 4: Discrimination between strongly folding (circles) and non-folding sequences (dots). $\Delta\epsilon_{10}$ is the energy gap between the native state and the second most stable compact self-avoiding conformation. T_x is the temperature at which the MC simulations are performed. The larger are $\Delta\epsilon_{10}$ and T_x, the more pronounced the global energy minimum is. The continuous line separates the two groups of sequences by minimizing the number of the folding and non-folding sequences in the non-folding and folding parts of the plot, respectively. The dashed line indicates the critical temperature, defined as the temperature below which almost no folding is observed [52]. T_x is determined for each sequence separately such that the native state had a high probability to be reasonably stable (see Fig. 3) [52].

The reason for the correlation between folding and stability is that significant portions of the potential energy surface of the model system are "rugged". In particular, the random collapsed state that is sampled in the three-stage random search (3SRS) mechanism (see below) is a multiminimum surface on which the search for the native state requires surmounting many intervening barriers. This can be done on a reasonable time scale only if the folding temperature is sufficiently high for there to be a significant probability of overcoming such barriers. However, at a high temperature, the majority of the random sequences have a ground state that is not stable; in other words, the Boltzmann probability of being in any of the excited states is too large unless a sizeable energy gap separates the native state from the excited states. As the temperature at which the folding simulations are done is near the midpoint of the thermodynamic transition temperature between the native and denatured states, the simulation temperature is high enough to overcome the barriers only for the strongly folding sequences with a particularly stable ground state . The transition temperature for the nonfolding sequences is so low that the 27-mer gets trapped in a metastable well. This qualitative argument only explains why the pronounced energy minimum is necessary for folding. The explanation for why it is also sufficient is provided by the 3SRS mechanism discussed below. It is likely that the necessity of the energy gap condition is general for reasonable lattice models and for real proteins, while its sufficiency may be of more limited applicability.

The importance of the temperature in the protein folding reaction and the relation between an energy gap and folding, which are clearly demonstrated by the 27-mer simulations [12, 52], have been discussed previously. Based on statistical mechanical arguments and spin glass theory, Bryngelson and Wolynes [17, 56] suggested that there are two temperatures that need to be considered in determining the folding properties of a sequence. One is the folding

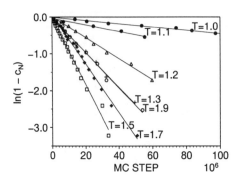

Figure 5: Kinetics of conversion of the denatured state into the native state for sequence 43 as a function of temperature. Kinetics of conversion of the denatured state into the native state for sequence 43 as a function of temperature. For each temperature, the probability, C_N, that the native state is reached in a given number of MC steps is estimated from 100 folding trials. The lines are linear least-squares fits to the points determined at the temperature as indicated on the plot. It can be seen that the results satisfy the simple unimolecular rate equation $dC_N / dt = kC_D$, where k is the rate constant, C_D is the probability of being in the denatured state. The line at $T = 1.0$ is linear in the whole time range explored (up to $400 \cdot 10^6$ MC steps where $C_N \approx 1$).

temperature and the other is the glass transition temperature. They suggested that the glass transition temperature corresponds to the temperature below which the chain is frozen into a random low energy conformation because it does not have enough energy to overcome the barriers separating such conformations. On this basis, they concluded that the temperature at which the sequence folds must be higher than the glass transition temperature. Further, it was shown that random sequences do not satisfy this condition and so would be likely to be trapped in metastable states [17, 56]. Bryngelson and Wolynes introduced specific biases toward the native state to make folding possible. The existence of such biases on the entire potential surface corresponds to the principle of "minimum frustration" [17, 56], which is closely related to the "consistency" or "harmony" principle proposed by Gõ and Abe [57]. One way of introducing the bias is by the use of associative-memory Hamiltonians [58, 59, 60, 61, 62] which have been employed successfully in a variety of applications; e.g., it was shown that the ratio between the folding and glass transition temperatures, whose maximization was assumed to lead to faster folding, is proportional to the ratio of the energetic separation of the native state from the denatured states and the range of energies corresponding to the denatured states [58].

Simulations using other simple lattice models confirmed that the pronounced global energy minimum is associated with rapid folding [38, 40, 63]. An additional confirmation came from the success of designing stable folding sequences by minimizing the energy of a given native state [35, 63, 64, 65].

3.2   Random sequences fold by the three-stage random search mechanism

The insights concerning the role of the temperature and the energy gap provided by the 27-mer computer experiment [52] and theoretical analyses [17] do not, in themselves, provide the specific mechanism by which a model resolves the Levinthal paradox. For this purpose, further examination of the results for the strongly folding sequences in the 27-mer was required [12, 54].

To explore the mechanism of folding, the density of states was determined as a function of the energy and the reaction coordinate (the number of native contacts) (Fig. 6); a related reaction coordinate, the number of residues in the native conformation, has been used previously [17]. If there were a nucleus of a small number of native contacts that would lead rapidly and with high probability to the native state, the fraction of native contacts would not be a good reaction coordinate; instead, the fraction of the contacts present in the nucleus should be used. However, a folding nucleus is not present in the model, confirming that the fraction of native contacts is a suitable reaction coordinate. From the density of states, the mean energy, entropy, and free energy for a given temperature were calculated (Fig. 7). Above the critical temperature ($T_c \approx 1$), the energy and entropy decrease smoothly as the chain approaches the native state. The free energy has a maximum corresponding to the transition region that separates the denatured and native states. This barrier, which makes the reaction a cooperative transition, is dominated by the entropic contribution, as can be seen from the temperature dependence of the free energy. Below the critical temperature, the reaction profile corresponding to the free energy becomes rugged [15, 17] and folding is much slower because the chain is likely to be trapped in one of the many local minima.

Analyses of individual trajectories for both strongly folding and non-folding sequences, as well as the calculated density of states and reaction profiles [12, 54], demonstrated that the sequences in the present model fold according to the three-stage random search (3SRS) mechanism at temperatures above 1.0 (Fig. 8). The time history of the folding process (Fig. 1b) shows that there is a rapid collapse in $\approx 10^4$ MC steps to a semi-compact random globule; *i.e.*, the number of contacts increases, the energy decreases, while the fraction of native contacts remains below 0.3. In this way, the total of $\approx 10^{16}$ random-coil conformations is effectively reduced to $\approx 10^{10}$ random semi-compact globule states. The fast collapse results from a large energy gradient (Fig. 1b) and the presence of many empty lattice points. In the second stage, which is rate limiting, the chain searches for one of the $\approx 10^3$ transition states. The transition region consists of all states from which the chain folds rapidly to the native state. The transition states are structurally similar to the native state, with 23–26 (80–95%) of the native contacts. Generally, the mean first passage time, τ, for finding any of the n states among the total of N states by a random search which explores r states per unit of time is $N/(n \times r)$. For the present model, $\tau \approx 10^{10}/(10^3 \times 1) = 10^7$, identical to the observed time scale. This indicates that the rate limiting stage in folding consists of a random search for a transition state in the semi-compact part of the phase space. In the third stage, the chain rapidly (within $\approx 10^5$ MC steps) attains the native conformation from any one of the transition states. The relationship of each of the three stages in the 3SRS-mechanism to other mechanisms is discussed in reference [4].

The second, rate-limiting stage is "random" in the sense that, over many trajectories, the microscopic states are occupied according to their Boltzmann probabilities and that there are many different microscopic states with comparable Boltzmann probabilities at the random-coil, random globule, and transition-state stages of folding. There is only a small difference between the folding and random non-folding sequences in the way they explore the phase space at the same absolute temperature. That is, above the glass transition temperature, the folding sequences tend to find their native states no more than an order of magnitude faster

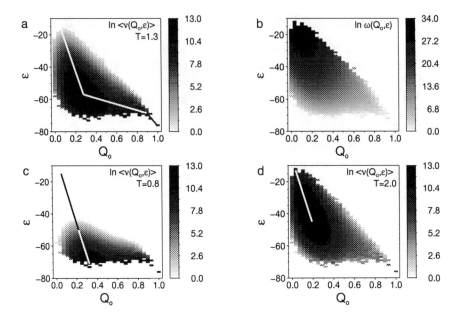

Figure 6: Density of states for a folding random sequence, as obtained from a long MC simulation. *a*, The logarithm of the average occupancy of the (Q_o, ϵ) bins, $\langle \nu(Q_o, \epsilon) \rangle$, at $T = 1.3$. Each bin spans $1/28$ Q_o units and 1 energy unit. The occupancy of a bin is the number of MC steps that remain or result in any of the conformations corresponding to the bin. The average is calculated from 20 independent MC sampling simulations of $50 \cdot 10^6$ steps each [12, 54]. The broken line indicates a typical folding pathway. *b*, The logarithm of the density of states, $\omega(Q_o, \epsilon)$. The density of states is calculated from $\langle \nu(Q_o, \epsilon) \rangle$ by the use of $\frac{\langle \nu(Q_o, \epsilon) \rangle}{\langle \nu(Q_o=1, \epsilon=\epsilon_o) \rangle} = \frac{\omega(Q_o, \epsilon)}{\omega(Q_o=1, \epsilon=\epsilon_o)} \frac{\exp[-\epsilon/(k_B T)]}{\exp[-\epsilon_o/(k_B T)]}$ where ϵ_o is the energy of the native state and k_B is the Boltzmann constant set to 1; because $\omega(Q_o = 1, \epsilon = \epsilon_o) = 1$, the density of states is $\omega(Q_o, \epsilon) = \frac{\langle \nu(Q_o, \epsilon) \rangle}{\langle \nu(1, \epsilon_o) \rangle} \exp(-\frac{\epsilon_o - \epsilon}{k_B T})$. The calculation is accurate because thermodynamic equilibrium at the present Q_o, ϵ resolution is achieved, as demonstrated by a small fractional error in $\langle \nu(Q_o, \epsilon) \rangle$ (less than 10% in the populated parts of the phase space). The summation of $\omega(Q_o, \epsilon)$ over all Q_o and ϵ results in $\approx 1.1 \cdot 10^{16}$ self-avoiding chains; this is in good agreement with the extrapolation of the exact enumerations for shorter chains: $\nu^{L-1}/12 = 2.2 \cdot 10^{16}$ where L is the number of monomers, $\nu = 4.68$ is the average number of monomer states, and division by 12 corrects for symmetry [74]. Semi-compact states are defined as the states with energy less than $-45k_B T$; summation over the appropriate region of $\omega(Q_o, \epsilon)$ yields $\approx 10^{10}$ such states. The transition states correspond to all the states with $0.8 \leq Q_o < 1$; there are $\approx 10^3$ such states. *c*, The average occupancy of the bins at a low T ($T = 0.8$) as calculated from $\omega(Q_o, \epsilon)$. The line shows the rapid collapse of a random coil chain into a random semi-compact frozen conformation. *d*, The calculated average occupancy of the bins at a high T ($T = 2.0$). The line shows a rapid collapse of the random coil chain into a region consisting of many interconverting semi-compact random states; the ground state is no longer stable so the chain spends most of its time in the entropically favored denatured states. In contrast, at $T = 1.0$, the native state occurs for $\approx 40\%$ of the time while still being kinetically accessible.

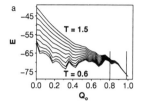 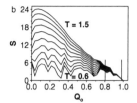 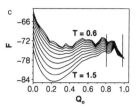

Figure 7: Reaction profiles as a function of the reaction coordinate for the folding random sequence at $0.6 \leq T \leq 1.5$. *a*, Energy, E. *b*, Entropy, S. *c*, Free energy, F. The transition state lies between the two vertical lines at $0.83 \leq Q_o \leq 0.96$. Profiles are calculated in temperature intervals of 0.1, using the partition function $Z(Q_o, T) = \sum_\epsilon \omega(Q_o, \epsilon) \exp(-\epsilon/kT)$. $E(Q_o, T) = \sum_\epsilon \omega(Q_o, \epsilon) \, p_\epsilon \, \epsilon$, $p_\epsilon = \exp(-\epsilon/k_B T)/Z(Q_o, T)$, $F(Q_o, T) = -k_B T \ln Z(Q_o, T)$, and $S(Q_o, T) = [E(Q_o, T) - F(Q_o, T)]/T$.

than the non-folding sequences [40, 52, 54]. However, in the neighbourhood of T_m, the midpoint of the folding transition, the non-folding sequences fold much slower. This is clearly different from the funnel hypothesis of protein folding which assumes that folding sequences fold because they have a single large folding funnel leading to the native conformation and that non-folding sequences do not fold because they have multiple pathways leading to several conformations [11].

The pronounced energy minimum is the necessary condition for the folding of a 27-mer on a lattice because it guarantees that the native state is stable above the critical temperature, where the rearrangements required in the rate limiting stage are energetically possible. It is also a sufficient condition because a random search of compact globules with random structures can rapidly find a transition state that folds to the stable native state in a short time. While a non-folding sequence may also fold slowly to its native state above the critical temperature, it would not be stable and, therefore, could not correspond to a real protein.

Surfaces can be constructed for which resolution of the Levinthal paradox is trivial (*e.g.*, a smooth descent to an energy minimum [57], or only local interactions stabilizing the native state [66], as in the helix-coil transition). However, this does not obviate the fact that the large size of the configuration space is a necessary condition for a paradox to exist. The 27-mer model satisfies this condition with 10^{16} configurations, while short oligomers that have been extensively studied on a two-dimensional square lattice [14, 38, 39, 46] may not; for example, in reference [46], simulations involving more than 10^5 MC steps were used to fold a 13-mer on a square lattice that has only $\approx 4 \cdot 10^4$ conformers. As was pointed out previously, the shape of the configuration space, as well as the number of conformers, is important [11, 52, 66]. The landscape of the 27-mer is clearly sufficiently complex to have a Levinthal paradox; otherwise all sequences would have folded rapidly to the stable native state.

The size of the search for the native state is greatly reduced when the chain is semi-compact as it is in real proteins [67]. Nevertheless, in the 27-mer model as in real proteins, a random search of a collapsed globule cannot find the native state in the observed time. It is the existence of a transition region, consisting of a large number of states, that reduces the search time to realistic values when combined with the search of the random compact

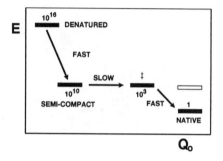

Figure 8: Three-stage random search mechanism of folding for the present model (see text). The numbers of the states were obtained from figure 6. The relative rates are obtained from 100 folding simulations (Fig. 2). The empty rectangle indicates the energy of the native state of a non-folding sequence; in the non-folding sequence, the ground state would not be populated at a temperature sufficiently high to avoid being trapped as in figure 6c. The other states of a non-folding sequence appear at essentially the same positions as the corresponding states of a folding sequence. It can be estimated that a real protein of 80 residues has $2.57^{79} \approx 10^{32}$ possible mainchain conformations of which $1.7^{79} \approx 10^{18}$ are semi-compact[67]. The number of the transition states can be extrapolated from a 27-mer as follows. In a 27-mer, 10^3 out of the 10^{10} semi-compact states are transition states; thus, in an 80-residue protein, approximately 10^6 out of the 10^{18} semi-compact states are likely to be transition states. According to a molecular dynamics simulation of native hydrated myoglobin at 300 K[75], there are 52 mainchain dihedral angle changes per 153 residues per 100 ps or 3 transitions per residue in 1 ns; conformational transitions in the semi-compact state are likely to be faster. Use of these numbers for an 80 residue protein that folds by the three-stage mechanism yields a rate determining step of 10^{12} transitions which would correspond to a folding time to a molten globule state of about 3 sec. This is close to the time scale observed in real proteins.

globule. Extrapolation of the folding time to real proteins suggests that the 3SRS-mechanism could be effective for small proteins (Fig. 8). However, the mechanism breaks down for long chains because the folding time is expected to increase exponentially with chain length; *i.e.*, the number of semi-compact states increases faster than the number of the transition states. Thus, a modification of the present mechanism is required for larger proteins.

It is likely that proteins existing early in evolution were small enough to fold according to the 3SRS-mechanism[68]. Since the pre-biotic and early biotic environment was hot, unusually thermostable proteins were required, such as those found in the most primitive bacteria that live at temperatures as high as 105°[69]. If so, the stability condition required a native state that is a very low energy minimum for which the folding problem was solved simultaneously. As evolution progressed, longer proteins evolved. These proteins had to fold on the same time scale. One way of achieving this is by evolving proteins with sequences that have a larger difference between the native and non-native contact energies than the random folding sequences of the present model. Such sequences would have an even more pronounced global minimum in their potential surfaces, in line with the "consistency principle" [57] and the "principle of minimal frustration" [56]. It is also in accord with the existence of a nucleus for folding [8], or the early appearance of secondary structural elements [7, 70], neither of which are found in the folding sequences of the present model. As a result, the collapse would not result in random semi-compact globules and the very favorable native contacts would lead more directly to a native-like molten globule state; *i.e.*, the folding pathway in figure 6a would approximate a straight line from the random-coil to the "native state". Such a mechanism has been observed in folding simulations of long chains with highly stable native states [13, 34, 71]. Actual proteins could use an intermediate mechanism that might vary with the external conditions.

The results of this study may have implications for the prediction of the structure of a protein from its amino acid sequence. The success of the 3SRS-mechanism in finding the pronounced global minimum on a potential surface suggests, at least for small proteins, that the bottleneck in structure prediction may be the derivation of a suitable potential function rather than the design of folding algorithms.

Acknowledgements

We are grateful to Aaron Dinner, Daša Šali, Oleg Ptitsyn, Alexander Gutin, Georgios Archontis, Amedeo Caflisch, Oren Becker, and Lloyd Dimitrius for discussions concerning the protein folding problem. A.Š. was a Fellow of The Jane Coffin Childs Memorial Fund for Medical Research. This investigation has been aided by a grant from The Jane Coffin Childs Memorial Fund for Medical Research (A.Š.), by David and Lucille Packard Fellowship (E.S.), and by a grant from the National Science Foundation and a gift from Molecular Simulations Inc. (M.K.). The computations were done on IBM RS/6000, Silicon Graphics Iris 4D, SUN Sparcstation, DEC Decstation, DEC Alphastation, and NeXT workstations.

References

[1] T. E. Creighton (ed.), *Protein Folding*, W.H. Freeman and Company, New York, 1992.

[2] K. Merz Jr. and S. Le Grand (eds.), in *The Protein Folding Problem and Tertiary Structure Prediction*, Birkhäuser, Boston, 1994.

[3] M. Karplus and E. Shakhnovich, Protein folding: Theoretical studies of thermodynamics and dynamics, p. 127–196. In T. E. Creighton (ed.), *Protein Folding*, W.H. Freeman and Company, New York, 1992.

[4] M. Karplus and A. Šali, Theories of protein folding, *Curr. Opin. Struct. Biol. in press*

[5] C. Levinthal, How to fold graciously, in *Mossbauer Spectroscopy in Biological Systems*, Proceedings of a Meeting held at Allerton House, Monticello, IL, P. Debrunner, J. C. M. Tsibris and E. Münck (eds.), University of Illinois Press, Urbana, p. 22–24, 1969.

[6] M. Karplus and D. L. Weaver, Protein folding dynamics: The diffusion-collision model and experimental data, *Prot. Science*, 3, p. 650–668, 1994.

[7] P. Kim and R. Baldwin, Intermediates in the folding reactions of small proteins, *Ann. Rev. Biochem.*, 59, p. 631–660, 1990.

[8] D. B. Wetlaufer, Nucleation, rapid folding, and globular intrachain regions in proteins, *Proc. Natl. Acad. Sci. USA*, 70, p. 697–701, 1973.

[9] K. M. Fiebig and K. A. Dill, Protein core assembly process *J. Chem. Phys.*, 98, p. 3475–3487, 1993.

[10] E. Shakhnovich, G. Farztdinov, A. M. Gutin and M. Karplus, Protein folding bottlenecks: A lattice Monte Carlo simulation, *Phys. Rev. Lett.*, 67, p. 1665–1668, 1991.

[11] P. E. Leopold, M. Montal and J. N. Onuchic, Protein folding funnels: A kinetic approach to the sequence-structure relationship, *Proc. Natl. Acad. Sci. USA*, 89, p. 8721–8725, 1992.

[12] A. Šali, E. I. Shakhnovich and M. Karplus, How does a protein fold?, *Nature*, 369, p. 248–251, 1994.

[13] V. I. Abkevich, A. M. Gutin and E. I. Shakhnovich, Specific nucleus as the transition state for protein folding: Evidence from the lattice model, *Biochem.*, 33, p. 10026–10036, 1994.

[14] C. J. Camacho and D. Thirumalai, Kinetics and thermodynamics of folding in model proteins, *Proc.Natl.Acad.Sci. USA*, 90, p. 6369–6372, 1993.

[15] E. I. Shakhnovich and A. M. Gutin, Formation of unique structure in polypeptide chains. Theoretical investigation with the aid of a replica approach, *Biophys. Chem.*, 34, p. 187–199, 1989.

[16] E. I. Shakhnovich and A. M. Gutin, Implications of thermodynamics of protein folding for evolution of primary sequences, *Nature*, 346, p. 773–775, 1990.

[17] J. D. Bryngelson and P. G. Wolynes, Intermediates and barrier crossing in a random energy model (with applications to protein folding), *J. Phys. Chem.*, 93, p. 6902–6915, 1989.

[18] A. Caflisch and M. Karplus, Molecular dynamics studies of protein and peptide folding and unfolding, *The protein folding problem and tertiary structure prediction*, K. Merz Jr. and S. Le Grand (eds.), Birkhäuser, Boston, p. 193–230, 1994.

[19] H. Frauenfelder and P. G. Wolynes, Biomolecules: Where the physics of complexity and simplicity meet, *Physics Today*, 47, p. 58–64, 1994.

[20] V. Daggett and M. Levitt, Protein folding — unfolding dynamics, *Curr. Opin. Struct. Biol.*, 4, p. 291–295, 1994.

[21] K. A. Dill, Folding proteins: finding a needle in a haystack, *Curr. Opin. Struct. Biol.*, 3, p. 99–103, 1993.

[22] H. S. Chan and K. A. Dill, The protein folding problem, *Physics Today*, 46, p. 24–32, 1993.

[23] G. D. Rose and T. P. Creamer, Protein folding: predicting predicting, *Proteins*, 19, p. 1–3, 1994.

[24] G. D. Rose and R. Wolfenden, Hydrogen bonding, hydrophobicity, packing and protein folding, *Annu. Rev. Biophys. Biomol. Struct.*, 22, p. 381–415, 1993.

[25] K. A. Dill and D. Stigter, Modeling protein stability as heteropolymer collapse, *Adv. Prot. Chem.*, in press 1995.

[26] M. Levitt, Protein folding, *Curr. Opin. Struct. Biol.*, 1, p. 224–229, 1991.

[27] R. A. Abagyan, Towards protein folding by global energy optimization, *FEBS Lett.*, 325, p. 17–22, 1993.

[28] J. Skolnick, A. Kolinski and A. Godzik, From independent modules to molten globules: Observations on the nature of protein folding intermediates, *Proc. Natl. Acad. Sci. USA*, 90, p. 2099–2100, 1993.

[29] C. L. Brooks III, M. Karplus and B. M. Pettit, *Proteins: A Theoretical Perspective of Dynamics, Structure and Thermodynamics*, John Wiley & Sons, New York, 1988.

[30] M. Levitt and A. Warshel, Computer simulation of protein folding, *Nature*, 253, p. 694–698, 1975.

[31] N. Gō and H. Abe, Noninteracting local-structure model of folding and unfolding transition in globular proteins. II Application to two-dimensional lattice proteins, *Biopolymers*, 20, p. 1013–1031, 1981.

[32] J. Skolnick and A. Kolinski, Simulations of the folding of a globular protein, *Science*, 250, p. 1121–1125, 1990.

[33] K. F. Lau and K. A. Dill, A lattice statistical mechanics model of the conformational and sequence spaces of proteins, *Macromolecules*, 22, p. 3986–3997, 1989.

[34] V. I. Abkevich, A. M. Gutin and E. I. Shakhnovich, Free energy landscape for protein folding kinetics: Intermediates, traps, and multiple pathways in theory and lattice model simulations, *J. Chem. Phys.*, 101, 6052, 1994.

[35] S. Ramanathan and E. Shakhnovich, Statistical mechanics of proteins with "evolutionary selected" sequences, *Physical Review E*, 50, p. 1303–1312, 1994.

[36] A. Dinner, A. Šali, M. Karplus and E. Shakhnovich, Phase diagram of a model protein derived by exhaustive enumeration of the conformations, *J. Chem. Phys.*, 101, p. 1444–1451, 1994.

[37] J. T. Ngo, J. Marks and M. Karplus, Computational complexity, protein structure prediction, and the Levinthal paradox, *The Protein Folding Problem and Tertiary Structure Prediction*, K. Merz Jr. and S. Le Grand (eds.), Birkhäuser, Boston, p. 433–506, 1994.

[38] H. S. Chan and K. A. Dill, Transition states and folding dynamics of proteins and heteropolymers, *J. Chem. Phys.*, 100, p. 9238–9257, 1994.

[39] C. J. Camacho and D. Thirumalai, Minimum energy compact structures of random sequences of heteropolymers, *Phys. Rev. Lett.*, 71, p. 2505–2508, 1993.

[40] N. D. Socci and J. N. Onuchic, Folding kinetics of proteinlike heteropolymers, *J. Chem. Phys.*, 101, p. 1519–1528, 1994

[41] E. M. O'Toole, Effect of sequence and intermolecular interactions on the number and nature of low-energy states for simple model proteins, *J. Chem. Phys.*, 98, p. 3185–3190, 1993.

[42] A. Kolinski and J. Skolnick, Monte Carlo simulations of protein folding. I Lattice model and interaction scheme. *Proteins*, 18, p. 338–352, 1994.

[43] D. A. Hinds and M. Levitt, Exploring conformational space with a simple lattice model for protein structure, *J. Mol. Biol.*, 243, p. 668–682, 1994.

[44] D. G. Covell, Lattice model simulations of polypeptide chain folding, *J. Mol. Biol.*, 235, p. 1032–1043, 1994.

[45] M. - H. Hao and H. A. Scheraga, Monte Carlo simulation of a first-order transition for protein folding, *J. Phys. Chem.*, 98, p. 4940–4948, 1994.

[46] R. Miller, C. A. Danko, M. J. Fasolka, A. C. Balazs, H. S. Chan and K. A. Dill, Folding kinetics of proteins and copolymers, *J. Chem. Phys.*, 96, p. 768–780, 1992.

[47] O. B. Ptitsyn, Protein folding: Hypotheses and experiments, *J. Prot. Chem.*, 6, p. 273–293, 1987.

[48] M. Harding, D. Williams and D. Woolfson, *Biochemistry*, 30, p. 3120–3128, 1991.

[49] E. I. Shakhnovich and A. V. Finkelstein, Theory of cooperative transitions in protein molecules. I. Why denaturation of globular protein is a first-order phase transition, *Biopolymers*, 28, p. 1667–1680, 1989.

[50] Z. - Y. Peng and P. S. Kim, A protein dissection study of a molten globule, *Biochemistry* 33, p. 2136–2141, 1994.

[51] D. A. Dolgikh, R. I. Gilmanshin, E. V. Brazhnikov, V. E. Bychkova, G. V. Semisotnov, S. Y. Venyaminov and O. B. Ptitsyn, α-lactalbumin: Compact state with fluctuating tertiary structure?, *FEBS Lett.*, 136, p. 311–315, 1981.

[52] A. Šali, E. I. Shakhnovich and M. Karplus, Kinetics of protein folding: A lattice model study of the requirements for folding to the native state, *J. Mol. Biol.*, 235, p. 1614–1636, 1994.

[53] J. Skolnick and A. Kolinski, Dynamic Monte Carlo simulations of a new lattice model of globular protein folding, structure and dynamics, *J. Mol. Biol.*, 221, p. 499–531, 1991.

[54] A. Šali, E. I. Shakhnovich and M. Karplus, Thermodynamics of protein folding: A lattice model study of folding to the native state, *In preparation*.

[55] J. D. Honeycutt and D. Thirumalai, The nature of folded states of globular proteins, *Biopolymers*, 32, p. 695–709, 1992.

[56] J. D. Bryngelson and P. G. Wolynes, Spin glasses and the statistical mechanics of protein folding, *Proc. Natl. Acad. Sci. USA*, 84, p. 7524–7528, 1987.

[57] N. Gō and H. Abe, The consistency principle in protein structure and pathways of folding, *Adv. Biophysics*, 18, p. 149–164, 1984.

[58] R. A. Goldstein, Z. A. Luthey-Schulten and P. G. Wolynes, Optimal protein-folding codes from spin-glass theory, *Proc. Natl. Acad. Sci. USA*, 89, p. 4918–4922, 1992.

[59] M. S. Friedrichs, R. A. Goldstein and P. G. Wolynes, Generalized protein tertiary structure recognition using associative memory Hamiltonians *J. Mol. Biol.*, 222, p. 1013–1034, 1991.

[60] M. S. Friedrichs and P. G. Wolynes, Toward protein tertiary structure recognition by means of associative memory Hamiltonians, *Science*, 246, p. 371–373, 1989.

[61] M. Sasai and P. G. Wolynes, Molecular theory of associative memory Hamiltonian models of protein folding, *Phys. Rev. Lett.*, 65, p. 2740–2743, 1990.

[62] M. Sasai and P. G. Wolynes, Unified theory of collapse, folding, and glass transitions in associative-memory Hamiltonian models of proteins, *Phys. Rev. A*, 46, p. 7979–7997, 1992.

[63] E. I. Shakhnovich, Proteins with selected sequences fold into unique native conformation, *Phys. Rev. Lett.*, 72, p. 3907–3910, 1994.

[64] E. I. Shakhnovich and A. M. Gutin, Engineering of stable and fast-folding sequences of model proteins, *Proc. Natl. Acad. Sci. USA*, 90, p. 7195–7199, 1993.

[65] E. I. Shakhnovich and A. M. Gutin, A new approach to the design of stable proteins, *Prot. Eng.*, 6, p. 793–800, 1993.

[66] R. Zwanzig, A. Szabo and B. Bagchi, Levinthal's paradox, *Proc. Natl. Acad. Sci. USA*, 89, p. 20–22, 1992.

[67] K. A. Dill, Theory for folding and stability of globular proteins, *Biochemistry*, 24, p. 1501–1509, 1985.

[68] E. E. Di Iorio, W. Yu, C. Calonder, K. H. Winterhalter, G. De Sanctis, G. Falcioni, F. Ascoli, B. Giardina and M. Brunori, Protein dynamics in minimyoglobin: Is the central core of myoglobin the conformational domain?, *Proc. Natl. Acad. Sci. USA*, 90, p. 2025–2029, 1993.

[69] K. O. Stetter, Life at the upper temperature border, In *Frontiers of Life*, J. K. Trân Thanh Vân, J. C. Mounolou, J. Schneider, C. McKay (eds.), Editions Frontières, Gif-sur-Yvette, France, p. 195–212, 1992.

[70] M. Karplus and D. L. Weaver, Protein-folding dynamics, *Nature*, 260, p. 404–406, 1976.

[71] A. R. Dinner, A. Šali and M. Karplus, Folding requirements for longer model proteins, *In preparation*.

[72] S. Miyazawa and R. L. Jernigan, Estimation of effective interresidue contact energies from protein crystal structures: Quasi-chemical approximation, *Macromolecules*, 18, p. 534–552, 1985.

[73] N. Metropolis, A. W. Rosenbluth, M. N. Rosenbluth, A. H. Teller and E. Teller, Equation of state calculations by fast computing machines, *J. Chem. Phys.*, 21, p. 1087–1092, 1953

[74] M. F. Sykes, Self-avoiding walks on the simple cubic lattice, *J. Chem. Phys.*, 39, p. 410–412, 1963

[75] R. J. Loncharich and B. R. Brooks, Temperature dependence of dynamics of hydrated

myoglobin. Comparison of force field calculations with neutron scattering data, *J. Mol. Biol.*, 215, p. 439–455, 1990

Folding Kinetics of
Protein Like Heteropolymers

Nicholas D. Socci and José Nelson Onuchic

Department of Physics-0319, University of California at San Diego, La Jolla, California
92093-0319, U.S.A.

Abstract

Using a simple three-dimensional lattice copolymer model and Monte Carlo
dynamics, we study the collapse and folding of proteinlike heteropolymers. The
polymers are 27 monomers long and consist of two monomer types. Although
these chains are too long for exhaustive enumeration of all conformations, it
is possible to enumerate all the maximally compact conformations, which are
$3 \times 3 \times 3$ cubes. This allows us to select sequences that have a unique global
minimum. We then explore the kinetics of collapse and folding and examine
what features determine the various rates. The folding time has a plateau over
a broad range of temperatures and diverges at both high and low temperatures.
The folding time depends on sequence and is related to the amount of energetic
frustration in the native state. The collapse times of the chains are sequence
independent and are a few orders of magnitude faster than the folding times,
indicating a two-phase folding process. Below a certain temperature the chains
exhibit glass-like behavior, characterized by a slowing down of time scales and
loss of self-averaging behavior. We explicitly define the kinetic glass transition
temperature (T_g), and by comparing it to the folding temperature (T_f), we find
two classes of sequences: good folders with $T_f > T_g$ and non-folders with
$T_f < T_g$.

1   Introduction

A great deal of work (both experimental and theoretical) has been done on the kinetics of
protein folding. One extremely useful theoretical technique is to study simple heteropolymer
models. The idea is to reduce the complex system of proteins in solution to its bare essentials,
leaving only the key features. The advantage of studying these simpler models is that an
in-depth analysis (sometimes even an exhaustive one) can be performed, yielding detailed
answers and information. This information should, in turn, provide insights into real proteins.

One class of model that is often used in theoretical polymer work is the lattice model.
Excluded volume is included by allowing only one monomer per site and by choosing a move
set that does not allow bond crossing. To study dynamics, the Monte Carlo algorithm with a
variety of move sets is used. Some of the earliest work using lattice models on proteins was
done by Gō and coworkers [1, 2] using two- and three-dimensional lattices to examine the
folding process. However, the interaction potential they used was somewhat unusual. The
native state was explicitly built into the potential. The energy of any given conformation

was determined by counting the number of native contacts, i.e., contacts found in the native structure. An attractive contribution to the energy was added for each native contact formed. This potential is somewhat unphysical, depending on an *a priori* knowledge of the native structure. Although much of this early work on lattice models was on simple cubic lattices, Skolnick and others [3, 4, 5, 6, 7] have used more complex lattices which are able to more faithfully represent the structure of actual proteins.

Rather than trying to model real proteins exactly, some have opted for simpler models which permit a more thorough analysis. Chan and Dill [8, 9, 10, 11] have used a two-dimensional simple cubic lattice model with two monomer types (a polar monomer, P, and a hydrophobic one, H). They studied short chains, which allowed them to do exhaustive enumeration to measure a variety of properties (both static and dynamic). For dynamics they used both Monte Carlo [9] and transfer matrix methods [10, 11]. By using short polymers, they were able to construct the full transfer matrix (this matrix determines the probability of one state transforming to another) and use it to solve exactly for the dynamics of the system. Although their model is simpler than an actual protein, it has yielded a wealth of interesting information and provided valuable insight into proteins and heteropolymers. Their models show a two-phase process similar to that found in proteins. There is a rapid collapse to compact states, followed by slower reconfiguring of the chains to the native structure. There have been a wealth of other studies for three-dimensional lattice polymer systems [12, 13, 14, 15, 16, 17, 18, 19] indicating the rich and interesting behavior of these systems.

In this work we use the three-dimensional simple cubic lattice model. The polymers will be 27 monomers long and consist of two monomer types. Monte Carlo dynamics will be used to study the collapse and folding kinetics. The chains are too long for exhaustive enumeration of all conformations but are short enough to permit exhaustive enumeration of all maximally compact configurations. This information will be used to determine the minimum energy structure (native state) which will allow us to measure the folding time from extended conformations. We will examine several different sequences and measure collapse and folding time as a function of temperature and sequence. One question to be addressed is which kinetic quantities are sequence dependent and which are sequence independent (*self-averaging*). In addition, we will examine how the glass transition affects the ability of a sequence to fold. A major goal is to define, as precisely as possible, various physically important quantities. Of particular importance will be the determination of the important time scales. One problem with Monte Carlo dynamic simulations is the relation between Monte Carlo steps and physical time. There is no simple connection; in fact, the precise relation may depend on the move set [10, 11]. To circumvent this problem, we will relate Monte Carlo steps to physical time by looking for the natural time scales in the problem, such as the collapse and the folding time. Using these time scales, we will then be able to define a kinetic glass transition temperature (T_g) of this model. In the past others have speculated that the relation between the folding temperature (T_f) and the glass temperature (T_g) would play an important role in protein folding. Bryngelson and Wolynes [20, 21] have proposed that in order for a chain to fold, the folding transition must occur before the glass transition of the system, and the optimal folding temperature would lie between T_f and T_g. Specifically, Wolynes and others state that to optimize folding potentials for structure prediction, one should maximize the ratio of the folding temperature to the glass temperature (T_f/T_g) [22, 23]. To calculate the glass transition, they used a random energy model assumption; i.e., for each given value of the degree of folding, the energies of the different conformation are independent random variables. In our work we will give a direct kinetic definition of the glass temperature that does not rely on this assumption, and show explicitly that the relative values of T_g and T_f will determine the folding properties of a given sequence.

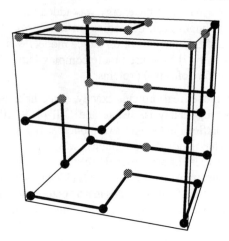

Figure 1: An example 27 length polymer on a three dimensional simple cubic lattice. The conformation is a maximally compact cube. The light and dark spheres represent the two different types of monomers. The sequence shown here is 013 and the conformation shown is the native (minimum energy) state.

2   Model and methods

The model used in this work is a three-dimensional lattice copolymer. Monomers that are connected along the chain are constrained to be nearest-neighbors on the lattice, and only one monomer is allowed per site. (This is the excluded volume condition.) The chain is then a self-avoiding walk on the lattice. The polymers are all 27 monomers long. The maximally compact state is a $3 \times 3 \times 3$ cube (see Fig. 1). It is easy to enumerate all the compact cubes, of which there are 103 346. If we choose a potential that favors the formation of contacts, then the minimum energy conformation will usually be a compact cube. Selecting such a potential enables us to determine the native structure of a given sequence by enumeration of the cubes, since for this simple model the native state is the lowest energy conformation. In addition, the degeneracy of the lowest energy state can be determined. Since we are interested in proteinlike polymers which have a "single" native state,[1] we will choose sequences with a non-degenerate ground state, i.e., those with only one lowest energy conformation.

We want a potential that will favor compact states and cause the chain to fold. The dominant force in protein folding is the hydrophobic effect [24]. This force is a many-body interaction between the hydrophobic side chains and the solvent (water). The main effect is to cause the chain to collapse and create a hydrophobic core. In our simulations we model this effect by using an attractive potential to collapse the chain. This potential favors the formation of contacts between any two monomers. However, we do not want a homopolymer, so the simplest possible interaction energy is dependent on whether the two monomers in contact are

---

[1]When we say a protein has a single native state we are ignoring the different conformations real proteins may have. Our model is too coarse to represent the slight differences between conformations of proteins.

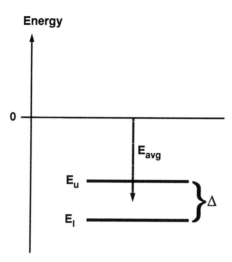

Figure 2: Energy level diagram. E_l and E_u are the contact energies used in specifying the potentials. E_{avg} represents the average drive for forming contacts or compacting the chain. Δ is the splitting in the energy levels and gives the heteropolymer character to the model. $E_l = E_{\mathrm{avg}} - \Delta/2$ and $E_u = E_{\mathrm{avg}} + \Delta/2$.

of the same type or not. The potential energy is given explicitly by

$$E = N_l E_l + N_u E_u, \tag{1}$$

where N_l is the number of contacts between monomers of the same type (like contacts) and N_u the number of contacts between monomers of different types.

Although it is easiest to write the energy function in terms of the E_l, and E_u variables, it is sometimes simpler to understand the behavior of the model by considering an equivalent set of parameters, E_{avg} and Δ, defined as follows:

$$
\begin{aligned}
E_{\mathrm{avg}} &= \frac{1}{2}\left(E_l + E_u\right) \\
\Delta &= \left(E_u - E_l\right).
\end{aligned}
\tag{2}
$$

Figure 2 shows a graphic representation of the two sets of parameters. E_{avg} represents the overall drive toward forming contacts or compacting the chain. If it is less than zero, contact formation will be favored. Δ determines the heterogeneity of the heteropolymer. In the limit that $\Delta = 0$ the model becomes a homopolymer. In this work, $E_{\mathrm{avg}} = -2$ and $\Delta = 2$, giving values -3 and -1 for E_l and E_u respectively.[2] These values insure that the chain will collapse rapidly. relative to the folding time, and that the minimum energy state will be a maximally compact cube for the sequences considered here.

To simulate the dynamics of folding we use a local move set Monte Carlo procedure (the details of which can be found in reference [17]). One must keep in mind that there is no

---

[2]The units of temperature and energy are such that $k_b = 1$. This still leaves an arbitrary scale factor since the only important quantity is the ratio of energy to temperature. I.e., we could have picked -200 and 200 for E_{avg} and Δ, multiplied all temperatures by 100 and the results would be the same. We have chosen small, integer values for convenience.

Table 1: The various sequences used in this paper. The last four (005, 006, 007, 013) were generated at random. Sequence 002 was optimized by Shakhnovich (Ref. [25]). Sequence 004 is a single monomer mutation of 005 ($B_{13} \rightarrow A$). Both 002 and 004 have the lowest energies possible for the potential used and have native states that are completely unfrustrated. $\tau_{\min}$ is the fastest folding time for each sequence. T_g is the glass transition temperature (calculated with a $\tau_{\max} = 1.08 \times 10^9$). T_f is the folding temperature calculated using the Monte Carlo histogram method. The numbers in parenthesis indicate the uncertainty of the last digit.

Run	Sequence	$E_{\min}$	$\tau_{\min}$	T_g	T_f
002	ABABBBBBABBABABABAAABBAAAAAAB	-84	2.0×10^7	1.00	1.285(15)
004	AABAABAABBABAAABABBABABABBB	-84	1.6×10^7	0.96	1.26(1)
005	AABAABAABBABBAABABBABABABBB	-82	2.3×10^7	0.98	1.15(2)
006	AABABBABAABBABAAAABABAABBBB	-80	5.2×10^7	1.07	0.95(6)
007	ABBABBABABABAABABABABBBABAA	-80	9.3×10^7	1.09	0.93(5)
013	ABBBABBABAABBBAAABBABAABABA	-76	9.7×10^7	1.01	0.83(5)

simple and direct connection between Monte Carlo steps and the physically relevant times scales of the system. One important result of this work is that we will determine the mapping between the physically important time scales such as the folding time and the computation time scales (Monte Carlo steps). This will be useful in later works in which we will study the thermodynamics of these systems where it will be necessary to know how long it takes for systems to reach equilibrium and explore conformation space. Once again, the precise connection between physical time (like the folding time) and Monte Carlo steps will depend on the details of the move set used. However, we expect that as long as the moves are chosen with care, that is, one attempts to make it as physically realistic as possible, then the qualitative features will remain the same. For example, the behavior of folding time as a function of temperature will look qualitatively the same although the exact folding time (number of steps) will vary.

3   Results and discussion

We study six sequences, all 27 monomers long. Four were selected by the following procedure. First a sequence was generated at random with the appropriate ratio of monomer types. We then enumerated all cubes, calculating the number of minimum energy states. Sequences with degenerate minimum energy states were rejected. From the remaining non-degenerate sequences we picked four which had a spread in energy of the native states from -82 to -76. One sequence was obtained by changing a single monomer in one of the original four; i.e., it is a single-site mutation, which lowered the ground state energy, from -82 to -84. The last sequence was taken from a paper by Shakhnovich [25] which gave a method for finding optimal sequences; it also has a ground state energy of -84.

Table 1 shows the various sequences along with some data for each. All six sequences have the same ratio of monomer types, roughly 50:50 (14:13, actually). For these simulations the value for the contact energies are -3 for monomers of the same type and -1 for unlike monomers. There are 28 non-covalent or *topological* contacts in the cube conformations, so the lowest possible energy is -84. Two of the sequences have this energy for their

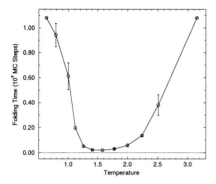
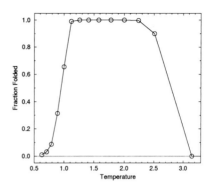

Figure 3: Mean folding times (A, left) and fraction folded (B, right) versus temperature for one sequence (sequence 002). Note all axes are linear scale and the time is in billions of Monte Carlo steps. The error bars (in figure A) are the *standard deviation of the mean*: that is, they are equal to the standard deviation of the folding-time distribution at a given temperature divided by the square root of the number of runs at that temperature. Note that the plateau at which the chains fold 100% of the time occurs at the temperature at which the chains fold the fastest.

minimum conformation. This corresponds to a completely "unfrustrated" ground state. By "unfrustrated" we mean that the ground state has no topological contacts between monomers of different types. The other three sequences have ground state energies higher than -84 and, consequently, their ground states have at least one weak topological contact and consequently are frustrated energetically.

We simulated the folding of these sequences and examined how the folding behavior depended on temperature and differed from sequence to sequence. For each sequence we started with a random, completely unfolded, initial conformation. Here, completely unfolded means that there are no contacts between any of the monomers. A temperature was selected, and the sequence was allowed to fold. Once the sequence found its folded state (which we detected by monitoring the energy), we stopped the simulations. The simulations were also stopped if the sequence did not find its folded state within τ_{max} steps. For the simulations in this work, $\tau_{max} = 1.08 \times 10^9$ Monte Carlo steps. This maximum time was picked both so that it was longer than the typical folding time of most sequences and to minimize the actual computer time used in the simulations. It is important to realize that any times longer than τ_{max} are undefined. Ideally, we would want to pick τ_{max} to be longer than any interesting and relevant physical or biological time scale. Since there is no simple connection between Monte Carlo steps and physical time, we cannot directly determine τ_{max}. We chose a first value for τ_{max} which seemed reasonable and then made sure that it was much longer than the folding time for the various sequences.

At each temperature we ran many simulations, each with a different random initial condition (always unfolded). We then calculated an average folding time (τ_f) from these runs. This time is the mean first passage time from the set of unfolded initial states to the folded state. Figure 3A shows τ_f as a function of temperature. We ran anywhere from 10 to 600 simulations at each temperature and calculated the average folding time. If the folded state was not found within τ_{max} steps, we averaged in τ_{max} for that run. The error bars are the standard deviation of the mean given by $\sigma/\sqrt{N}$, where σ is the standard deviation of the distribution of folding times and N is the number of runs at that temperature. It is important to note that since we average in $\tau_{\max}$ when the chain does not fold, the error bars are not as meaningful at temperatures where the folding time approaches $\tau_{\max}$ and may be much larger at these temperatures. In particular, at high and low temperature the points equal $\tau_{\max}$ with zero error. That is simply due to the fact that at those temperatures the simulations never found the folded state. Figure 3B shows the fraction of times the folded state was found as a function of temperature. We observe three different temperature regions, similar to those found in two-dimensional lattice simulations [9, 11]. Above a temperature of ~ 3 and below $\sim .65$, the chains did not fold within $\tau_{\max}$ steps. Between these temperatures the folding time drops rapidly to approximately 2×10^7–5×10^7. The fraction of runs that find the folded state increases sharply from 0 to 1 in this temperature range. In this middle temperature range there is a maximum plateau in the fraction folded with a minimum plateau in the folding time. At temperatures where the chain folds rapidly, it also finds its native state 100% of the time. The transition from the fast folding regime to the slow folding are fairly sharp in particular the low temperature transition. Note, at temperatures where the simulations did not find the folded state all the time, the τ_f shown in Fig. 3A is a lower bound to the actual mean first passage time since, has previously mentioned, $\tau_{\max}$ was averaged in when the chain did find the native state.

At low temperatures (around $T \approx 1$) the system is beginning to slow down, kinetically, and is now getting trapped in local *meta*-stable states. Even though we expect, at these low temperatures, the free energy to have a very pronounced minimum at the native state, the system is unable to reach it within a reasonable time. This region is often referred to as the glass phase. We can define a temperature at which the system undergoes a kinetic glass transition characterized by the slowing down of various times, such as the folding and compaction times. The autocorrelation time of the system would also increase in this temperature region, indicating that the chain was locally trapped. We define the glass transition temperature (T_g) as the temperature at which the folding time is half way between $\tau_{\max}$ and $\tau_{\min}$ (where $\tau_{\min}$ is the fastest folding time observed). Using this definition we get $T_g \approx 1$. Note that the definition of glass temperature is not the usual thermodynamic definition of temperature. It is not determined by the inverse of the derivative of entropy with respect to energy ($1/T_g = \partial S/\partial E$) at the point where the entropy "vanishes" [26]. A difficulty with this definition is its relation to the kinetics of the system. The idea is that as a system is taken out of equilibrium, the time it takes to relax back will increase as the temperature gets closer to T_g. To avoid this kind of assumption, we have given a kinetic definition for T_g in which we will explicitly look for a slowing down of the system. We would expect the precise value of T_g to depend on the moves used and the choice of $\tau_{\max}$. Therefore we will not focus on the exact value but on some approximate value and a relative comparison of this value for different sequences. Later we will compare T_g to another important temperature, the folding temperature (T_f), and we will discover a key relation between the two. Additionally T_g depends on the value of $\tau_{\max}$; that is, it will depend on how long we run our simulations. This is a subtle but extremely important fact to remember when studying finite sized systems. When talking about glass-like behavior of a finite system the notion of glass-like depends on the time scale you are looking at. If you wait long enough the chain will always find the native state. To speak of a physically meaningful glass transition one must define the physical time scales of interest. The time scales of importance here are related to the minimum folding time of a good folding sequence. We want to examine our system on a time scale that is reasonable greater then the minimum folding time. For our simple system there is no obvious greater time to pick. We picked a time that was roughly two orders of magnitude greater than the fastest folding time observed in this system.

The two regions in which the chain fails to fold are qualitatively very different. At high temperatures the energy differences between conformations becomes negligible so all conformations have roughly equal probabilities. The chain is randomly exploring the conformation space. It takes a long time to find the native state by random search due to the vast number of conformations. The free energy is dominated by the entropic term so the native state is no longer the global minimum. At low temperatures the energy differences between states becomes important and the folded state is the global minimum free energy. The problem now is that the barriers between states are too high and at low temperatures there is a very small probability for crossing them. For compact conformations many moves will involve the breaking of contacts which at low temperatures becomes unlikely. In particular, moves that break more than one contact are much less probable than those that break only one. Instead of a random search the chain is now forced in to a very narrow kinetic pathway consisting of those steps with very small free energy barriers. The chain gets trapped in the many local minima.

If we were willing to wait long enough the system would eventually fold. Since our system is finite, the system always has a finite nonzero probability to find the native state. The same is true for the high-temperature case. However, one must remember that at those temperatures the folded state is not the free energy minimum and is therefore not stable. For example, consider the following two temperatures: 2.24 and 1.12. The folding time for these two temperatures is roughly the same. At the higher temperature (as we will see shortly) the chain spends almost zero time in the folded state (less than 0.04%). At the lower temperature the chain spends roughly 77% of the time in the folded state. When we speak of folding time, this is simply the time it takes the chain to find the native conformation. There is another important factor here: Namely, is the folded state stable thermodynamically? We will address this issue at the end of this paper, where we see that it is not enough that a chain find its native state in a short time, but it must do so at temperatures where the native state is thermodynamically stable.

Let us return to the question of how long is too long to wait for a sequence to fold. Too long is in general determined by other time scales in the system. For proteins, there are a number of biologically relevant time scales, the lifespan of the organism for example. Other more important time-scales would be the aggregation time or the time for proteolysis. In a cell, unfolded proteins (or protein that did not fold fast enough) would be subject to either aggregation or proteolysis. Proteins that do not fold fast enough on these time scale can be considered not to fold at all. Since we are studying a simple artificial system there is no *a priori* time scale to pick, other than limits on the simulation (computer) time. One of the problems with Monte Carlo dynamics is that there is no easy way to "calibrate" them, that is to make a connection between Monte Carlo steps and "real" physical or biological time. What we have done here is to define the relevant time scale as the folding time (or the compaction time) for a good folding sequence and make sure we ran simulations for long enough that we could see the the variation of folding time as a function of temperature.

We have examined the folding (and compaction) time as a function of temperature for one sequence. We now would like to see how this function varies from sequence to sequence. Figure 4 show a plot of the folding time and compaction time versus inverse temperature for several sequences. The compaction time is simply the number of steps it takes for an unfolded state to reach a maximally compact cube. In addition, we also show a time to reach a nearly compact state, which we define to be a conformation with 25 (out of 28) contacts. The behavior of the compaction time as a function of temperature is similar to that of the folding time, but chains compact much faster than they fold. This behavior is similar to what is believed to occur in real proteins in which the chain first folds rapidly to a compact state and

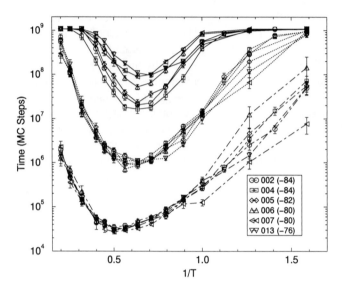

Figure 4: Folding and collapse times versus inverse temperature for all sequences, plotted on a semi-log scale. The top set of solid lines are the folding times, the middle set of dotted lines are the times to compact to a cube and the bottom set are the times to compact to a partially compact (25 contacts) conformation. The legend shows the energy of the native states.

then rearranges itself to the native structure. From this figure we notice two very interesting features of this model. First the compaction time is sequence independent. All six sequences have roughly the same compaction time for temperatures above T_g. In contrast the folding time is highly sequence dependent. At a temperature of roughly 1.6 ($1/T \approx .63$) there is a difference of nearly an order of magnitude between the fastest and slowest folding sequence. The folding time is also roughly correlated with the energy of the folded state. The lower the energy, the faster the folding time. However, the relation between the energy of the native state and the folding time is not a simple one. For example the two sequences with the lowest energy folded states (sequence 002 and 004, see Table 1) have different folding times. The difference is slight but sequence 004 has a consistently faster folding time at all temperatures. Sequence 005, which is a single monomer mutation of 004, has a higher ground state energy (−82), but its folding times are very close to those of the lower energy sequence 002. There also appears to be a fairly large difference between the sequences that have energies below −81 and those that have energies above.

Note that the collapse time is always much faster than the folding time for all sequences. Even sequences that fold slowly collapse as rapidly as the fast-folding ones. This sequence-independent property of the collapse time is often referred to as a *self-averaging* property; it does not depend on the specifics of the sequence but rather on the general character of the ensemble of sequences. It is important to remember here that we are choosing a restricted ensemble of sequences though, namely the subset of sequences with a particular ratio of monomer types (a ratio of 14:13). Sequences that contain a different composition of monomers may have different collapse times than the sequences used here. The folding time is not self-averaging; i.e., it depends on the sequence. So we can view the kinetics of folding as a two-stage process. The first involves a rapid collapse of the polymer. The nature of this collapse is sequence independent. We can picture the polymer in this collapsed state as fluctuating about various compact cube states. This picture has been advanced previously by others [27]. The next step is a medium-to-slow event in which the polymer searches for the minimum energy state among the compact states. The time it takes for the polymer to find its minimum state depends on the specifics of the sequence. The two-phase collapse with two distinct time scales has also been observed for real proteins [28, 29, 30]. The first phase is a rapid collapse in which a hydrophobic core is formed. We should expect this collapse to be independent of the specific sequence, depending on the ratio of hydrophobic to hydrophilic monomers. This collapsed state then undergoes rearrangement to the folded structure of the specific sequence. The collapse time below the glass temperature loses its self-averaging property. Examining Fig. 4 we see that below $T_g \approx 1$ the collapse time is no longer sequence independent. In the glass region we would expect the kinetics to depend on the details of the energy surfaces and these details will be sequence dependence. This is expected of a system exhibiting glassy behavior. Note how this contrasts with the high temperature limit, where the collapse times remain sequence independent even as they approach $\tau_{\max}$.

At this point one may be tempted to conclude that we have two types of sequences: Fast folders and slow folders. However this is not the case. In reality what we have are sequences that fold and sequences that do not. In order to see this we need to look at the thermodynamics of these systems. In particular we need to look at the thermodynamic stability of the native state as a function of temperature. To do so, we performed a series of thermodynamic runs using the same Monte Carlo algorithm described above. The system was equilibrated by first running it for 100 million steps, which is on the order of the folding time for most of the sequences. Care must be taken at low temperatures since near the glass transition the system will slow down; i.e., the auto-correlation time will diverge. We looked at temperatures above T_g to avoid this problem. We calculate the following thermodynamic quantity:

$$P_{\mathrm{nat}}(T) = \frac{e^{-E_{\mathrm{nat}}/T}}{Z}, \tag{3}$$

where E_{nat} is the energy of the native state and Z is the partition function. This quantity is the probability that the system is in the native state; that is, it is folded. We define the folding temperature as the temperature at which $P_{\mathrm{nat}}(T_f) = 0.5$; that is when the folded state is half occupied. Note that $P_{\mathrm{nat}}(T) > 0.5$ is a sufficient condition that the native state be the global minimum of the free energy. Four sequences were used, each with a different minimum energy ranging from -84 to -76. Several simulations were run at a number of different temperatures. Figure 5 shows the results. In addition to running simulations at different temperatures, we also used the Monte Carlo histogram method [31] to calculate the function $P_{\mathrm{nat}}(T)$ at temperatures other then the simulation temperature. Using histograms collected from simulations run at $T = 1.58$, we were able to calculate P_{nat} for all temperatures, extrapolating into the glass region. These lines are plotted along with the points calculated from the standard Monte Carlo runs.

The folding temperature, T_f, varies with the value of the minimum-energy state. The lower the minimum energy the higher the folding temperature. More importantly we see that the two lower energy sequences have folding temperatures above the glass temperature, T_g, while the others have $T_f < T_g$. At T_g the lowest energy sequence (which also folds the fastest) is 90% in the native state. The highest energy sequence has a native state population of only 15%. At temperatures at which the folded state of the high-energy sequence is thermodynamically

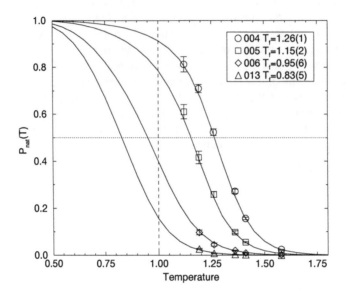

Figure 5: $P_{\text{nat}}(T)$ for several sequences. T_f is defined to be the temperature at which $P_{\text{nat}}(T_f) = .5$ The points were calculated using the standard Monte Carlo procedure. The solid lines are *not* fits to the data. They were calculated using the Monte Carlo Histogram Method (Ref. [31]), which enables one to calculate thermodynamic quantities at temperatures other than the simulation temperature. Two of the sequences have folding temperatures above T_g, the others have temperatures below T_g. The vertical line at $T = 1$ indicates the glass transition point. The legend shows the folding temperatures, the numbers in the parenthesis indicate the uncertainty in the last digits.

stable this state is not kinetically accessible. Therefore we would say this sequence does not fold. In order for a sequence to be foldable it must meet two conditions. First, it must have a reasonably fast folding time, where by reasonable we mean on the relevant (biological) time scales, and second, the folding temperature must be above the glass temperature. The analogous situation would be a polypeptide which had a folding temperature below the freezing point of the solvent. Such a protein would not be considered foldable.

The sequences we have examined so far are all 2-letter code sequences (they have two monomer types). The best value for the ratio T_f/T_g is approximately 1.30, which is somewhat smaller than one would expect. It turns out by adding a third monomer type, one can obtain a better folding sequence with a higher ratio of folding to glass temperature. The sequence was designed by taking one of the unfrustrated sequences (002 in this case). An examination of the minimum energy cube (the native state) reveals that it can separated into non-interacting domains. For sequences 002 there are 4 domains of size 11, 10, 3, and 3. What we did was keep the 11 and 10 domains fixed and assigned the third monomer type to the two 3 size domains. Since, these domains do not interact in the native state, the energy of this state is *unchanged*. However, the addition of this third monomer type changes the energy of the other conformations, specifically it changes some of the strong bonds (between like monomer

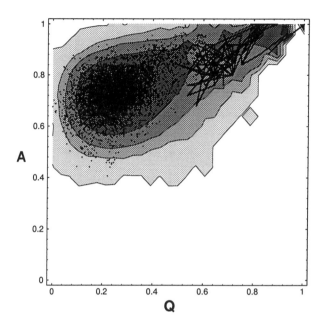

Figure 6: This figure show a transition trajectory projected onto the QA place. The time span is roughly 25% of the folding time which is approximately 3×10^6 MC steps. The temperature of the simulation was set to the folding temperature ($T_f = 1.51$). The sequence was a 3-letter code variant of sequence 002 (ABABBBCBACBABABACACBACAACAB). The trajectory is superimposed on a contour plot of the free energy with the levels spanning the range from -67.5 to -82.5 in increments of 2.5. The initial part of the trajectory is shown as a series of disconnected points while the final 10^5 MC steps, the transition event is shown as with series of line segments connecting the points.

types) but incorrect (i.e. non-native bonds) to weak bonds (unlike monomers). This removes many low energy states, several of which were traps, slowing down the folding time. The folding time for this sequence was almost an order of magnitude faster than the corresponding 2-letter code sequence. Additionally, the folding temperature increased from 1.29 to 1.51 so that $T_f/T_g \approx 1.6$.

Finally, in figure 6, we show a folding trajectory superimposed on a plot of the free energy for this 3-letter code sequence. The free energy is calculated using the Monte Carlo histogram technique and is plotted along the QA plane. Q is the percentage of *native* contacts and A is the percentage of correct bond angles present in the structure. These two coordinates give a measure of overlap a given conformation has with the native state. Q is a more global measure and individual Monte Carlo steps can change it by approximately 0.18. A is a more local measure (it however, does not uniquely identify the ground state) and is changed less by a single step, roughly 0.08. The trajectory is approximately 3×10^6 MC steps or roughly 25% of the folding time for this sequence at this temperature ($T = T_f = 1.51$). The initial part of the trajectory is shown has disconnected points the density roughly corresponding to the frequency a given value of QA is seen. The last 10^5 MC steps are shown as a connected line and indicated the actual transition event. In some cases the transition even can be as small as 3000 MC steps or if trapping occurs in the transition region it can be much longer. However, the transition time is much shorter than the folding time. Recently, the simulation results for the 3-letter code have been connected to the mechanism for folding for real proteins [19]. Although in its early stages, these results provide a guideline for relating folding simulations for these simple models with real protein data. Wolynes addresses this point in detail in his contribution to this volume.

4   Conclusions

Using a simple lattice model and Monte Carlo dynamics we have studied the kinetics (and some thermodynamics) of proteinlike heteropolymer folding. Our results are related to other works on simple model systems and also match some of the properties of the folding real proteins. We find that our models display a two-stage folding behavior. First there is a rapid collapse to a compact state, followed by a slower stage in which the collapsed state rearranges itself to the native structure. We find that the folding time has a minimum plateau at intermediate temperatures and diverges at both high and low temperatures. The same is true for the collapse time. In this work we have examined the folding behavior as a function sequence and have discovered several interesting results. The collapse time and the glass temperature are both sequence independent (self-averaging) quantities. The folding time and temperature are both sequence dependent. The folding time correlates approximately with the energy of the native state: The lower this energy the faster the chain folds. This is consistent with the results found by Shakhnovich [25] that the larger the energy gap of the native state the better the sequence folds. We did not measure the gap, since there is no clear or simple definition of the gap in our system. Another way to view this result is that sequences with unfrustrated native states (native states with no bad contacts) fold best; i.e., we want to minimize energetic frustration of the ground state. However, we expect that this may be a property of these simple systems and that in more complex systems other forms of frustration (geometric or energetic frustration of conformations other than the native state) may play an important role. This starts to become apparent when we switch from the 2- to 3-letter code sequences. One would then expect that systems with reduced frustration should give rise to a large number of conformations that are rapidly connected kinetically to the native state (rapid compared to the folding time) or, as first proposed by Leopold and others [27], a "dominant folding funnel".

An important point we have tried to stress is the issue of time scales, in particular the relevant physical time scales for this system and for protein folding in general. We note that there was no simple way to connect the computation time (Monte Carlo steps) to physical time. Rather than attempt to do so, we simply ran our simulations for a reasonable number of steps and then observed the folding time for the system. It is this folding time that now becomes the key time scale. For example, when we say a sequence does not fold what we mean is that is does not fold within a time that is over an order of magnitude greater than the folding time for the fast sequences. Since we are looking at finite systems we know that they will all fold given enough time. What is important is whether they fold in a reasonable time where reasonable is the folding time for the faster sequences. For real proteins, this time scale would be some suitable biological time.

By examining the behavior of folding time versus temperature we defined the glass transition temperature of this system. Below this temperature the kinetics slow down, causing the folding time to increase rapidly. Also the collapse times lose their self-averaging property and are now dependent on sequence. Most importantly we observed that for the slow-folding sequences the folding temperature (the temperature at which the native state is half populated) is below the glass temperature. This indicates that these sequences will never fold since at temperatures where the native state is thermodynamically stable it is kinetically inaccessible.

Good folding sequences have T_f greater than T_g. It has been suggested by others [22, 23] that a good design principle for optimizing folding would be to maximize the ratio T_f/T_g. We observe this result explicitly in our simulations.

Perhaps the most interesting observation is that even simple systems such as these display a wide variety of complex and intriguing properties, many of which are shared by real proteins. This is particularly compelling in that one can much more easily study these simple systems and understand their behavior in great detail. By examining slightly more complex models we hope to understand how much of protein behavior is unique to proteins and how much is shared by the general class of heteropolymer systems. Hopefully, as we already have attempted recently [19], much of the apparent complexity of proteins will be understandable in the context of simpler model system.

Acknowledgments

We would like to gratefully acknowledge the computational assistance of A. Schweitzer. We thank S. Skourtis, K. A. Dill, and H. S. Chan for interesting and helpful discussions. We also thank J. Song and A. Schwartz for careful reading of and enlightening comments on the manuscript. N. D. S. is a Chancellor's Fellow at UCSD. J. N. O. is a Beckman Young Investigator. This work was funded by the Arnold and Mabel Beckman Foundation and by the National Science Foundation (Grant No. MCB-9316186). J. N. O. is in residence at the Instituto de Física e Química de São Carlos, Universidade de São Paulo, São Carlos, SP, Brazil during part of the summers.

References

[1] Y. Ueda, H. Taketomi, and N. Gō, Studies on protein folding, unfolding, and fluctuations by computer simulations. ii. a three-dimensional lattice model of lysozyme, *Biopolymers*, 17, 1531–1548, 1978.

[2] N. Gō, Protein folding as a stochastic process, *J. Stat. Phys.*, 30, 413–423, 1983.

[3] J. Skolnick and A. Kolinski, Dynamic monte carlo simulations of globular protein folding/unfolding pathways. I. Six-member, greek key β-barrel proteins, *J. Mol. Biol.*, 212, 787–817, 1990.

[4] A. Sikorski and J. Skolnick, Dynamic monte carlo simulations of globular protein folding/unfolding pathways. II. α-helical motifs, *J. Mol. Biol.*, 212, 819–836, 1990.

[5] J. Skolnick and A. Kolinski, Dynamic monte carlo simulations of a new lattice model of globular protein folding, structure and dynamics. *J. Mol. Biol.*, 221, 499–531, 1991.

[6] A. Kolinski, M. Milik, and J. Skolnick, Static and dynamic properties of a new lattice model of polypeptide chains, *J. Chem. Phys.*, 94, 3978–3985, 1991.

[7] A. Kolinski and J. Skolnick, Discretized model of proteins. I. Monte Carlo study of cooperativity in homopolypeptides, *J. Chem. Phys.*, 97, 9412–9426, 1992.

[8] H. S. Chan and K. A. Dill, Polymer principles in protein structure and stability, *Annu. Rev. Biophys. Biophys. Chem.*, 20, 447–490, 1991.

[9] R. Miller, C. A. Danko, M. J. Fasolka, A. C. Balazs, H. S. Chan, and K. A. Dill, Folding kinetics of proteins and copolymers, *J. Chem. Phys.*, 96, 768–780, 1992.

[10] H. S. Chan and K. A. Dill, Energy landscapes and the collapse dynamics of homopolymers, *J. Chem. Phys.*, 99, 2116–2127, 1993.

[11] H. S. Chan and K. A. Dill, Transition states and folding dynamics of proteins and heteropolymers, *J. Chem. Phys.*, 100, 9238–9257, 1994.

[12] E. M. O'Toole and A. Z. Panagiotopoulos, Monte Carlo simulation of folding transitions of simple model proteins using a chain growth algorithm, *J. Chem. Phys.*, 97, 8644–8652, 1992.

[13] E. M. O'Toole and A. Z. Panagiotopoulos, Effect of sequence and intermolecular interactions on the number and nature of low-energy states for simple model proteins, *J. Chem. Phys.*, 98, 3185–3190, 1993.

[14] C. J. Camacho and D. Thirumalai, Kinetics and thermodynamics of folding in model proteins, *Proc. Natl. Acad. Sci. USA*, 90, 6369–6372, 1993.

[15] E. I. Shakhnovich, Proteins with selected sequences fold into unique native conformations, *Phys. Rev. Lett.*, 72, 3907–3910, 1994.

[16] A. Šali, E. Shakhnovich, and M. Karplus, Kinetics of protein folding—a lattice model study of the requirements for folding to the native state, *J. Mol. Biol.*, 235, 1614–1636, 1994.

[17] N. D. Socci and J. N. Onuchic, Folding kinetics of proteinlike heteropolymers, *J. Chem. Phys.*, 101, 1519–1528, 1994.

[18] J. D. Bryngelson, J. N. Onuchic, N. D. Socci, and P. G. Wolynes, Funnels, pathways and the energy landscape of protein folding: A synthesis, In Press: *Proteins: Struct. Funct. Genet.*

[19] J. N. Onuchic, P. G. Wolynes, Z. Luthey-Schulten, and N. D. Socci, Towards an outline of the topography of a realistic protein folding funnel, In Press: *Proc. Natl. Acad. Sci.*

[20] J. D. Bryngelson and P. G. Wolynes, Spin glasses and the statistical mechanics of protein folding, *Proc. Natl. Acad. Sci. USA*, 84, 7524–7528, 1987.

[21] J. D. Bryngelson and P. G. Wolynes, Intermediates and barrier crossing in a random energy model with applications to protein folding, *J. Phys. C*, 93, 6902–6915, 1989.

[22] M. Sasai and P. Wolynes, Molecular theory of associative memory hamiltonian models of protein folding, *Phys. Rev. Lett.*, 65, 2740–2743, 1990.

[23] R. A. Goldstein, Z. A. Luthey-Schulten, and P. G. Wolynes, Optimal protein-folding codes from spin-glass theory, *Proc. Natl. Acad. Sci. USA*, 89, 4918–4922, 1992.

[24] K. A. Dill, Dominant forces in protein folding, *Biochemistry*, 29, 7133–7155, 1990.

[25] E. I. Shakhnovich and A. M. Gutin, Engineering of stable and fast-folding sequences of model proteins, *Proc. Natl. Acad. Sci. USA*, 90, 7195–7199, 1993.

[26] B. Derrida, Random-energy model: an exactly solvable model of disordered systems, *Phys. Rev. B*, 24, 2613–26, 1981.

[27] P. E. Leopold, M. Montal, and J. N. Onuchic, Protein folding funnels: Kinetic pathways through compact conformational space, *Proc. Natl. Acad. Sci. USA*, 89, 8721–8725, 1992.

[28] K. Kuwajima, The molten globule state as a clue for understanding the folding and cooperativity of globular-protein structure, *Proteins*, 6, 87, 1989.

[29] K. Kuwajima, *Current Opinion in Biotechnology*, 3, 462, 1992.

[30] R. L. Baldwin, *Current Opinion in Structural Biology*, 3, 84, 1993.

[31] A. M. Ferrenberg and R. H. Swendsen, New Monte Carlo technique for studying phase transitions, *Phys. Rev. Lett.*, 61, 2635–2638, 1988.

Energy Landscape and Folding Mechanisms in Proteins

Zhuyan Guo and David Thirumalai

Chemical Physics Program, Institute for Physical Science and Technology, University of Maryland, College Park, MD 20742, U.S.A.

Abstract

We present theoretical ideas for protein folding mechanisms and correlate these with the topography of the underlying energy landscape. The studies show that for foldable sequences a fraction of initial population of molecules reach the native state by a specific collapse process making folding and collapse synchronous. The remaining fraction approach the native conformation by a three stage multipathway kinetic mechanism. We also show that in the folding process very few low energy states are visited. These model studies demonstrate a remarkable property that in finite time scales some of the basins corresponding to low energy native like state are explored repeatedly. Implications of these results for other disordered systems (such as finite dimensional short range spin glass models) are also outlined.

1   Introduction

Recent theoretical progress in protein folding indicates that the distinction between sequences that fold in finite time scale (to be referred to as foldable sequences from here on) and those that do not can be understood if the underlying energy landscape can be properly characterized [1]. This perspective, based on understanding the energy landscape characterizing proteins, has provided a picture of the kinetics of protein folding that is drastically different from the conventional scenario [2]. According to the conventional picture of protein folding the native conformation is reached from the denatured state in such a way that successive stages of foldingindexfolding mechanisms yield conformations that are increasingly native-like [2]. Schematically one can indicate this as

$$U \rightleftharpoons I_1 \rightleftharpoons I_2 \rightleftharpoons \cdots N \qquad (1)$$

where I_1, I_2 etc are possible intermediates with I_2 having more native character than I_1 and so on. The energy landscape perspective, which has been suggested based on extensive studies of several minimal models, offers a drastically different scenario. According to this "new view" [3] of protein folding there are multiple pathways that lead the protein to the native conformation from an ensemble of denatured states. Although the clearest manifestation of the multiple pathway picture is most evident in the early stages of folding it is clear that even in the late stages there are many paths that could lead to the native state [4]. A direct consequence of this is that the transition state for folding of the protein is not unique and this represents a drastic departure from the old view [5].

Another crucial finding that has resulted from off-lattice simulations of minimal models is that there are pathways to the folded conformation that are synchronous with the collapse process itself [6]. This process, which has been referred to as the specific collapse, occurs in such a way as to produce the correct overall topology, and is triggered by the formation of a critical nucleus. Once the critical nucleus is formed then the transition to the native state is a downhill process that occurs very rapidly [6, 7]. The specific collapse process leading to a well defined topology does not occur in homopolymers because entropy arguments show that the probability of this process is very small. In contrast the guiding forces in proteins, that render the native conformation stable, can overcome the entropy loss leading to the formation of the native conformation by the specific collapse process. In fact if the basin of attraction corresponding to the native conformation is very large, then the specific collapse leading directly to the native conformation can occur with overwhelming probability [6, 8]. In this case protein folding would appear kinetically to be a two state process i.e. "all or none" and the time scale for folding would only be of the order of several $msec$ [9].

Since the quantitative aspects of folding kinetics can be largely explained in terms of the underlying rugged energy landscape it is instructive to devise numerical techniques to probe aspects of the potential energy surface that are explored in time. In the next section we present a summary of the folding mechanisms in foldable sequences of proteins. In section 3, we introduce methods that can be used to finger print the topography of the energy landscape. The major advantage of the method is that it can be readily used in standard simulation methods. Here we apply the method to expose the conformational states that are explored in a model protein whose ground state is a hairpin conformation. The paper is concluded in section 4 with additional remarks.

2   Folding mechanisms

The statistical mechanics of protein folding, which is based on detailed studies of analytical and simulation of minimal models, has revealed that there are several possible mechanisms for a protein to reach the native [5]. Nevertheless it has proven useful to decipher the generic mechanisms that are usually operative in foldable systems. By foldable we mean those systems that reach the native conformation on biological time scale which is of the order of a second or less. In order to uncover the folding mechanisms we studied in detail the approach to the native conformation of certain off-lattice minimal models of proteins [6]. This study was partly inspired by the observation that in a variety of proteins (barnase, cytochrome c, hen lysozyme, ribonuclease A, and interlukin) the folding kinetics as revealed by amide proton exchange studies is multiphasic involving multiple pathways [10]. We have theoretically proposed the origin of this complex kinetics using a combination of computational methods [6] and scaling arguments [9]. Here we provide a brief summary of our findings.

The kinetics approach to the native conformation starting from a denatured state was inferred from the distribution of first passage time

$$P_{FP}(t) = \frac{1}{N} \sum_{k=1}^{N} \delta(t - \tau_{1k}) \qquad (2)$$

where τ_{1k} is the first time kth trajectory reaches a conformation resembling the native one, and N is the number of independent trajectories monitored in the simulation. The experimentally related quantity (related to the protection kinetics seen in hydrogen exchange labeling experiments) is the fraction of unfolded molecules at time t which can be written as

$$P_u = 1 - \int_0^t P_{FP}(s)ds \tag{3}$$

For the model system, whose native state is a β-barrel structure, we find that over a range of temperature $P_u(t)$ can be adequately described by [6]

$$P_u(t) = a_f(T)\exp(-k_f t) + a_s(T)\exp(-k_s t) \tag{4}$$

where $k_f \gg k_s$. Note that both the amplitudes and the rates are explicitly temperature dependent. The characterization that generically folding simultaneously involves a very fast process and a slow process is in complete accord with hydrogen exchange labeling experiments.

Our simulations have very clearly uncovered the origins of the fast and slow processes seen in theoretical models and in experiments. By analyzing the dynamical behavior of several individual trajectories we have discovered that the fast process corresponds to a nucleation mechanism [6]. This implies that once a critical nucleus is formed the folding is extremely rapid [6, 9]. The results of our computations clearly reveal that the critical nucleus occurs early in the folding process. The nature of the critical nucleus is such that they actually lead to the formation of a mobile topology preserving native like structures. The subsequent rearrangement to the native state is in all probability too fast to be resolved by standard experiments. Finally it should be stressed that only a fraction ($\propto a_f(T)$) of the initial population of molecules follows this direct pathway by undergoing a specific collapse to the native structure. The size of the critical nucleus can be inferred by assuming that driving force for forming a compact native structure is the effective attractive hydrophobic interactions that buries the nonpolar groups. This allows us to write the free energy of a droplet with N_R residues as [11]

$$\Delta F(N_R) \approx -\frac{\epsilon_H}{2} f_H^2 N_R^2 + 4\pi\gamma a^2 N_R^{2/3} \tag{5}$$

where ϵ_H is an effective hydrophobic interaction, f_H is the fraction of hydrophobic residues in the sequence, γ is the surface tension, and a is the size of an amino acid residue. Minimization of $\Delta F(N_R)$ yields the size of the critical nucleus

$$N_R^* \sim (8\pi\gamma a^2/3f_H^2\epsilon_H)^{3/4} \tag{6}$$

Using standard range of values for γ, ϵ_H, and f_H yields $N_R^* \approx$ (12-18) residues. These numbers are consistent with our simulations of a 46-mer minimal protein model.

The slow process described by an effective rate constant k_s applies to the fraction of molecules that do not reach the native conformation by a specific collapse process. We have discovered that the molecules that reach the native conformation by this mechanism are described by a three stage multipathway mechanism [11, 12]. In the first stage, the molecule collapses rapidly in a non-specific manner to one of an ensemble of compact structures. Subsequently there is a random diffusive search among the compact structures. As this process continues the molecule reaches one of the many native-like structures due to the guiding force present in foldable sequences. The native-like structures have between (60-80)% of native contacts. The last stage involves activated transitions from these native-like structures via a multiple transition state to the native state. It is because of the activated transitions folding for these molecules that follow the indirect process is slow. Surprisingly the effective free energy barrier separating the native-like structures and the native conformation is small. For our model system $\langle \Delta F^{\ddagger} \rangle \sim 6k_B T_f$ where T_f is the folding temperature.

The origin of such small barriers in protein folding can be understood by using scaling arguments [9]. Let us assume that the free energy distribution of native like states is a Gaussian.

There are rough analogies between the behavior of minimal protein models and Potts glasses and minimally frustrated random energy models that can be used to rationalize this assumption. Since the pathways connecting the native-like structures and the native state are independent it follows that the distribution of barrier heights is also Gaussian. The dispersion in the distribution which gives the average free energy barrier height must scale as $\langle \Delta F^{\ddagger} \rangle \sim \sqrt{N}$. These arguments can be further developed to show that the folding time for these indirect pathways at $T = T_f$ for large N should go as

$$\tau_f \propto k_s^{-1} \sim \tau_0 \exp(\langle \Delta F^{\ddagger} \rangle / k_B T_f) \sim \tau_0 \exp(\alpha^{-1}\sqrt{\bar{N}}) \tag{7}$$

where $\alpha = T_f / T_g$. This shows that for large α folding is very rapid as discovered first by Bryngelson and Wolynes [5]. For the 46-mer $T_f / T_g \approx 1.3$ and this in turn leads to $\langle \Delta F^{\ddagger} \rangle \approx 5.2 k_B T_f$ which is in good agreement with simulation results. The estimate for the height of the free energy barrier at $T = T_f$ for $N = 27$ for a three letter model protein with $\alpha = 1.6$ is $\langle \Delta F^{\ddagger} \rangle \sim 3.3 k_B T_f$ using Eq.(7). This estimate is in very good agreement with the simulation results of Onuchic *et al.* [13].

3   Finger Print of the Energy Landscape

It is anticipated that the potential energy surface of a complex system such as proteins is rough containing many minima that are separated by barriers of varying heights [4]. Several theoretical [15, 16] as well as experiments lend support to this notion. Let us assume that the temperature of the system is such that $k_B T$ is sufficiently larger than several high energy barriers. In order to illustrate the basic idea behind our method we assume that $k_B T$ is larger than all the barriers. Assume that one has generated a long simulation trajectory (using MD, MC or other type of dynamics) at the temperature T. Start from an initial configuration labelled a. With this as the initial condition minimize the energy of the structure. In our simulations this is done using conjugate gradient technique. This process of minimization would map the initial configuration to a local minimum α. Denote the coordinates of all the particles corresponding to the minimum α as $\vec{x}_{imin}^a(0)$. Let $\vec{x}_i^a(t)$ be the trajectory at the temperature of interest starting from the initial condition labelled a. If the minimum energy structure starting with the initial configuration $\vec{x}_i^a(t)$ is obtained this minimum may or may not be different from the one labelled α. In any event let $\vec{x}_{imin}^a(t)$ be the coordinates of the minimum energy structure that the configuration $\vec{x}_i^a(t)$ maps onto. Now consider the measure

$$\Delta(t) = \{ \frac{1}{N} \sum_{i=1}^{N} [\vec{x}_{imin}^a(t) - \vec{x}_{imin}^a(0)]^2 \}^{1/2} \tag{8}$$

It is instructive to analyze the expected behavior of $\Delta(t)$. If $\vec{x}_{imin}^a(t)$ maps onto the same minimum as $\vec{x}_{imin}^a(0)$, namely the one labelled α, then $\Delta(t) \equiv 0$. It follows, therefore, that if $\Delta(t) \neq 0$ then the coordinates $\vec{x}_{imin}^a(t)$ belong to another distinct minimum. The time for which $\Delta(t)$ remains constant then gives the residence time in a given minimum. The time dependent "spectrum" generated by $\Delta(t)$ is then a way of fingerprinting the energy landscape.

In order to probe the energy surface that is explored by the proteins we have used the measures in Eq. (8) in the context of low friction Langevin Simulations [11]. The model used for this study is a 22-mer formed using three letter code. The native conformation for this sequence used (described elsewhere [11]) is a hairpin bead. The energy of the native conformation is $E_N = -10.6\epsilon_H$ where ϵ_H is the unit of energy that gives the strength of the hydrophobic interaction [11, 17]. In addition to using Eq.(8) which gives the structural

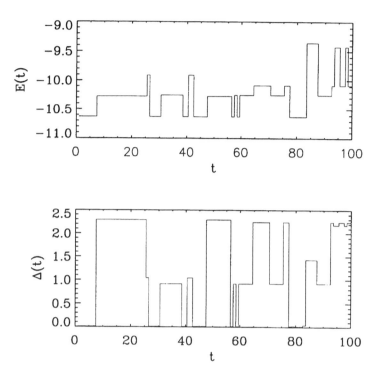

Figure 1: This figure shows the measures used to fingerprint the energy landscape in proteins. The top panel shows the minimum energy corresponding to the various basins of attraction as a function of time. The energy is measured in units of an effective hydrophobic interaction, ϵ_H, and time is measured in reduced units with one unit being roughly $2nsec$. The energy of the native state with a hairpin conformation is $-10.6\epsilon_H$[11]. The simulation temperature is $T = 2T_f$. The bottom panel gives $\Delta(t)$ (cf Eq.(8)) as a function of t in units of σ^2 where σ is the measure of length. These figures establish that in this 3-letter 22-mer minimal model only a small number of basins with native like structures are repeatedly explored in the finite duration time scale.

characterization in the basin that is being visited, we have also calculated the energy $E(t)$ of the basin. The calculations were done at $T = 0.4k_B/\epsilon_H$ which is $2T_f$ the folding transition temperature [11]. It should be pointed out that visited corresponds to choosing specific low energy conformations.

In figure 1 plots of $E(t)$ and $\Delta(t)$ as a function of time are shown. For the purpose of converting t into real time one can assume our unit of time corresponds to about $2nsec$. It is interesting that the system only visit very few states on the time scale of about $200nsec$. Since the measure used here unambiguously determines whether the same basin or a distinct basin is visited one can directly read off from $\Delta(t)$ the exact number of conformational states explored in the time scale plotted. Such a counting would not be possible using $E(t)$ alone because several distinct structures could give the same value for $E(t)$. From figure 1 it is clear that in the course of our simulation only about 10 distinct conformations have been explored at $T = 2T_f$ on the time scale of about $200nsec$.

It is remarkable that in this short time scale the chain *repeatedly* visits the same basin of attraction several times. For example the basin with $\Delta(t) \approx 2.3$ is visited five times implying that this conformation is *connected* to the native conformation by perhaps only very small barriers. It should be emphasized that in a truly disordered system such repeated visiting of basins of attraction is very unlikely. In contrast our findings here suggest that in proteins, which are modeled here to produce well defined three dimensional structures, structures that are well separated from the native conformation which are explored often play an essential role. In order to elucidate the nature of these 10 distinct conformations we have analyzed their structural characteristics. We find that all these have considerable native character. Thus these foldable sequences have the property that the native conformation is separated by a *manifold of native-like structures* and the average energy of separation is the stability gap. This aspect for sequences that reach the native state rapidly was noted first by Bryngelson and Wolynes [17], and was was demonstrated explicitly in minimal models sometime ago by Honeycutt and Thirumalai [18]. In this study we have for the first time demonstrated the dynamic significance of these native like states in determining folding kinetics.

4   Conclusions

It is now becoming increasingly clear that in order to fully understand the kinetics approach to the native conformation of protein from a denatured state it is necessary to characterize the nature of native-like conformations and their connectivity to the native state as well as to more disordered structures. Theoretical ideas in this context have lead to testable mechanisms for protein folding. There appears to be little doubt that the basic tenants of such mechanisms (described briefly here) are valid for real proteins as well. In fact several recent experiments indeed suggest that generically this is what is observed in experiments. Furthermore, scaling arguments [9] and other ideas based on the correspondence principle [13], have made connections between model proteins and the kinetics expected in large single domain proteins explicit. The theoretical picture presented here and elsewhere also suggests that a complete elucidation of protein folding kinetics will require probes of fast folding events which are thought to take place on the order of $10^{-6}sec$.

From a purely theoretical view point the representation of proteins by minimal models offers a remarkable contrast to the other disordered systems studied in condensed matter physics [20, 21]. One example of this provided here is the small number of relevant states (or basins of attraction) that are explored by the system. In contrast, at least in infinite range models of spin glasses [20], it is believed that there are a very large number of symmetry unrelated pure states that are present in the ordered (spin glass) phase. Since these differ only insignificantly in free energies it follows that in any finite system many of these would be visited in a simulation of long enough time scale and the chances of recurrence are small due to entropic reasons. On the other hand in the model systems that we have studied here only very few conformations are visited. More importantly the same basin of attraction is traversed repeatedly in finite simulation time scales. These results may have implications for short range spin glass models as well. For example it may be that finite dimensional short range spin glasses may not be as frustrated as the Sherrington-Kirkpatrick (SK) model and may behave in a similar way to foldable minimal protein models.

References

[1] P. G. Wolynes, J. N. Onuchic and D. Thirumalai, *Science*, 267, 1619, 1995.

[2] P. S. Kim and R. L. Baldwin, *Ann. Rev. Biochem.*, 51, 459, 1982.

[3] R. L. Baldwin, *Nature*, 369, 183, 1994.

[4] C. J. Camacho and D. Thirumalai, *Proteins: Struc., Func. Gen.*, in press, 1995.

[5] J. D. Bryngelson *et al.*, *Proteins: Struc., Func. Gen.*, in press, 1995.

[6] D. Thirumalai and Z. Guo, *Biopol. Res. Comm.*, 35, 137, 1995.

[7] V. I. Abkevich, A. M. Gutin and E. I. Shakhnovich, *Biochemistry*, 33, 10026, 1994.

[8] T. R. Sosnick, L. Mayne, R. Hiller, and S. W. Englander, *Nat. Struc. Biol.*, 1, 149, 1994.

[9] D. Thirumalai, *J. Phys. press. I*, submitted January, 1995.

[10] For a review see S. Radford and C. Dobson, *Proc. Phil. Soc. B*, London. in press, 1995.

[11] Z. Guo and D. Thirumalai, *Biopolymers*, in press, 1995.

[12] C. J. Camacho and D. Thirumalai, *Proc. Natl. Acad. Sci. USA.*, 90, 6369, 1993.

[13] J. Onuchic, P. G. Wolynes, Z. Schullan, and N. Socci, *Proc. Natl. Acad. Sci. USA.*, in press, 1995.

[14] H. Frauenfelder, S. G. Sligar, and P. G. Wolynes, *Science*, 254, 1598, 1991.

[15] R. Elber and M. Karplus, *Science*, 235, 318, 1987.

[16] J. Straub and D. Thirumalai, *Proc. Natl. Acad Sci. USA.*, 90, 809, 1993.

[17] J. Straub, preprint, 1995.

[18] J. D. Bryngelson and P. G. Wolynes, *J. Phys. Chem.*, 93, 6092, 1989.

[19] J. D. Honeycutt and D. Thirumalai, *Proc. Natl. Acad. Sci. USA.*, 87, 3526, 1990.

[20] K. Bindov and A. P. Young, *Rev. Mod. Phys.*, 58, 801, 1976.

[21] T. Garel, H. Orland, and D. Thirumalai, in *New Developments in Theoretical Studies of Proteins*, R. Elber (ed.), World Scientific, in press, 1995.

Topological Aspects of Protein Folds

Resonator Driven Protein Folding:
The Implication of Topology
for Protein Structure and Folding

J. Bohr*, H. Bohr[†] and S. Brunak[†]

* Physics Department, Building 307, The Technical University of Denmark, DK-2800 Lyngby, Denmark

[†] Center for Biological Sequence Analysis, Building 206, The Technical University of Denmark, DK-2800 Lyngby, Denmark

Abstract

An analysis of the geometrical nature of the protein backbone is presented resulting in a winding topology for the peptide chain. The relationship to the writhing number used in knot diagrams of DNA is discussed. The winding state defines a long range order along the backbone of a protein and long-range excitations will exist (twist'ons). Energy can be pumped into these excitations, either thermally, or by an external force. A mechanism for the folding of proteins occur when the amplitude of a twist excitation becomes so large that it is more energetically favorable to curve the backbone. It is proposed that protein folding is a resonance phenomena.

1 Introduction

The length of the polypeptide chain of globular proteins is much longer than typical diameters of the molecules. Yet, with the possible exception of some very short proteins, the polypeptide chain never displays a knotted topology [1, 2]. Thus, the disparity between different protein folds [3, 4, 5, 6] cannot be due to differences in their knot topology. Rather, the number of possible different protein structures is indeed limited by a "knot preventing mechanism". In this paper we address what further reduction of the phase space one may infer from topological arguments, and we present a model for the phenomenon of protein folding based on winding.

We view protein folding not primarily as a phase transition driven by entropy [7, 8, 9, 10, 11], but rather as a transition leading to a catastrophic event. Only folded structures which are stabilized by hydrogen bonds, disulphide bridges, *ect.* can maintain a significant fraction of folded proteins in balance with unfolded chains. Although, the proposed mechanism for initiation of folding of polypeptide chains is general, the biological evolution of living organisms selects proteins with the ability to acquire stable conformations. Initiation of protein folding is *not* a conventional rate-determining nucleation process, but a fast seeding that precedes the rate-determining step [12, 13, 14]. Unfolding of proteins is not the reverse process of the catastrophic event leading to the folding. Rather, it is changes in the external conditions (temperature, solvents, *ect.*) that are responsible for the destabilization of the folded protein.

There have been earlier attempts in molecular biology to apply topological methods in structural analysis of macromolecules. Most studies have investigated supercoiled DNA [15, 16, 17], and differential geometrical aspects of biological membranes [18, 19]. For circular DNA it was possible to utilize the concepts of twist, writhing and linking to establish a conservation law [16, 17, 20], and for membranes to obtain a comprehensive differential geometrical analysis of phase, vesicle formation, and critical exponents [21, 22]. Further, topological methods have been applied to protein structures for the purpose of energy minimization [23, 24, 25, 26, 27]. In this paper we argue that topological constraints can lead to a deterministic model of folding. In contrast to earlier views, topological folding may not necessarily lead to a folding path that minimize the sum of self-interactions. Rather, the physical reason for folding to follow topological constraints is the interaction of a protein with its environment.

2 Winding

Next we investigate the winding of the protein backbone. By this, we refer to the ubiquitous winding phenomena which may be observed in everyday life when dealing with items such as telephone cords, water hoses in gardens, pump hoses at self service gas stations *etc*. Basically, unless these tubes are handled with great care, their unwinding requires large motions in the space of the tube. The point of view put forward in this paper is that, as the protein folds in interaction with its environment (e.g. *in vivo*), such large motions of the protein backbone are unlikely. This is in contrast to spin-glass and lattice models which are based on self-interactions [11, 28]. Notice, that it would be a lot easier to wind the water-hose on the reel in the garden if there was no gravity. This is of course not physical.

An illustration of what we mean by winding is shown in figure 1. The first part, a), shows a straight tube which has zero winding. The winding of the tube is defined as the number of rotations the end of the tube has made relative to the other end. This number is determined by the path of the tube. But, winding cannot be calculated as a continuous measure depending uniquely on the local geometrical progression of the curve. This is illustrated in figures 1b and 1c, where two nearly identical approximately flat structures are depicted. While, one is not winded (fig. 1b), the other is winded by two turns (4π), (fig. 1c). At first, it is therefore not possible to assign an unambiguous winding to a shortened path such as the one displayed in figure 1d.

A consequence of the above consideration is that in order to assign winding to a polypeptide backbone it is necessary to know what path the backbone has taken during folding. But, this folding pathway is most often unknown. Instead one must work with protein backbones that are extended to form a closed curve (or are extended to infinity). The winding of the backbone can thereafter be found as the *linking* of the curve. The linking of a closed curve is topological conserved. Below we discuss the relation between linking, twisting, and writhing [29].

3 Twistons

Associated with a particular path of the backbone is a geometrical orientation. It is normal practice to define a ribbon, or a frame, by assigning a vector-field for this purpose. Nevertheless, even in the absence of a ribbon, a vector-field can be defined. Observing a line drawn by a pencil on an elastic tube one may easily be convinced about this. For a tube with rotational symmetry the incremental twist equals the torsion of the curve, equation (1), as such a geometrical-frame minimizes the twist energy. In equation (1), $\vec{r}$ is a vector representation of the curve and the

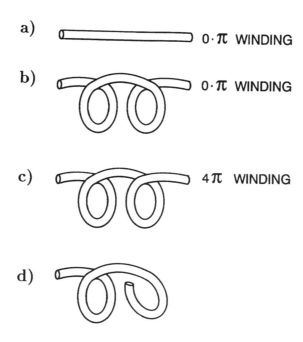

Figure 1: Examples of winding considerations, a) a straight tube with no winding, b) an almost flat double loop structure with zero winding; the two loops have opposite chirality, c) an almost flat double loop structure with 4π winding; the two loops have identical chirality. For a shortened structure such as the one depicted in d), it is not possible to say whether it is a part of b) or c), and hence it is not possible to assign an unambiguous winding to it).

primes denote derivatives. Notice, that the above geometrical frame may be different from the physical frame imposed by the backbone itself due to additional twist of the physical backbone.

$$\frac{\vec{r}' \times \vec{r}'' \cdot \vec{r}'''}{|\vec{r}' \times \vec{r}''|} \tag{1}$$

As there is a geometrical frame with long range order, twist excitations of the backbone will exist. Figure 2a shows an example of two solitons. In the limit where the backbone is considered to have continuous symmetry, the twistons displayed in figures 2b and 2c are the lower lying excitations. A pair of solitons may have a relatively low creation energy, but such pairs do not destroy the long range order, as they consist of an equal amount of clockwise and counterclockwise twist. The twist mode present depends on the boundary conditions at the two ends.

The basic consideration for linking the winding property and the protein folding problem may be addressed in two conjectures: *(a)* the path of the segments of the polypeptide chain trace out a "simple motion", *(b)* the backbone does not rotate unnecessary. The physical reason for this is that proteins do not fold in vacuum but rather in a viscous aqueous medium. Often they also interact with carbohydrates, other proteins and membranes.

The twistons are long range collective excitations over an entire protein folding domain. The polypeptide backbone will begin to bend at a certain amplitude of the local twist. The

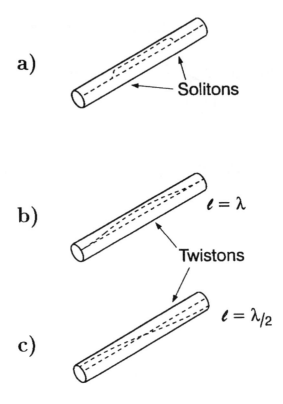

Figure 2: Three examples of twist excitations displayed on a tube. a) Solitons, local increment (or decrement) in the twist amplitude. Two solitons of opposite twist have no long range implication for the twist amplitude. b) and c) show collective twist excitations over the entire tube. We call such excitations twistons. b) and c) have different boundary conditions.

twist mode will involve non-zero values for the dihedral angle ω and therefore be rather stiff. The characteristic time involved can be much shorter than the characteristic time associated with the random motion of the unfolded backbone.

In general a change in the dihedral angles, ϕ and ψ will lead to a change in the path of the backbone [30]. In contrast, a change in the twist maintain the path of the backbone. A twist mode therefore involves strained chemical bonds. However, the dihedral rotations ψ_{i-1} and ϕ_i are almost coaxial (see fig. 3). However, such a rotation, and counter rotation, does not have any long range implication for the twist of the backbone and thus does not interfere with long wavelength twist modes.

4   Resonator driven transition

We hypothesize that the phase transformation of a protein from the unfolded structure to the folded structure is initiated by excitations of long wavelength twistons of the backbone which

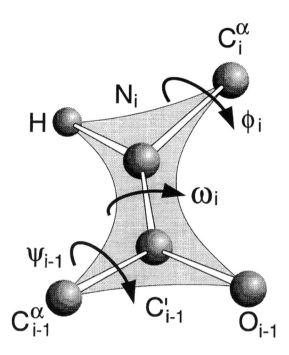

Figure 3: Part of the polypeptide backbone depicting the dihedral angles ψ, ϕ, and ω. The shaded area is approximately planar.

become unstable in favor of curvature. The nature of the transition may be characterized as being catastrophic rather than entropic. By this we mean that the primary reason for the transition is not a change in entropy. The excitation of the twist mode is pumped to a higher and higher level. A resonator is responsible for this pumping of the twist mode. The resonator must continuously be re-energized such; for thermal fluctuations by contact with the thermal bath. Almost literately, the initial folding of the protein can be thought as being analogous to the famous collapse of The Tacoma Narrows Bridge in Seattle, 1940. Twist modes of the bridge are excited by strong winds. Eventually, the amplitude of the twist modes becomes so large that the bridge fractures. The bridge did not have the option, that proteins do, to form folded structure.

What is the "pump"? At this point we shall restrict the discussion to making it plausible that such a resonator exists by mentioning a set of alternative possibilities. It could originate from thermal vibrations or rotations in the sidechains. It could originate from the rhythm of the ribosome translational process, from fluctuating carbohydrates, or from external molecules such as chaperonins [31].

A number of unique features follow from the scenario of a pumped transition. The resonance would be sensitive to the length of the polypeptide chain. This is consistent with protein folding domains all being of roughly the same length [32, 33]. For example, insulin is synthesized as a single chain which is folded before it is cleaved into its constituents being 21 and 30 amino acids long [34]. Carbohydrates with large masses can define folding domains by constraining the twist modes. Protein folding can be promoted by pauses in the ribosome

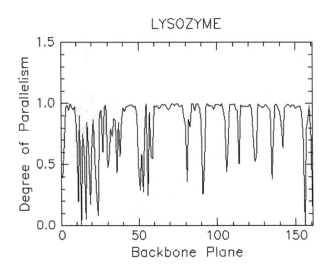

Figure 4: The degree of parallelism in lysozyme between the geometrical frame associated with the backbone path and the planes defined by the backbone atoms, see fig. 3. The frequently observed values of nearly 1 reflect the almost prefect parallelism found in α helices.

translation process if halts [35, 36, 37, 38] are engineered to come after a particular part of the peptide chain has been completed. It is natural to interpret this phenomenon as a means of selection of length, see below in the summary. The part of the protein which would first begin to fold will depend on the twist mode, and on the detailed location of the different amino acids (the bridge broke at the 1/4 point — corresponding to maximum torsion). This means that the protein folding path to a large extend would be deterministic and that folding could be a fast process. Finally, winding symmetries and conservation laws will exist, depending on the twist mode.

5   Linking and writhing

The heuristic description of the winding state of a protein can be extended to a more well founded continuous measure using differential geometry and knot theory [39]. The topological conserved winding is given by the linking number of a closed curve. Define a ribbon as the geometrical frame where the twist is equal to the torsion of the curve. A linking number of zero means that if one cut the ribbon (with a scissor) along a central line, one will end up by two non-interwoven ribbons. If the linking number is ± 1 you will end up by two ribbons that are linked as links in a chain.

The linking number, L, is related to the writhing number, W, and the total twist, T, through the White theorem

$$L = W + T \qquad (2)$$

The vectors $\vec{t}$, $\vec{v}$, and $\vec{v}^{\perp}$ define a right-handed frame of the curve; $\vec{t}$ being a unit vector parallel to the velocity $\vec{r}'$. The total twist can then be calculated as

$$T = \frac{1}{2\pi} \int_0^l \vec{v}^{\perp} \cdot d\vec{v} \qquad (3)$$

and the writing as

$$W = \frac{1}{4\pi} \int \int_{c \times c} \frac{\partial \vec{e}}{\partial s_1} \times \frac{\partial \vec{e}}{\partial s_2} \cdot \vec{e} \, ds_1 \, ds_2 \qquad (4)$$

where

$$\vec{e} = \frac{\vec{r_2} - \vec{r_1}}{| \vec{r_2} - \vec{r_1} |} \qquad (5)$$

Writhing can be formed on the expense of twist. This may commonly be observed in double twisted telephone cords. A concept that was introduced in discussions of circular supercoiled DNA [15, 16, 17, 29], and has been suggested to be associated with protein folding as well [23, 26, 27].

How to calculate the writhing along the backbone of the protein? Writhing must be calculated as a double integral [23], a fact that otherwise have been ignored in studies of proteins [26, 27]. Two fundamental problems arise. One being the issue of how to extend the backbone into a closed curve, and the other being concerned with the fact that the position of the curve is known at discrete points as given by X-ray or NMR measurements. In the limit $\omega_i = 0$, the polypeptide backbone consists of planar plates joined together at the C_α atoms by the two other dihedral angles. Due to the relatively free rotations of these planes, which in particular is the case when glycine is involved, one cannot calculate the winding state solely by inspecting the planes. Firstly, between each pair of planes there is a right/left twist ambiguity. And as the rotations often are large it is not adequate to let the right/left question be settled simply by which angles are smallest. Secondly, the unfolded state is unknown. A given physical representation of the ribbon is not necessarily untwisted in the unfolded state. But, in contrast, the geometrical frame described above can provide us with a way of calculating meaningful linking numbers. Notice, that the sign of torsion (1) and the chirality is determined by the right/left handedness of the local frame. However, for backbone geometries where the chirality is a global property, the chirality becomes associated with the sign of the writhing (see fig. 1).

It is interesting to compare the orientation of the planes of atoms with the geometrical frame of the folded structure as it provides us with information about the preferences of the folded structure. For this purpose the backbone is characterized by a set of points that are midpoints between the C_α atoms, and the successive planes defined by normal vectors given by $\vec{O_i C_i'} \times \vec{N_i C_i'}$. The coarse grained mesh of points on the backbone leads to some sign errors in calculating the geometrical frame. A 1 Å random motion leads to about 4 sign changes in every 100 residues. In figure 4 the absolute value of the scalar product of the vector of the geometrical frame and the normal of the physical plane is shown for lysozyme (7LZM). The absolute value of the scalar product is not sensitive to sign errors. For lysozyme it is very close to 1 for the majority of the residues; there is a high degree of parallelism between the geometrical frame and the physical planes. The reason for this is due to the relative rigidity of the α-helix structures which are abundant in lysozyme. Figure 5 shows the result obtained for porin (2POR). The tendency to parallelism between the geometrical frame and the physical frame is less clear, because of the lower degree of rigidity of the β-strands, which are abundant in porin. In porin the sign is alternating most of the time. This reflect the alternating orientations of atomic planes making up the β-strands. It shows an inherent problem with winding since such a behaviour is consistent with a collapse of a spiral where the period is reduced to two residues. As such, it could explain the frequently observed alternating motif

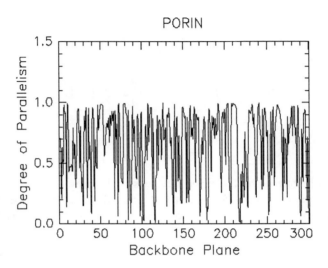

Figure 5: The degree of parallelism in porin between the geometrical frame associated with the backbone path and the planes defined by the backbone atoms (see fig. 3).

between α-helices and β-strands as seen in tim-barrels [40]. We will not further develop this point of view here, but stress the ambiguity it leaves.

6   Summary

One of the paradoxes in our current understanding of protein folding is how fast it really goes. For example it has been estimated that the time required to sample all possible conformations would be 10^{77} years [1]. In reality, many proteins fold in a fraction of a second. The hypothesis for protein folding presented in this paper is consistent with fast folding as the phase space is not searched for possible conformations.

The geometrical winding of polypetide backbones has been considered and it has been shown that long wavelength excitations exist. Simple conjectures for the process of protein folding lead to constrains for the winding of the backbone of the folded state of proteins. But as the unfolded structure of the polypeptide chain is unknown no unique winding can be prescribed. It is hypothesized that the transition from the unfolded state to the folded state of a protein is due to a catastrophic transition, when a twist mode of the protein backbone becomes unstable to curvature. Energy is driven into the twist mode by a resonator.

References

[1] T. E. Creighton, *Protein, Structure and Molecular Properties*, 2nd edition, Freeman, New York, 1993.

[2] M. L. Mansfield, Are there knots in proteins?, *Nature Structural Biology*, 1, 213-214, 1994.

[3] J. Richardson, The anatomy and taxonomy of protein structure, *Adv. Prot. Chem.*, 34, 167-339, 1981.

[4] C. Chothia, Proteins: One thousand families for the molecular biologist, *Nature*, 357, 543-544 1992.

[5] C. Chothia and A. V. Finkelstein, The classification and origins of protein folding patterns, *Ann. Rev. Biochemistry*, 59, 1007-1039 1990.

[6] J. U. Bowie, R. Luthy and D. Eisenberg, A method to identify protein sequences that fold into a known three-dimensional structure, *Science*, 253, 164-170, 1991.

[7] C. B. Anfinsen and H. A. Scheraga, Experimental and theoretical aspects of protein folding, *Adv. Prot. Chem.*, 29, 205-300, 1975.

[8] T. E. Creighton, Conformational restrictions on the pathway of folding and unfolding of the pancreatic trypsin inhibitor, *J. Mol. Biol.*, 113, 329-341 1977.

[9] D. B. Wetlaufer and S. Ristow, Acquisition of 3-dimensional structure of proteins, *Annu. Rev. Biochem.*, 42, 135-158, 1973.

[10] R. L. Baldwin, Intermediates in protein folding reactions and the mechanism of protein folding, *Ann. Rev. Biochem.*, 44, 453-475, 1975.

[11] P. G. Wolynes, Spin glass ideas in the protein folding problem, in *Spin glasses and biology*, D. L. Stein (ed.), World Scientific Press, New York 1990.

[12] R. L. Balwin, How does protein folding get started?, *Trends Biochem. Sci. Pers. Ed.*, 11, 6-9, 1986.

[13] P. E. Wright, H. S. Dyson and R. A. Lerner, Conformation of peptide fragments of proteins in aqueous solution: Implications for initiation of protein folding, *Biochemistry*, 27, 7167-7175, 1988.

[14] J. P. Waltho, V. A. Feher, G. Merutka, H. S. Dyson and P. E. Wright, Peptide models of protein folding initiation sites. 1. Secondary structure formation by peptides corresponding to the G- and H- helices of myoglobin, *Biochemistry*, 32, 6337-6347, 1993.

[15] F. H. Crick, Linking numbers and nucleosomes, *Proc. Natl. Acad. Sci. U. S. A.*, 73, 2639-2643, 1976.

[16] F. B. Fuller, The writhing number of a space curve, *Proc. Natl. Acad. Sci. U. S. A.*, 68, 815-819, 1971.

[17] F. B. Fuller, Decomposition of the linking number of a closed ribbon: A problem from molecular biology, *Proc. Natl. Acad. Sci. U. S. A.*, 75, 3557-3561, 1978.

[18] W. Helfrich and W. Harbich, in *Physics of Amphiphilie layers*, D. Langevin and N. Boccasa (eds.), 58, Springer, Berlin 1987.

[19] H. Bohr and J. H. Ipsen, Differential geometry and topology of biological membranes, in *Characterizing Complex Systems*, H. Bohr (ed.), World Scientific, Singapore 1989.

[20] J. H. White, Self-linking and the Gauss-integral in higher dimensions, *American J. of Math.*, 91, 693-728, 1969.

[21] W. Helfrich, Elastic properties of lipid bilayers: Theory and possible experiments, *Z. Naturforsch.*, 28c, 693-703, 1973.

[22] R. E. Goldstein and S. Leibler, Model for laminar phases of interacting lipid membranes, *Phys. Rev. Lett.*, 61, 2213-2216, 1988.

[23] M. Levitt, Protein folding by restrained energy minimization and molecular dynamics, *J. Mol. Biol.*, 170, 723-764, 1983.

[24] S. Rackovsky and H. A. Scheraga, Differential geometry and polymer conformations I, *Macromolecules*, 11, 1168, 1978.

[25] S. Rackovsky and H. A. Scheraga, Differential geometry and polymer conformations II, *Macromolecules*, 13, 1440, 1980.

[26] P. De Santis, S. Morosetti and A. Palleschi, Topological aspects of the conformational transformations in polypeptides and proteins, *Biopolymers*, 22, 37-42, 1983.

[27] S. Chiavarini, P. De Santis, S. Morosetti and A. Palleschi, Topological aspects of confor-

mational transformations in proteins, *Biopolymers*, 23, 1547-1563, 1984.

[28] E. I. Shahknovich, Proteins with selected sequences fold into unique native conformation, *Phys. Rev. Lett.*, 72, 3907-3910, 1994.

[29] W. F. Pohl, DNA and Differential Geometry, *Math. Intelligence*, 3, 20-27, 1980.

[30] A. M. Lesk, *Protein Architecture*, Oxford University Press, Oxford 1991.

[31] M. Gething and J. Sambrook, Protein folding within the cell, *Nature*, 355, 33-45, 1992.

[32] J. Janin and S. Wodak, Structural domains in proteins and their role in the dynamics of protein function, *Prog. Biophys. Molec. Biol.*, 42, 21-78, 1983.

[33] J. R. Garel, Large multi-domain and multi-subunit proteins, in *Protein Folding*, T. E. Creighton (ed.), Freeman, New York 1992.

[34] J. Kendrew, *The Encyclopedia of Molecular Biology*, Blackwell Science, Oxford 1994.

[35] P. M. Sharp, and W. Li, Codon usage in regulatory genes in *Escherichia coli*, *Nuc. Acids Res.*, 10, 7737-7749, 1986.

[36] P. M. Sharp, T. M. F. Tuohy and K. R. Mosurski, Codon usage in yeast: cluster analysis clearly differentiates highly and lowly expressed genes, *Nuc. Acids Res.*, 14, 5125-5143, 1986.

[37] I. A. Purvis, J. Bettany, T. C. Santiago, J. R. Coggins, K. Duncan, R. Eason and A. J. Brown, The Efficiency of folding of some proteins is increased by controlled rates of translation *in vivo* — A hypothesis, *J. Mol. Biol.*, 193, 413-417, 1987.

[38] S. L. Wolin and P. Walter, Discrete nascent chain lengths are required for the insertion of presecretory proteins into microsomal membranes, *J. Cell. Biol.*, 121, 1211-1219, 1993.

[39] L. H. Kauffman, *Knots and Physics*, World Scientific, Singapore 1991.

[40] C. Branden and J. Tooze, *Introduction to protein structure*, Garland Publishing Inc, New York 1993.

Chirality in Protein Structure

Timothy W. F. Slidel and Janet M. Thornton

Biomolecular Structure and Modelling Unit, Department of Biochemistry and Molecular Biology, University College London, Gower Street, London WC1E 6BT, United Kingdom

Abstract

It is well known that the intrinsic chirality of the L-amino acid is reflected in the chirality of the α-helices and β-strands of protein structure. In turn, this chirality influences that of secondary structure aggregates such as the $\beta\alpha\beta$ motif, which exhibits a strong preference for right-handedness. Occasionally, when examining a protein structure, a motif with unusual chirality is found. Such a motif might contain residues that are central to the function of a protein or may indicate the presence of an important structural anomaly such as an incorrect chain tracing. Clearly, an understanding of the chirality of these motifs is desirable. In this report we discuss protein structure chirality in general and present the results of an analysis of the chirality of some structural motifs.

1 Introduction

I call any geometrical figure, or group of points, chiral, and say it has chirality, if its image in a plane mirror, ideally realized, cannot be brought to coincide with itself [1]. An object is therefore defined as chiral if it has no inverse symmetry elements.

The appearance of chirality throughout nature, its origin, and the possible relationships between molecular chirality and the morphological chirality found in higher organisms have fascinated science for more than a century. Pasteur [2] showed that many organic molecules exist in enantiomeric pairs, with identical physical and chemical properties but with the opposite sign of optical rotation. He also found that laboratory experiments produced equal numbers of left- and right-handed molecules, whereas biological processes gave only one enantiomer, leading him to propose the existence of a chiral force in nature. The tetrahedral model for the orientation of the four valences of the carbon atom [3, 4] gave the molecular basis for Pasteur's observations. Subsequently Fischer [5], through his studies of proteins and sugars, characterised chemically two enantiomeric series of amino acids. He found that in living organisms biochemistry is dominated by the L-amino acids. He postulated that the underlying asymmetry of amino acids was extended into larger structures resulting in the formation of chiral products and eliminating the need for Pasteur's chiral force. However, the origin of this asymmetry remains a mystery.

Protein structure chirality can be divided into two main types: *topological* chirality and *geometric* chirality. The former relates to the inter-connectivity (*intrinsic topology*) of a polypeptide chain and to the realisation of this connectivity in 3D space (its *extrinsic topology*), whereas the latter relates only to the spatial disposition of a polypeptide backbone (i.e., its *geometry*). The chirality of the amino-acids can also be classed as geometric chirality.

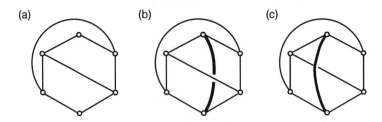

Figure 1: The graph form of protein topologies. (a) A planar (achiral) graph. (b) and (c) The nonplanar, chiral L and D topologies respectively[8].

1.1 Topological chirality

The intrinsic topology of an object relates only to its connectivity, regardless of any other properties such as length or angle. Thus, two polypeptide backbones have the same intrinsic topology since in this context they are simply line segments. However, if inter-residue cross-links (such as disulphide bonds) are included as part of a protein's intrinsic topology then the situation becomes more complex.

The intrinsic topology of a cross-linked polypeptide can be represented in the form of a "graph" (Fig. 1a) in which points (or vertices) represent cross-linked residues and lines (or edges) between points indicate that they are connected by a cross-link and/or a segment of polypeptide chain [6]. Topological chirality occurs when such a graph cannot be rearranged and presented in a planar form without edges crossing since two mirror image forms (or *topological enantiomers*) of the graph then exist (Fig. 1b and 1c) [8]. Such a graph and the corresponding protein's topology are called "nonplanar". The two enantiomeric forms have identical intrinsic topology but can be distinguished by their difference in extrinsic topology, i.e., by the relative disposition of the crossed edges. Therefore, with knowledge of a protein's primary structure and any cross-links one can determine whether a protein is topologically chiral or achiral but to find out to which enantiomer a topologically chiral protein corresponds its 3D structure must also be known.

Recent analyses of topological chirality in proteins have involved three types of cross-link:

a) disulphide bonds [7, 8, 9]
b) covalently bound cofactors, e.g., haem groups [10]
c) hydrogen bonds [11]

Topological chirality in disulphide bond containing proteins has important implications for algorithms that attempt to predict tertiary structure from the primary structure of such proteins, since these algorithms must be able to deduce which topological enantiomer the folded protein will adopt. Since the difference between topological enantiomers depends on the global fold of a protein there is no reason to expect a preference for one enantiomer over the other. Fortunately, the above analyses have shown that topological chirality induced by disulphide bond connectivity is very rare in proteins, only two examples have been found so far [9]. In two other analyses of disulphide bond connectivity Kikuchi *et al.* [12, 13] use a different definition of nonplanarity that is not strictly topological in nature. Thus, the majority of proteins that they class as "nonplanar" are in fact topologically achiral in three-dimensions. They term such proteins "pseudononplanar" and introduce the term "loop chirality" to describe the isomerism that occurs in them. A second form of topological chirality can result if

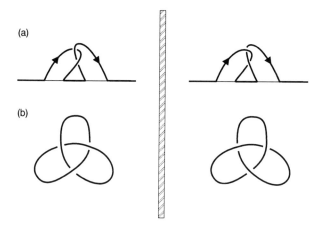

Figure 2: Loop and knot chirality. (a) Mirror-image interlinked loops. Thick lines represent the polypeptide backbone and thin lines represent inter-residue cross-links. (b) Mirror-image trefoil knots.

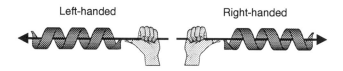

Figure 3: The sense, or hand of a helix. The fingers of the hand curl round the same way as the helix when the thumb points from N- to C-terminus.

topologically interlinked loops or knots occur in a protein (Fig. 2). The origin of this chirality lies purely within extrinsic topology (these entanglements have planar graphs). However, a recent analysis found that these structures do not occur within the disulphide connectivity of proteins [7].

The additional cross-links formed by covalently bound cofactors such as haem groups and metal ions make protein topologies more complex; under these circumstances topological chirality is more prevalent [10]. Again, there is no reason to expect a particular enantiomeric preference (and indeed none is found [10]). Knowledge of this kind of connectivity usually requires detailed information about a protein's three-dimensional structure. Therefore, the observed topological chirality is not as fundamental a property as that induced by disulphide bond connectivity.

The topological chirality induced by the third type of cross-link above (hydrogen bonds) is so dependent on a protein's local geometry that the distinction between topological chirality and geometric chirality becomes blurred. However, Mao *et al.* [11] have shown that not all geometrically chiral hydrogen bonded α-helices are topologically chiral.

An understanding of protein structure topology and topological chirality is important in the context of protein folding since a lower incidence of nonplanar and nontrivial extrinsic

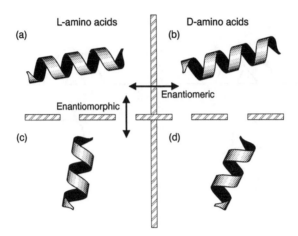

Figure 4: The four possible helical forms in protein structure. (a) and (b) or (c) and (d) are true mirror images of one another whereas (a) and (c) have opposite helical sense but the same amino acid type. (a) and (b) are enantiomers whereas we refer to (a) and (c) as enantiomorphs. In analyses of geometric chirality in proteins we are interested primarily in the relative frequency of occurrence of the two L-amino acid enantiomorphs.

topologies is clearly related to earlier formation of the corresponding cross-links in the protein folding process.

1.2   Geometric chirality

The topology of a linear polypeptide chain may be trivial but its Euclidean geometrical properties (i.e., the way it is arranged in 3D space) are far from it. On the contrary, we see a huge variety of ways in which such a chain can bend and twist into a stable structure. Many segments of polypeptide chain adopt helical geometries. Clearly, the geometry of a helical path in space is chiral (i.e., a helical path has geometric chirality). The two mirror image forms of a helical path can be distinguished by their helical "sense" or "hand" (Fig. 3). In protein structure there are, in principal, four possible helical forms (Fig. 4). We refer to helical forms of similar construction and the same amino-acid type as isomorphs. To distinguish between true mirror image isomers (commonly called enantiomers) and isomorphic helical forms of opposite hand we will refer to the latter as enantiomorphs.

The asymmetry of the L-amino acids has a profound influence on the geometry of proteins. In the same way that asymmetric steps produce only one hand of spiral staircase, the L-amino acids give rise to the right-handed α-helices and left-handed β-strands of protein secondary structure [14]. A good measure of chirality at this structural level is the Cα atom virtual torsion angle "α" since it indicates the sign and magnitude of the local torsion along the polypeptide backbone (Fig. 5) [15, 16, 17]. A recent analysis of these values gave a mean value of +49.3° for α-helices and -166.4° for β-strands (T. W. F. Slidel, unpublished results) indicating low-to-moderate right-handed torsion and high left-handed torsion respectively. When viewed along the chain, the *left-handed torsion* in β-strands appears as a *right-handed twist* since one instinctively observes the twist in the overall plane of the hydrogen bonds rather than associating pairs of hydrogen bonds from opposite sides of a β-strand (Fig. 6).

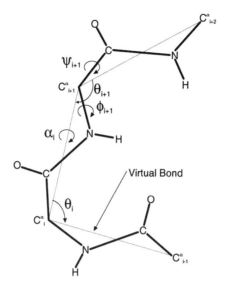

Figure 5: Polypeptide chain angles. The α torsion angle is a good measure of secondary structure chirality.

The preferred helical sense of β-strands and α-helices is transferred, to some degree, when secondary structures aggregate to form supersecondary structures or structural motifs. It is usually possible to define a helical path through such a motif that passes along the central axis of sequential secondary structures and joins them together. The handedness of this path can then be used to distinguish between the two enantiomorphs of the motif. The classic example of a structural motif that has a preferred enantiomorph is the $\beta\alpha\beta$ motif (Fig. 7). This motif is found almost exclusively in its right-handed form [18, 19]. The occurrence of a left-handed $\beta\alpha\beta$ motif is so unusual that it may indicate the evolutionary conservation of some vital feature. This can be seen clearly in the serine proteinase subtilisin which has evolved a left-handed $\beta\alpha\beta$ motif that positions histidine 64 in a catalytic triad with serine 221 and aspartic acid 32 (See Color plate 13, page xxvi). One of the factors that affects the helical sense of structural motifs is the angle at which α-helices and β-strands pack together. About 50% of α-helices pack together at a left-handed angle of approximately 50° and about 25% pack at a more shallow right-handed angle of 20° [20]. This is due to the arrangement of the side chains around the helices and the way these side chains pack together [20, 21]. In accordance with their right-handed twist, β-strands form β-sheets with a right-handed twist (when viewed along the strands). Adjacent β-strands are related by a left-handed rotation of approximately 25° [22]. In general, when α-helices pack onto β-sheets, they lie parallel to the β-strands because the two surfaces have similar asymmetry [23]. The chirality of the secondary structures "cancels out" in this case to give a symmetrical result. A combination of the above geometrical preferences, together with other conformational factors and the preferred right-handed twist of isolated extended chain [14] may result in a preferred handedness for many structural motifs. Efimov has examined a variety of these motifs (see [24] for a review) and in most cases found that they have a preferred hand, for example, the "$\alpha\alpha$-corner" has a preference for "right-handedness" (as defined in [25]).

In some cases the chirality of structural motifs can be inherited into tertiary structure. One of the most striking examples of this occurs in the "β-barrel" structure of triosephosphate

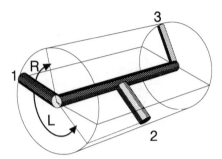

Figure 6: The local, left-handed torsion along a β-strand appears as a right-handed twist when viewed along the strand. Points 1, 2, and 3 define a left-handed helix. But the relationship between every second point (e.g., 1 and 3) defines a right-handed one.

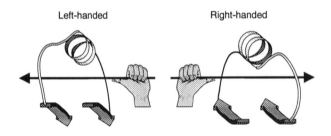

Figure 7: The helical sense, or handedness of a $\beta\alpha\beta$ motif.

isomerase (Fig. 8). Due to the consistent handedness of the $\beta\alpha\beta$ motifs in this protein, the chain winds around the barrel in an anticlockwise direction (when viewed from the C-termini of the β-strands). However, chiral preferences are not generally observed at tertiary structure level in globular proteins since by this stage the asymmetric influence of the L-amino acids is too dilute. This influence has all but disappeared at domain and quaternary structure levels. A new structural hierarchy with different rules begins at this stage, where globular proteins play the role of the amino acids. Without intrinsic constraints on their symmetry these new building blocks are able to form helical assemblies of either hand.

2   An analysis of structural motif handedness

In view of their pivotal position in the protein structure hierarchy we feel that an understanding of the chirality of structural motifs is important. Previous investigations, discussed above, have been carried out by visual inspection of motifs. This can be time consuming if many motifs are involved, as is often the case with today's large structure databases. The assignment of helical sense to motifs can also become highly subjective in cases where it is difficult to define (Fig. 9). Therefore, in the following analysis we use an algorithm which was developed to determine the handedness of generic structural motifs in an efficient and consistent way (T. W. F. Slidel and J. M. Thornton, submitted for publication).

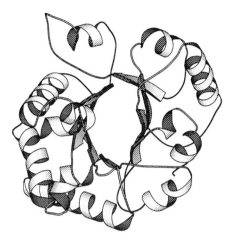

Figure 8: A MOLSCRIPT[30] diagram of triosephosphate isomerase (PDB code 5TIM [31]) showing how the chain winds into a barrel in an anticlockwise direction (when viewed from the C-termini of the β-strands).

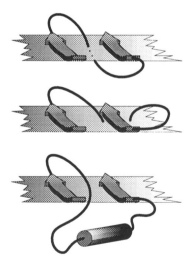

Figure 9: Examples of motifs whose helical sense is difficult to classify as right-handed or left-handed.

2.1 Method

The chirality of the following three types of structural motif was analysed:

- parallel strand $\beta\alpha\beta$ motifs: two parallel β-strands connected by a segment of chain containing an α-helix and no β-strands.
- parallel strand $\beta c\beta$ motifs: two parallel β-strands connected by a segment of chain containing no α-helices or β-strands.
- $\alpha\alpha\alpha$ motifs: three sequential α-helices.

These were extracted from a non-homologous dataset of 271 protein chains (which was derived from PDB [26] structures using the method of Orengo *et al.* [27]). Coordinate and secondary structure assignment data for these chains were extracted from the output of the DSSP program [16]. The program DBSHEET [28] was used to determine, from the hydrogen bonding patterns of a β-sheet, whether two β-strands contained in that β-sheet were parallel or anti-parallel.

A computer program called GCCP (geometric chirality classification program) (T. W. F. Slidel and J. M. Thornton, submitted for publication) was used to classify each motif into one of the following categories:

- Right-handed: the motif has a right-handed helical swirl (Fig. 7).
- Left-handed: the motif has a left-handed helical swirl (Fig. 7).
- Other: the motif cannot be classified as left- or right-handed (Fig. 9).

The program incorporates an algorithm that can determine the handedness of generic structural motifs comprising three segments of protein chain: two outer segments ("axes") and a central segment (the "cross-over") that connects them together. For example, two β-strands connected by a segment containing an α-helix (i.e., a $\beta\alpha\beta$ motif).

Conceptually this algorithm determines the handedness of a motif in the same way one might do so visually. That is, it:

a) Defines a frame of reference based on the axes
b) Locates the Cα atoms in the crossover within this frame of reference and thereby assigns each one a code that describes its position.
c) Simplifies the resulting sequence of position codes to give the handedness of the motif.

The frame of reference is based on three sets of surfaces (Fig. 10a) which intersect and divide the 3D space around a motif into eighteen "zones". The surfaces are generated from the coordinates of the Cα atoms in the axes. This process results in a frame of reference that is appropriate for even the most convoluted of motifs. The Cα atoms in the crossover are located in the frame of reference simply by calculating on which side of each surface each atom lies. The handedness of the motif is then obtained by removing extraneous information from the sequence of position codes assigned to the Cα atoms.

2.2 Results

Table 1 shows the results of the above analysis for the three motif types.

2.3 Discussion

Previous analyses have shown that parallel strand $\beta\alpha\beta$ motifs have an almost exclusive preference for right-handedness [18, 19]. In the analysis of Sternberg and Thornton [18] 57 out of the 60 observed motifs (95%) were found to be right-handed and two could not be assigned a hand. Table 1 shows that the current automated analysis found 271 right-handed $\beta\alpha\beta$ motifs out of a total of 286 (95%). Therefore, even when a wider variety of

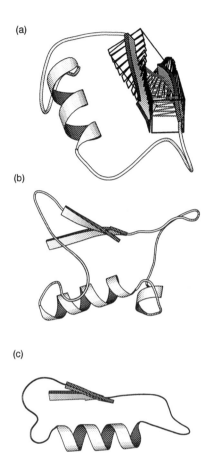

Figure 10: MOLSCRIPT[30] diagrams of the three left-handed $\beta\alpha\beta$ motifs found in this analysis. (a) Residues 44-94, chain E, from subtilisin (PDB code 1CSE[29]). This diagram also shows the surfaces which form the frame of reference by which the sense of a motif is defined. (b) Residues 444-516 from lipase (PDB code 1THG[32]). (c) Residues 109-150, chain A, from asparaginase type II (PDB code 3ECA[33]). All three motifs contain functionally important residues in their crossovers.

protein structures is considered the same degree of preference for right-handed $\beta\alpha\beta$ motifs is observed. The three left-handed motifs found are shown in figure 10. In each case there are functionally vital residues in the crossovers of these motifs. Therefore, it seems likely that the handedness of these motifs has been tolerated in order to preserve functional integrity.

In a previous analysis of $\beta c \beta$ motif handedness Sternberg and Thornton [22] found 15 instances of this motif, 13 of which (87%) were right handed (two could not be assigned a hand). As shown in table 1, the current analysis found 42 motifs, of which 33 (79%) were right-handed. Therefore, as for the $\beta\alpha\beta$ motifs there is still a clear preference for right-handedness. The difference in percentages may be attributable to the inclusion of 3_{10} helices in the coil region between the two strands of the $\beta c \beta$ motif in this analysis. It may also be due

Table 1: Classification of motif chirality into three categories: right-handedness (R), left-handedness (L), and other (O).

Classification code	Frequency of occurrence	Percentage occurrence
$\beta\alpha\beta$ motifs		
R	271	94.8
L	3	1.0
O	12	4.2
Total	286	100.0
$\beta c\beta$ motifs		
R	33	78.6
L	3	7.0
O	6	14.3
Total	42	100.0
$\alpha\alpha\alpha$ motifs		
R	112	32.2
L	126	36.2
O	110	31.6
Total	348	100.0

to statistical fluctuations arising from the small number of $\beta c\beta$ motifs available in the previous analysis. Again, it seems likely that the occurrence of exceptional left-handed $\beta c\beta$ motifs will be attributable to conservation of functionally important residue positions.

The striking preference for right-handedness in the above motifs has been attributed to the left-handed twist of β-sheets (when viewed edge-on) [18, 22] and to the preferred right-handed twist of extended chain together with the right-handedness of the α-helices [19].

In contrast to the β-motifs, table 1 shows that there is no distinct preference for the handedness of three linked α-helices. However, it is important to point out that there are no constraints on the inter-helix angles in these motifs. Clearly, given that the two outer helices are not necessarily parallel (as they are in the above β-motifs), one would not necessarily expect any preference in this case. We are currently looking at these motifs in more detail to see if there are any correlations between the metric properties of the chain and its handedness.

3   Conclusions

We have discussed many of the chiral features of protein structure. In particular we have presented a preliminary analysis of structural motif handedness using an automated method. A full analysis is currently in progress and will be published in the near future. We believe that an understanding of this and other types of chirality in proteins will be beneficial within the fields of protein structure prediction, modelling and verification.

References

[1] W. T. Kelvin, *Baltimore Lectures on Molecular Dynamics and the Wave Theory of Light*, C. J. Clay (ed.), London, p. 439, 618-619, 1904.

[2] L. Pasteur, *Researches on molecular asymmetry* (1860), Alembic Club Reprint 14, Edinburgh, 1948.

[3] J. A. Le Bel, Sur les relations qui existent entre les formules atomiques des corps organiques, et le pouvoir rotatoire de leurs dissolutions, *Bull. Soc. Chim. Fr.*, 22, p. 337-347, 1874.

[4] J. H. van't Hoff, Sur les formules de structure dans l'espace, *Arch. Neerl. Sci. Exactes Nat.*, 9, p. 445-454, 1874.

[5] K. Freudenberg, Emil Fischer and his contribution to carbohydrate chemistry, *Advances in Carbohydrate Chemistry*, 21, p. 1-38, 1966.

[6] G. M. Crippen, Topology of Globular Proteins, *J. Theor. Biol.*, 45, p. 327-338, 1974.

[7] C. J. Benham and M. S. Jafri, Disulfide bonding patterns and protein topologies, *Protein Sci.*, 2(1), p. 41-54, 1993.

[8] B. Mao, Molecular topology of multiple-disulfide polypeptide-chains, *J. Am. Chem. Soc.*, 111(16), p. 6132-6136, 1989.

[9] B. Mao, Topological chirality of proteins, *Protein Sci.*, 2, p. 1057-1059, 1993.

[10] C. Z. Liang and K. Mislow, Topological chirality of proteins, *J. Am. Chem. Soc.*, 116(8), p. 3588-3592, 1994.

[11] B. Mao, K. Chou and G. M. Maggiora, Topological analysis of hydrogen bonding in protein structure, *Eur. J. Biochem.*, 188, p. 361-365, 1990.

[12] T. Kikuchi, G. Nemethy and H. A. Scheraga, Spatial geometric arrangements of disulfide-crosslinked loops in nonplanar proteins, *J. Comput. Chem.*, 10(3), p. 287-294, 1989.

[13] T. Kikuchi, G. Nemethy and H. A. Scheraga, Spatial geometric arrangements of disulfide-crosslinked loops in proteins, *J. Comput. Chem.*, 7(1), p. 67-88, 1986.

[14] G. N. Ramachandran and V. Sasisekharan, Conformation of polypeptides and proteins, *Adv. Prot. Chem.*, 23, p. 283-437, 1968.

[15] R. Srinivasan, R. Balasubramanian and S. S. Rajan, Some new methods and general results of analysis of protein crystallographic structural data, *J. Mol. Biol.*, 98, p. 739-747, 1975.

[16] W. Kabsch and C. Sander, Dictionary of protein secondary structure-pattern-recognition of hydrogen-bonded and geometrical features, *Biopolymers*, 22(12), p. 2577-2637, 1983.

[17] C. Chothia, Coiling of b-pleated sheets, *J. Mol. Biol.*, 163(1), p. 107-117, 1983.

[18] M. J. E. Sternberg and J. M. Thornton, On the conformation of proteins, the handedness of the β-strand-α-helix-β-strand unit, *J. Mol. Biol.*, 105, p. 367-382, 1976.

[19] J. S. Richardson, Handedness of crossover connections in β-sheets, *Proc. Natl. Acad. Sci. USA*, 73(8), p. 2619-2623, 1976.

[20] C. Chothia, M. Levitt and D. Richardson, Helix to helix packing in proteins, *J. Mol. Biol.*, 145(1), p. 215-250, 1981.

[21] F. H. C. Crick, The packing of α-helices, simple coiled coils, *Acta Cryst.*, 6, p. 689-697, 1953.

[22] M. J. E. Sternberg and J. M. Thornton, On the conformation of proteins, the handedness of the connection between parallel β-strands, *J. Mol. Biol.*, 110, p. 269-283, 1977.

[23] J. Janin and C. Chothia, Packing of α-helices onto β-pleated sheets and the anatomy of α/β proteins, *J. Mol. Biol.*, 143, p. 95-128, 1980.

[24] A. V. Efimov, Favored structural motifs in globular-proteins, *Structure*, 2(11), p. 999-1002, 1994.

[25] A. V. Efimov, New supersecondary protein-structure — the $\alpha\alpha$-corner, *Mol. Biol.*, 18(6),

p. 1239-1251, 1984.

[26] F. C. Bernstein, T. F. Koetzle, G. J. B. Williams, E. F. Meyer, M. D. Brice, J. R. Rodgers, O. Kennard, T. Shimanouchi and M. Tasumi, The Protein Data Bank, A computer-based archival file for macromolecular structures, *J. Mol. Biol.*, 112, p. 535-542, 1977.

[27] C. A. Orengo, T. P. Flores, W. R. Taylor and J. M. Thornton, Identification and classification of protein fold families, *Protein Eng.*, 6(5), p. 485-500, 1993.

[28] E. G. Hutchinson, DBSHEET computer program, Department of Biochemisty and Molecular Biology, University College London, London, 1991

[29] W. Bode, E. Papamokos and D. Musil, The high-resolution x-ray crystal-structure of the complex formed between subtilisin carlsberg and eglin-c, an elastase inhibitor from the leech *hirudo-medicinalis* — structural analysis, subtilisin structure and interface geometry, *Eur. J. Biochem.*, 166(3), p. 673-692, 1987.

[30] P. J. Kraulis, MOLSCRIPT, a program to produce both detailed and schematic plots of protein structures, *J. Appl. Crystallogr.*, 24, p. 946-950, 1991.

[31] R. K. Wierenga, M. E. M. Noble, G. Vriend, S. Nauche and W. G. J. Hol, Refined 1.83 Åstructure of trypanosomal triosephosphate isomerase crystallized in the presence of 2.4 M ammonium sulfate — a comparison with the structure of the trypanosomal triosephosphate isomerase-glycerol-3-phosphate complex, *J. Mol. Biol.*, 220(4), p. 995-1015, 1991.

[32] J. D. Schrag and M. Cygler, 1.8 Årefined structure of the lipase from *geotrichum-candidum*, *J. Mol. Biol.*, 230(2), p. 575-591, 1993.

[33] A. L. Swain, M. Jaskolski, D. Housset, J. Rao and A. Wlodawer, Crystal-structure of *escherichia-coli L-asparaginase*, an enzyme used in cancer-therapy, *Proc. Natl. Acad. Sci. USA*, 90(4), p. 1474-1478, 1993.

Packing Within And Between Protein Subunits Defined By Internal Cavities

Simon J. Hubbard and Patrick Argos

European Molecular Biology Laboratory, Postfach 10.2209, Meyerhofstrasse 1, D-69012 Heidelberg, Germany

Abstract

An analysis of internal cavities within protein structures has been undertaken, including cavities within and between domains in given polypetide chains and between protein subunits. Objective parameters for the delineation of protein packing defects are defined in terms of probe distances to elicit consistent detection of cavities and their constituent waters. We report a number of basic findings common to all cavity types as well as a number of features that distinguish cavity subclasses from one another. Cavities are non-artefactual and independent of the method of structure determination, resolution and refinement. Despite a general increase with protein size, the total cavity volume remains only a small fraction of the total protein volume, although cavities are nearly always found in proteins of size greater than 100 residues. The mobility of cavity-defining surface atoms are reduced relative to their environments. Classifying cavities by their solvation state (i.e. solvated or "empty"), we find solvated cavities to possess a much more polar surface whilst "empty" cavities are predominantly hydrophobic, the former also extending up to larger volumes. The two cavity types also exhibit different amino acid type and secondary structural preferences. Solvated cavity waters are necessary to satisfy the local hydrogen bonding potential, are well hydrogen bonded, and occupy a similar volume to that in bulk solvent. Inter-subunit and inter-domain cavities are on average larger than the intra-domain cavities. Inter-domain and inter-subunit cavities occupy a much larger fraction of the respective inter-domain and inter-subunit surfaces than do intra-domain cavities relative to the surface buried in the folded protein. These results provide useful guidelines for protein modelling and design.

1 Introduction

Protein structures pack with a very high efficiency, comparable to the tight packing observed in small inorganic crystals [1]. This widely held truth has lead to many approaches to solve elements of the protein folding problem, recently reviewed by Richards and Lim [2]. Folding proteins is in effect a distance problem, since one of the goals of good packing is to reduce the distances between atoms to achieve a compact, globular structure. Cavities, therefore, might be viewed as the very antithesis of optimal atomic packing. Yet, they have been documented in tertiary structures of proteins determined by crystallography [3, 4, 5] and either contain solvent molecules or are apparently empty. Since these defects may well be destabilising to proteins, their presence can be expected for some structural/functional reasons. However, their role in protein structures is at present largely unknown, and therefore a re-evaluation of their morphology and characteristics is worthwhile and could well prompt discovery of their etiolology.

There have been a number of theoretical studies of cavities and their associated waters in the literature [6, 7, 8, 9]. These works have detailed a number of basic features common to cavities, including their size, distribution and polarity. Cavities have also been studied indirectly by several experimental groups who attempt to "fill" or "create" them in protein cores by means of site-directed mutagenesis [10, 11, 12, 13, 14]. It has not been straightforward to predict the effects of such mutations on protein stability, though generally, introducing cavities has been to some extent destabilising. One T4 phage lysozyme mutant contained a cavity sufficiently large to sequester a benzene molecule despite its central location 7 Å from the protein surface [15].

Numerous computational methods for defining "cavities" and regions of poor packing have been reported [7, 9, 16, 17, 18, 19]. Many of these are only suited for graphical and visual purposes, and are not fully objective to provide statistics regarding cavity characteristics. However, the method of Connolly [16] analytically defines the accessible and molecular surface of all a protein's atoms and delineates all unique surface components including those of cavities as well as their associated volumes. Rashin [7] extended the more approximate Shrake and Rupley method [20] to define surface components and hence cavities, while Kleywegt and Jones [19] use a grid-point "filling" approach to estimate cavity volumes and surface defining atoms.

2 Cavity definition

2.1 What is a cavity?

Kleywegt and Jones [19] supply some useful definitions for "cavities". A cavity or "void" is entirely closed by its surrounding atoms whilst an "invagination" is only closed when a probe of certain size is reached. A "pocket" is a surface cleft which never becomes a true cavity. Some of these effects are illustrated in Figure 1. Small probes allow invaginations near the surface to be completely accessible (Figure 1A) whilst with a larger probe (Figure 1B) a cavity is formed as the probe can no longer pass the lip of the cleft. At a still larger size (Figure 1C), the probe can no longer enter the cleft and the cavity is missed entirely.

Hence, as made salient previously [10], defining cavities is a non-trivial exercise. Nevertheless, cavities, clefts, pockets and invaginations are likely to be important biologically, for example, as ligand binding sites, micro-environments for catalytic reaction, or "gateways" for passage of small molecules through the protein. They must also affect the overall stability of the protein and hence, by inference, its function. Therefore it is critical to ascertain optimal parameters with which to define consistently packing defects and their constituent solvent.

2.2 Finding packing defects in structures

We have selected the MSP program suite of Connolly [16, 21], as it is widely used and tested, produces exact analytical cavity and protein volumes as well as a list of all contributing atoms, requires no initial seeding points, and is not dependent on a relatively large number of user-definable parameters. The program lists individual atomic contributions to the unique surface

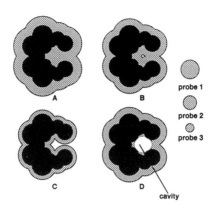

Figure 1: A planar depiction of cavity definition with differing probe size. The accessible surface through which the probe centroid passes when rolled over the atomic van der Waals surface of the protein in black is shown with another solid line for probes 1, 2 and 3 in A, B and C respectively. A true cavity (void) is detected for the middle probe size only. The molecular surface perimeter of this cavity is shown in D and bounds the white cavity volume.

components delineated from 1 to n, where 1 is the atomic (external) accessible surface and 2 to n represent cavities. Atomic contributions to the respective surfaces are further classified as accessible, contact, re-entrant and molecular [16]. The Cartesian centre and volume of each component are also output. We refer in this work to the more appropriate molecular surface since the accessible surface tends to zero for cavities only slightly larger than the defining probe size. Heteroatoms such as cofactors, inhibitors and ligands were not included in the calculations, although all cavities determined were checked for their presence, which prompted the deletion of such cavities (other than those containing water) from the statistics. The atomic van der Waals radii were taken from [7].

When present in the Brookhaven entry [22], waters were assigned to cavities using a grid point placement method described in detail previously [8]. Briefly, from their Cartesian centre, cavities are filled with cubic grid points at a separation of g Å and all solvent atoms within g Å of any cavity grid point are assigned to that cavity. Cavities without waters were deemed "empty". If no waters or solvent were listed in the Brookhaven databank entry, all cavities for that protein were classed as "unknown". It should be noted that our definition of "empty" is dependent on researchers who determine positions for water molecules but do not place any in the considered cavity. However, it may be possible that the cavity contains some solvent, albeit transiently. Nonetheless, if we observe significant trend differences between solvated and "empty" cavity types, then our classification would be justified.

2.3   Consistency of cavity detection

2.3.1   Methods

To define cavities with likely biological significance, a consistent protocol is required. Hence we investigated the cavities in a set of 5 groups of structures determined for the same protein; they are listed in Table 1, either determined by different laboratories, different methods or under somewhat different crystallisation conditions. *A priori* it can be expected that any

Table 1: Cavity consistency data set. Brookhaven PDB identifiers [22] are listed for the 5 proteins groups studied.

Protein structural group	Broohkaven PDB identifiers					
Bovine pancreatic trypsin inhibitor	4PTI	5PTI	6PTI	7PTI	9PTI	
Interleukin 1-β	1I1B	2I1B	4I1B			
Bovine Trypsin	1NTP	1TLD	1TPA	1TPO	1TPP	2PTC
	2PTN	3PTB	3PTN	4PTP		
Hen egg-white lysozyme	1LYM	1LYZ	1LZT	2LYM	2LYZ	2LZT
	3LYM	3LYZ	4LYM	4LYZ	5LYZ	6LYZ
	7LYZ	8LYZ				
Sperm whale myoglobin	1MBC	1MBD	1MBI	1MBN	1MBO	2MB5
	4MBN	5MBN				

significant disparity between the different determinations of the same structure is a likely result of experimental error or the over-sensitivity of techniques used to delineate conformational statistics. Hence, the presence of cavities that are not consistently observed in equivalent spatial positions over such a series of structures are doubtful and they would be less likely to play any biologically significant structural or functional role. Since most cavity detection methods are dependent on the size of the probe used to define them, it is necessary to select a probe size that will yield consistent and meaningful cavities. In this study we used 5 probe radii (1.2, 1.25, 1.3, 1.35 and 1.4 Å) to examine the effects of different probe sizes on cavity detection.

Using the method of McLachlan [23], the protein backbone atoms in each of the 5 groups were globally superimposed prior to cavity calculation. Subsequently delineated cavities were then equivalenced into groups with a single-linkage clustering algorithm such that any two cavities containing any two grid points less than g Å apart were deemed spatially and structurally equivalent. The grid points were assigned as described previously using values of g between 0.5 and 1.0 Å depending on the size of the protein group and number of cavities within it. Consistency values were assigned to all sets of equivalent cavities by dividing the number of cavities in each set by the number of structures in the associated protein group, producing values between 0 and 1. Each individual cavity was assigned the consistency value of its set.

The detection of cavities was also examined as a function of a number of conformational parameters related to the protein and the cavities. The volume of the cavity, the mean accessible surface of the cavity-defining residues, and the mean RMSD (Root Mean Square Deviation) of residues at each cavity surface-contributing residue position in the global superposition were calculated for comparative purposes.

2.3.2 Cavity detection

In the 5 structural families a total of 67 cavity equivalence sets were found, although not all spanned the complete probe size range. Figure 2 shows the degree of consistency of cavity detection in the independent protein structure determinations. In Figure 2A, the number of cavities with a minimum consistency of 0.9 is plotted against probe size. A peak is noted at 1.30 Å suggesting this to be the optimal probe radius for consistent cavity detection; however,

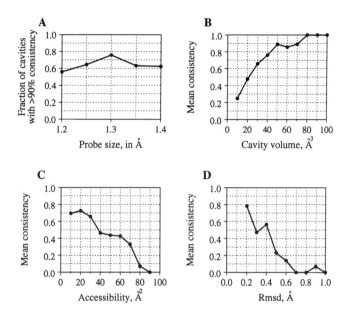

Figure 2: Consistency of equivalent cavity detection in several structure determinations of the same protein. The fraction of cavities with a consistency of at least 0.9 is plotted in A against the defining probe size. The mean consistency of equivalenced cavity groups is plotted against cavity volume in B, against mean cavity atom accessible surface in C, and against the mean RMSD of cavity-defining residues in the global superposition of the structures in D.

a range of probe sizes may be used to avoid missing small cavities of possible interest. Larger probe sizes will find large cavities and not detect smaller cavities, particularly those containing water. Conversely, small probes may "open up" true cavities to the external surface or find very small defects that are a likely result of structural determination error or over-sensitivity of the detecting method. For example, cavity groups with a mean volume less than that of a single water (11.5 Å^3) are detected on average with only a 0.25 consistency.

The dependence of consistency on the cavity conformational parameters is clear (Figures 2B-2D). Larger cavities are more consistently detected, particularly when they are more "buried" i.e. closer to the protein core and further from the external surface. Cavities from regions containing structurally and topologically equivalent atoms with high RMSD after superposition are less consistently detected. Indeed the mean RMSD for cavity-defining residues is about the same as that for buried residues, suggesting that cavities are at least as rigid as the rest of the protein core and do not impart thermal instability to their surroundings. Similar trends were observed for the individual probe sizes studied, albeit less smooth.

2.3.3 Buried water detection

In general, water-containing cavities were detected with greater consistency (mean 0.84) over the 22 solvated cavity sets found where at least one cavity contained water. The corresponding value for "empty" sets is 0.38. Only 3 of the 22 solvated equivalence sets contained both empty and solvated cavities, the others being all solvated. In the former, the majority of cavities were empty and the hydrophobic nature of the cavities' surfaces were conserved, suggesting erroneously placed solvent. For example in the lysozyme structures, one cavity detected with a 1.20 Å probe contained a single water whilst all the others in the set were empty, and yet the cavity itself has a 100% apolar surface. Nonetheless, the conservation of cavity water is strong; in 73% of the equivalent sets even the number of waters found in each member was absolutely conserved. One large trypsin cavity consistently contained 6 waters. These results concur with the similar observations by other workers [24, 25].

3 General Properties of cavities

We have studied some of the general properties of cavities within single subunits, within and between domains of single protein chains and between protein subunits. A single probe size of 1.25 Å was selected for cavity delineation since it was able to identify successfully the highest relative yield of buried waters in a subset of 10 protein structures [8], a criteria that should be met for such an analysis. This probe size is a compromise between the most optimal (1.30 Å) for consistency of detection and those chosen by other workers [7]. The following sections summarise the general cavity characteristics observed.

3.1 Datasets studied

The protein datasets studied for the general analysis of intramolecular [8] and interdomain and intersubunit cavities [26] are published elsewhere. The intramolecular dataset contained 121 protein chains, while the multi-domain dataset was represented by 30 structures and the multi-subunit proteins were 52 in total. No two chains or proteins possessed a sequence identity greater than 40% to any other for each individual cavity grouping.

3.2 Resolution, refinement and structure determination

Are cavities artefactual? Could the packing defects be a result of error in structure determinations at low resolution? Figure 3A shows a plot of the total cavity volume per residue *versus* the resolution of the X-ray diffraction data taken from the 121 protein intramolecular cavity dataset. Clearly, there is no appreciable effect on the cavity volume. This lack of correlation with resolution is also found for total cavity volume, total cavity surface and total cavity surface per residue as well as for the inter-domain and inter-subunit cavities. Similar results are obtained when considering R-factors instead of resolution and structures determined by nuclear magnetic resonance spectroscopy. R-factors measure the closeness of calculated and observed X-ray diffraction intensities. It is concluded that proteins do display packing defects and therefore cavities are non-artefactual.

Errors in a structure determination can nonetheless have subtle effects on the size and indeed "existence" of individual cavities, especially small cavities. Additionally, the placement of solvent is affected by structure quality. Accordingly, for studies dealing with differences between solvated and "empty" cavities, only structures with resolution 2.0 Å or better where at least one water was observed per two protein residues, were considered; these requirements mitigated misclassification of cavity solvation state. These data subsets were constituted by 57 protein chains for the intramolecular studies and 19 multidomain and 18 oligomeric proteins for the intermolecular investigations.

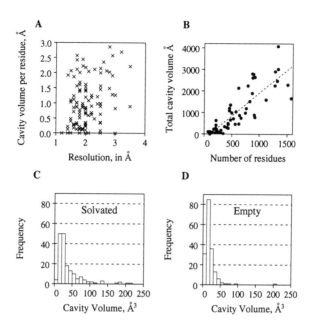

Figure 3: Cavity volumes in proteins of the intramolecular dataset. The total cavity volume per residue is plotted as a function of structure resolution in A, and the total cavity volume as a function of protein size (number of residues) in B. The distributions of solvated and "empty" cavity volumes are plotted in C and D respectively.

3.3 Cavity volume and protein size

The total cavity volume found in protein structures correlated with the total number of residues in a molecular unit. This relationship is illustrated in Figure 3B where cavities of all types are included. The relationship between total cavity volume and protein size is approximately linear, with the best fit to a straight line obtained when considering molecules, either mono- or multimeric, rather than individual domains or single subunits from multimers. Proteins exhibit on average about 2.0 Å^3 per residue of cavity volume.

The distribution of observed intramolecular cavity volumes of water-containing and "empty" cavities are illustrated in Figures 3C and 3D. Solvation clearly permits larger cavities as previously noted [7], although generally both solvated and "empty" cavities rarely exceed 100 Å^3 in volume. It is presumed that waters allow larger defects since they in effect reduce the void size and act as hydrogen bonding protein atoms whilst "empty" cavities can only be accommodated below a certain size. Indeed, only one "empty" cavity, found in the hemoglobin (Brookhaven code 4hhb), exceeded 100 Å^3 in volume over the high resolution subset.

3.4 Cavity polarity and waters

The distribution of cavity surface polarity (defined as the fraction of polar atom surface contributing to a given cavity surface) is plotted for both solvated and "empty" cavities in Figure 4. Solvated cavity surface is uniformly more polar, observed both for intra- and intermolecular cavities. In the intramolecular dataset, solvated cavities have a mean polarity

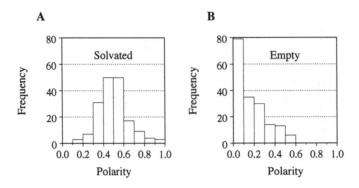

Figure 4: Distributions of cavity surface polarity. Histograms of the distribution of cavity surface polarity are plotted for solvated cavities (A), and "empty" cavities (B), over the intramolecular data set.

of 0.50, compared to only 0.16 for "empty" cavities. Obviously, hydrogen bonding partners are required for the trapped waters, or waters are present to satisfy the hydrogen bonding potential of the surrounding protein atoms. This observation provides a simple criteria to predict the likely solvation state of unknown cavities, an alternative to computationally intensive calculations reported elsewhere [27].

Considering the solvent itself, we find that in the majority of cases solvated cavities contain only one or two waters. However, in all instances, the waters are quite well packed, occupying an average volume of around 27 Å^3 per water, a value close to the 30 Å^3 volume they occupy in bulk solvent. Consequently, we observe that cavities *per se* do not impose unreasonable constraints upon their constituent waters.

3.5   Cavity surface constitution

The contribution to the cavity molecular surface of main and sidechain groups and residues in particular secondary structural conformations are detailed in Table 2. Similar data were obtained for inter-cavities (not shown). Comparisons are shown relative to the characteristics of accessible and buried protein surfaces. Solvated and "empty" cavities display distinct differences in their respective constitution, with the former being derived from a larger fraction of polar mainchain groups than all the other surfaces. The "empty" cavities however are mainly composed of non-polar sidechain groups. Furthermore, the two cavity classes exhibit secondary structural preferences. "Empty" cavity surface is dominated by residues from helices and strands as defined from the atomic coordinates by the DSSP algorithm of Kabsch and Sander [28], whilst solvated cavity surface has a higher contribution from coil residues. This result is explained by the highly non-polar surface of secondary structural elements themselves where helix and sheet surface is on average 70% non-polar. Hence, most "empty" cavities are the result of non-optimal packing of hydrophobic side chain groups at interfaces of secondary structural elements, whilst solvated cavities are the product of non-ideal packing amongst all protein atoms and especially those near the protein surface where coil segments generally appear. Since residues in loops are near the surface and easily accessible to solvent, this result comes as no surprise.

Table 2: Percentage contributions of atom types to atomic surfaces

Surface type	mainchain	sidechain	polar	non-polar	helix	strand	coil
accessible	29	71	40	60	25	18	57
buried	40	60	35	65	28	34	38
solvated cavity	45	55	46	54	18	31	51
empty cavity	20	80	14	86	41	41	18

3.6   Relative position of cavities

Using the protrusion index method of Taylor [29], an equimomental ellipsoid was defined about the protein shapes. Utilising the resulting principle axes for each protein, a set of 10 similarly shaped ellipsoids were derived, each containing successive groups of 10% of the protein atoms; exposed atoms laid within the outer ellipsoidal shell and were assigned a value of 9, while atoms in the innermost core were assigned score 0. The relative position of internal cavities can then be classified (protrusion index 0 to 9) by the particular ellipsoid within which they lie. This was performed for all proteins in our intramolecular dataset, first using all the atoms to define the initial equimomental ellipsoid, and then using only totally buried atoms. The latter procedure avoided the bias of outer ellipsoidal shells containing more exposed atoms, and hence, fewer cavities.

The distributions of cavity protrusion indices of solvated and "empty" cavities (for both calculations) are shown in Figure 5. There is a clear trend for cavities to be in the innermost protein core (protrusion indices 0-2). This trend, although somewhat attenuated, is maintained when considering only buried atoms to define the ellipsoid series. A simple explanation for this result is that cavities near the surface are more likely to be "popped out", becoming clefts on the accessible surface. However, the results from using only totally buried atoms maintain the trend, particularly for "empty" cavities. Indeed, in both distributions, "empty" cavities have a lower mean protrusion index than their solvated counterparts. This may be due to the more hydrophobic nature of the core, and the relatively large distance waters would have to travel to reach such defects.

One hypothesis to explain this phenomenon centres around protein folding, during which cavities may be "trapped" as the secondary structures and side chains coalesce. Cavities formed transiently, further from the core, during folding would be easier to eliminate whilst "core" defects might be carried through to the final fold. Certainly, protein cores are more rigid and dense than their accessible surfaces, and this would be expected to contribute to cavity formation.

3.7   Hydrogen bonding of cavity atoms and solvent

The hydrogen bonding of cavity-defining polar atoms and cavity waters was analysed. Polar hydrogens were built onto all polar atoms using the definitions of Baker and Hubbard [30]. A hydrogen bond was acceptable if the acceptor-donor distance was less than 3.6 Å and the angle at the hydrogen (or antecedent-donor-acceptor) was between 90-180°. On average, polar atoms contributing to solvated cavities were seen to be well hydrogen bonded, making on average 1.7 bonds per atom, although more than 50% of these were to water. By comparison, polar atoms contributing to "empty" cavities formed just over 1 hydrogen bond per atom, although these

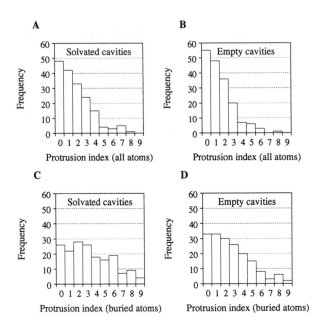

Figure 5: Distributions of cavity protrusion indices in the intramolecular database. Histograms of the distributions of cavity protrusion indices are plotted (ellipsoids based on all protein atoms) for solvated cavities (A), and "empty" cavities (B). The same statistics are shown in C and D defining the ellipsoids with only fully buried atoms.

bonds were almost exclusively made to other protein atoms rather than to outside solvent. This illustrates the need for solvation to satisfy the hydrogen bonding potential of the cavity surface-defining atoms. Though these results were obtained from the high resolution subset of the intramolecular data set, the same trends were displayed for the intercavity data sets.

The cavity waters themselves are also well hydrogen bonded, typically making 3 or 4 bonds per water, in agreement with other studies [9, 30]. Coupled with the result that they are not "over-packed" in cavities, cavity waters are not under strain and can satisfy the bulk of their hydrogen bonding potential within a space typical of bulk solvent.

3.8 Mobility of cavity-defining atoms

By considering the atomic temperature factors (B-values) derived from crystallographic refinement, we evaluated the relative mobility of cavity-defining atoms and associated solvent. The temperature factors effectively measure the size of a sphere in which atom centres can vibrate. The mean B-values were calculated for the accessible and totally buried atoms of each protein, with cavity-defining atoms excluded; buried atoms were defined as all those with zero accessibility to the solvent. The mean cavity-defining atomic B-values were then expressed as a number of standard deviations from these former global means (NSDMs). Similar calculations were performed for the cavity waters. The results are summarised in Figure 6 for the intramolecular cavities extracted from the intermolecular dataset. The distributions of NSDM values for cavity atoms relative to the buried means are broadly Gaussian, with the following

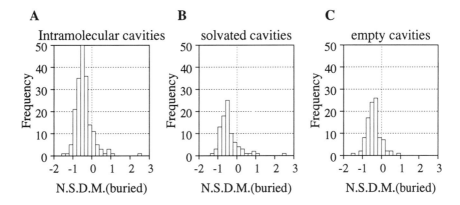

Figure 6: Distributions of the number of standard deviations from a given mean for the average temperature factors of cavity-defining atoms. Distributions are shown with respect to the mean temperature factors of all buried atoms in each protein for all intramolecular cavity atoms (A), intramolecular solvated cavity atoms (B), and intramolecular "empty" cavity atoms (C).

mean values of -0.42, -0.43 and -0.41 for all intramolecular, solvated and "empty" cavities respectively. Thus, cavity-defining atoms of all intramolecular cavity types are consistently less mobile than their immediate environments, implying that the packing defect does not allow or encourage an increased mobility in the surrounding atoms. This result is consistent with the proposal of Lee [31], who suggests that mutation of a rigid local environment in the protein core will result in the greatest destabilisation of a protein when a large hydrophobic residue is substituted by a smaller one. In native protein folds, the core is more rigid than the surface, and the protein is unable to rearrange its atoms locally to fill a possible packing defect. Indeed, cavities may be viewed as a result of the intrinsic inflexibility of the surrounding residue types leading to implicit "unpackability" of the local environment. The extra rigidity of the atoms surrounding the defect not only reflects the inflexibility and high atomic density of the environment but also mitigates any destabilisation. Interestingly, we observe strong linear correlations [26] between the amino acid preferences calculated for "empty" cavities and the flexibility prediction parameters of Karplus and Schulz [32], in support of this conclusion.

The mobility of the cavity waters was also analysed by comparing their mean B-values to those of the buried, cavity-defining and bulk solvent atoms. The distributions of the cavity water B-values were spread quite uniformly about the mean values of their respective cavity-defining atoms (not shown), indicating that cavity waters are on average about as mobile as their protein environment. However, they were typically much less mobile than the bulk solvent as would be expected, with a mean NSDM value of -1.36 over all cavity waters.

4   Interdomain and intersubunit cavities

Thus far, we have discussed general properties of cavities primarily found within single protein chains. Some of the distinguishing features of cavities that lie between domains within one chain and those between subunits within an oligomeric molecule have also been considered. Domain and subunit interfaces could well place different constraints on their attendant cavity properties. The results given subsequently were elicited from the second intermolecular dataset of protein structures where intradomain, interdomain and intersubunit cavities are fully distinguished. An understanding of the packing features at these interfaces is likely critical to such areas as domain-domain motions and the "docking problem".

4.1   Cavity size and polarity

The volumes of the three cavity subclasses (intradomain, interdomain and intersubunit) were compared. There is a noticeable increase in average volume from intradomain to interdomain to intersubunit, with the solvated cavities on average larger than the "empty" ones. The mean volumes observed were 39.8, 43.8 and 86.5 $Å^3$ for solvated cavities and 18.5, 27.1 and 28.1 $Å^3$ for "empty" cavities in the three respective subclasses. The same trend was noted when considering the entire intermolecular dataset and just the high-resolution subset. Interestingly, the ratio of solvated to "empty" cavity volume increases from 1.25 to 1.83 to 2.23 for intradomain to interdomain to intersubunit cavities. The correspondence between the increase in average volume and the higher preponderance of water-containing cavities at higher order surface types would be expected.

The basic polarity trend of solvated-hydrophilic/empty-hydrophobic is conserved for the higher order surface cavities, albeit somewhat attenuated. The intradomain "empty" cavities have a mean polarity of 0.14, whilst the interdomain and intersubunit display 0.20 and 0.26 respectively. This may be a result of the increased hydrophilicity of the interfaces relative to the buried surface in a folded protein [33], or to stabilisation requirements in interacting with the solvent prior to forming the full multimeric unit.

4.2   Comparative packing at interfaces

A simple estimate of the packing quality for the different surface types was obtained by calculating the fraction of a given surface occupied by cavity surface. Intradomain, interdomain and intersubunit cavity surfaces were considered and the surface buried upon domain folding acted as a "reference" surface for the intradomain cavities, while domain-domain and subunit-subunit interface surfaces were used to normalise the respective cavity surfaces. The distributions of these estimates of complementarity are plotted in Figure 7. Quite clearly, interfaces between domains and subunits are not as well packed as the buried surface within single domains. The mean percentage of buried domain surface occupied by cavity surface over the intermolecular protein cases is 2.8%, as compared to 9.6 and 10.7% for the respective interdomain and intersubunit cases. Optimal packing is clearly not achieved generally at protein interfaces. Indeed, only 10% of the multidomain proteins studied were without any cavities at their domain interfaces, and 77% of the multimeric proteins possess some intersubunit cavity surface.

The high observation of poor interfacial packing is tempered by the increased fraction of interface that are solvent filled. Indeed 77% of the interdomain cavity volume is provided by water-containing cavities whilst "empty" cavities constitute only 2.3 and 3.0% of the interdomain and intersubunit interface surfaces respectively. The important role that waters play in mediating molecular recognition between protein units has implications for prediction methods attempting to dock such elements. The native fit between two interacting surfaces is not the most optimal geometrically, as implied by Shiochet and Kuntz [34, 35], and that Connolly's original proposal to solve the docking problem on geometrical grounds alone [36], may be an insufficient treatment. These caveats may also apply to various other forms of macromolecular recognition.

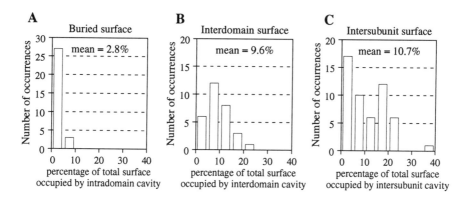

Figure 7: Distributions of the total cavity surface expressed as a fraction of its reference surface. The plots show intradomain cavity surface as a fraction of a domains' total buried surface upon folding (A), interdomain surface as a fraction of interdomain interface surface (B) and intersubunit cavity surface as a fraction of intersubunit interface (C).

4.3   A role for inter-cavities?

The observation that protein interfaces are non-optimally packed leads us to a number of hypotheses concerning cavities and their roles in protein structure and function.

1. The mutational pressure at protein interfaces leads to a greater cavity density. Domains are independent folding units and can tolerate many mutationally prone loops at their surfaces, yielding varying interfaces and more cavities. Within domains themselves, the core cannot tolerate so many mutations and cavities are correspondingly fewer.
2. Domains evolved and developed before multidomain and multimeric proteins and have subsequently optimized packing with few cavities. Because domains are used as building blocks for higher-order structure appearing later in evolution, there has been insufficient time to achieve the same level of packing between them. Thus, the looser packing between domains and subunits is simply a result of the "packing history" of the protein in question.
3. Interface cavities are structurally and/or functionally more important to accommodate, for instance, conformational changes when multimeric proteins interact with substrates or generally require flexibility such as in allostery. The intradomain cavities would be fewer because such motions are generally undesirable for stability of the overall fold, though a small proportion of intradomain cavities could also serve functional purposes.

5   Concluding remarks

5.1   Engineering, modelling and design

The results presented here concerning cavity detection, size, polarity, and constitution provide a basic set of guidelines for protein engineers and modellers to evaluate any packing defects in the context of those observed in native proteins. Notably, cavities should be defined carefully by use of optimal probe sizes. Since very small cavities close to the surface are poorly conserved in independent structure determinations of the same protein, they should be viewed with caution. Very large cavities are rarer and are more often water-filled. A polarity of 0.20

provides a simple guideline below which any putative cavity would be expected to be "empty". Cavity waters should be afforded several good hydrogen bonds to protein atoms and not be overly squeezed into the cavity volume. Solvated cavities are also less frequent between the hydrophobic surfaces of secondary structural units. Indeed some residue types, such as the large basic residues arginine and lysine, are very rarely found at cavity surfaces. Cysteine residues, although commonly buried, are also relatively rare at cavity surfaces and in almost all instances do not form disulphide bonds. In general, a guideline of 3 Å^3 per residue is suggested for the maximum permissible cavity volume in a protein model; native proteins in our database almost never exceed this value. Cavities should also be expected in proteins above 100 residues in size.

5.2   Functional roles

The relative fraction of cavities that are definitely involved in some functional role in proteins is unknown and a subject of further investigation. However, some cavities have already been implicated in protein function such as domain-domain movements [7]. Cavities are also believed to play a role in the passage of small ions, facilitating movements of catalytically-involved waters for the serine proteinases [37, 38]. They may also play some ligand binding role such as the large intermolecular uteroglobin cavity suggested to bind progesterone [39].

We have noted some preliminary evidence to support the hypothesis that cavities are critical in domain-domain rigid body motions. Taking proteins from a recent review classifying a number of motions as either predominantly "hinge" (rotational) or "shear" (translational) [40], corresponding proteins common to our datasets were analysed. We observed that the "shear" classified proteins exhibited a higher fraction of interdomain cavity surface than all proteins in the multidomain data set, which may be necessary to permit such motion. It is assumed that cavities would not be prerequisite to hinge motions. A theoretical examination of this putative functional role is in progress.

Acknowledgements

The authors would like to acknowledge Jaap Heringa for assistance in production of non-redundant protein datasets. This work was in part supported by an Institutional EC Human Capital and Mobility Grant ERBCHBGCT930241 to P. A. and S. J. H. and in part from a grant from the German Bundesministerium für Forschung und Technologie (FG5-1075 to P. A.).

References

[1] F. M. Richards, The interpretation of protein structures: total volume, group volume distributions and packing density, *J. Mol. Biol.*, 82, 1-14, 1974.

[2] F. M. Richards and W. A. Lim, An analysis of packing in the protein folding problem, *Quart. Rev. Biophysics*, 26, 423-498, 1994.

[3] B. P. Schoenborn, Structure of alkaline metmyoglobin-xenon complex, *J. Mol. Biol.*, 45, 297-303, 1969.

[4] R. F. Tilton, I. D. Kuntz and G. A. Petsko, Cavities in proteins: structure of metmyoglobin-xenon complex solved to 1.9 Å, *Biochemistry*, 23, 2849-2857, 1984.

[5] R. K. Wierenga, M. E. M. Noble and R. C. Davenport, Comparison of the refined crystal structure of liganded and unliganded chicken, yeast and trypanosomal triosephosphate isomerase, *J. Mol. Biol.*, 224, 1115-1126, 1992.

[6] M. L. Connolly, Atomic size packing defects in proteins, *Int. J. Peptide Protein Res.*, 28, 709-713, 1985.

[7] A. A. Rashin, M. Iofin and B. Honig, Internal cavities and buried waters in globular proteins, *Biochemistry*, 25, 3619-3625, 1986.

[8] S. J. Hubbard, K.H. Gross and P. Argos, Intramolecular cavities in globular proteins, *Protein Eng.*, 7, 613-626, 1994.

[9] M. A. Williams, J. M. Goodfellow and J. M. Thornton, Buried waters and internal cavities in monomeric proteins, *Protein Science*, 3, 1224-1235, 1994.

[10] A. E. Eriksson, W. A. Baase, X.J. Zhang, D. W. Heinz, M. Blaber, E. P. Baldwin and B. W. Matthews, Response of a protein to cavity creating mutations and its relation to the hydrophobic effect, *Science*, 255, 178-183, 1992.

[11] A. E. Eriksson, W. A. Baase, and B. W. Matthews, Similar hydrophobic replacements of Leu99 and Phe153 within the core of T4 lysozyme have different structural and thermodynamics consequences, *J. Mol. Biol*, 229, 747-769, 1993.

[12] J. T. Kellis Jr., K. Nyberg, D. Sali and A. R. Fersht, Contribution of hydrophobic interactions to protein stability, *Nature*, 333, 784-786, 1988.

[13] V. G. H. Eijsink, B. W. Dijkstra, G. Vriend, J. R. van der Zee, O. R. Veltman, B. van der Vinne, B. van den Burg, S. Kempe and G. Venema, The effect of cavity-filling mutations on the thermostability of *Bacillus stearothermophilus* neutral protease, *Protein Eng.*, 5, 421-426, 1992.

[14] J. T. Pedersen, O. H. Olsen, C. Betzel, S. Eschenberg, S. Branner and S. Hastrup, Cavity mutants of Savinase^{TM}, *J. Mol. Biol.*, 242, 193-202, 1994.

[15] A. E. Erikson, W. A. Baase, J. A. Wozniak and B. W. Matthews, A cavity-containing mutant of T4 lysozyme is stabilised by buried benzene, *Nature*, 355, 371-373, 1992.

[16] M. L. Connolly, Solvent-accessible surfaces of proteins and nucleic acids, *Science*, 221, 709-713, 1983.

[17] C. M. W. Ho and G. R. Marshall, Cavity search: an algorithm for the isolation and display of cavity-like binding regions, *J. Comput. Aided. Mol. Des.*, 4, 337-354, 1990.

[18] J. S. Delaney, Finding and filling protein cavities using cellular logic operations, *J. Mol. Graphics*, 10, 174-177, 1992.

[19] G. J. Kleywegt and T. A. Jones, Detection, delineation, measurement and display of cavities in macromolecular structures, *Acta. Cryst.* D50, 178-185, 1994.

[20] A. Shrake and J. A. Rupley, Environment and exposure to solvent of protein atoms. Lysozyme and insulin, *J. Mol. Biol.*, 79, 351-371, 1973.

[21] M. L. Connolly, The molecular surface package, *J. Mol. Graphics*, 11, 139-141, 1993.

[22] F. C. Bernstein, T. F. Koetzle, G. J. B. Williams, E. F. Meyer Jr., M. D. Brice, J. D. Rodgers, O. Kennard, T. Shimanouchi and M. Tasumi, The Protein Data Bank: A computer based archival file for macromolecular structures, *J. Mol. Biol.*, 112, 535-542, 1977.

[23] A. D. McLachlan, Gene duplications in the structural evolution of chymotrypsin, *J. Mol. Biol.*, 128, 49-79, 1979.

[24] U. Sreenivasan and P. H. Axelsen, Buried water in homologous serine proteinases, *Biochemistry*, 31, 12785-12791, 1992.

[25] X.J. Zhang and B. W. Matthews, Conservation of solvent-binding sites in 10 crystal forms of T4 lysozyme, *Protein Science*, 3, 1031-1039, 1994.

[26] S. J. Hubbard and P. Argos, Cavities and packing at protein interfaces, *Protein Sci.*, 3, 2194-2206, 1994.

[27] R. C. Wade, M. H. Mazor, J. A. McCammon and F. A. Quiocho, A molecular dynamics study of thermodynamic and structural aspects of the hydration of cavities in proteins,

Biopolymers, 31, 919-931, 1991.

[28] W. Kabsch and C. Sander, Dictionary of protein structure: pattern recognition of hydrogen bonded and geometrical features, *Biopolymers*, 22, 2577-2637, 1983.

[29] W. R. Taylor, J. M. Thornton and W. G. Turnell, An ellipsoidal approximation of protein shape, *J. Mol. Graphics*, 1, 30-38, 1983.

[30] E. N. Baker and R. E. Hubbard, Hydrogen bonding in globular proteins, *Prog. Biophys. Mol. Biol.*, 44, 97-179, 1984.

[31] B. Lee, Estimation of the maximum change in stability of globular proteins upon mutation of a hydrophobic residue to another of a smaller size, *Protein Sci.*, 2, 733-738, 1993.

[32] P. A. Karplus and G. E. Schulz, Predition of chain flexibility in proteins, *Naturwissenschaften*, 72, 212-213, 1985.

[33] P. Argos, An investigation of domain and subunit interfaces, *Protein Eng.*, 2, 101-113, 1988.

[34] B. K. Shiochet and I. D. Kuntz, Protein docking and complementarity, *J. Mol. Biol.*, 221, 327-346, 1991.

[35] B. K. Shiochet and I. D. Kuntz, Matching chemistry and shape in molecular docking, *Protein Eng.*, 6, 723-737, 1993.

[36] M. L. Connolly, Shape complementarity at the hemoglobin $\alpha 1$-$\beta 1$ interface, *Biopolymers*, 25, 1229-1247, 1986.

[37] J. S. Finer-Moore, A. A. Kossiakoff, J. H. Hurley, T. Earnest and R. M. Stroud, Solvent structure in crystals of trypsin determined by X-ray and neutron diffraction, *Proteins Struct. Func. Genet.*, 12, 203-222, 1992.

[38] A. A. Kossiakoff, M. D. Sintchak, J. Shpungin, and L. G. Presta, Analysis of solvent structure in proteins using D_2O-H_2O solvent maps: pattern of primary and secondary hydration of trypsin, *Proteins*, 12, 223-236, 1992.

[39] I. Morize, E. Surcouf, M. C. Vaney, Y. Epelboin, M. Buehner, F. Fridlansky, E. Milgrom and J. P. Mornon, Refinement of the $c222_1$ crystal form of oxidized uteroglobin at 1.34 angstroms resolution, *J. Mol. Biol.*, 194, 725-739, 1987.

[40] M. Gerstein, A. M. Lesk and C. Chothia, Structural mechanisms for domain movement in proteins, *Biochemistry*, 236, 1067-1078, 1994.

Protein Modelling and Docking

Modelling and predicting α-helical transmembrane structures

William R. Taylor and David T. Jones [1]

Division of Mathematical Biology, National Institute for Medical Research, The Ridgeway, Mill Hill, London NW7 1AA, U.K.

Abstract

Integral membrane proteins (of the α-helical class) are of central importance in a wide variety of vital cellular functions. Methods are reviewed, for the prediction of the location of transmembrane segments in sequence data and for the positioning of these helices in a given fold based on hydrophobic moments and preference parameters. Recent efforts on the more fundamental problem of predicting the fold of the protein, based on the lipid exposure of the helices, are outlined.

1 Introduction

A fundamental feature of the organisational structure of living processes is the enclosure of cellular and sub-cellular spaces by phospholipid bilayer membranes. Little would be achieved by this strategy if communication and selective transport could not occur across the membranes. This flow is almost entirely controlled by integral membrane proteins about which little is known structurally. The few structures that are available suggest a general basic form composed of bundles of α-helices that span the membrane and pack together with their axes approximately normal to the plane of the membrane. Examples include the bacteriorhodopsin proton pump which consists of a seven helix bundle and the light-harvesting complex from plants which is a more complex combination of multiple chains and numerous chromophores (haems, etc.). This general expectation that transmembrane structures will be helical has been unsettled, however, by the solution of the structure of porin which is a large 16-stranded antiparallel β-barrel in which the strands run across the membrane. A βα-structure may also possibly exist in the actylcholine receptor [30] in which five helices surround the channel and may themselves be encircled by a β-sheet (similar to that seen in some toxins).

The paucity of structural data on this class of protein has resulted in greater empahasis being placed on structure prediction. In principle, the prediction of α-helix membrane proteins should be easier than the prediction of globular proteins: there is only one type of secondary structure and all helices pack with a common alignment across the membrane. The resulting constraints on both the length and the hydrophobic nature of these helices make their detection from sequence data a relatively simple matter — compared to, say, secondary structure prediction (Section 2). A single sequence, however, provides little further guide as to how the helices

---

[1] Also at: Biomolecular Structure Unit, Dept. Biochemistry, University College London, Gower St., London WC1E 6BT, UK.

0-8493-4009-8/96/$0.00+$.50

should be packed relative to one another and this has confined most predictive work to the modelling-by-homology approach (Section 3). However, with a family of sequences, variable hydrophobic residues can be identified which are indicative of lipid exposure. The degree of exposure of each helix then places a constraint on its position in the fold, allowing some progress to be made (Section 4).

2 Chain topology prediction

2.1 Topogenic signals

Recent studies [32, 19, 17] have indicated the presence of topogenic signals in integral membrane proteins, i.e. sequence patterns which correlate with the topology of the membrane-spanning segments. The most evident of these signals is the prevalence of positively charged residues in the interior (cytoplasmic) loops which is now familiarly known as the "positive inside rule" [32].

These topogenic signals can be used to improve the quality of transmembrane helix prediction, and can also be used to evaluate the plausibility of predicted integral membrane structures. The first attempt to rationally incorporate topogenic signals into a prediction scheme for bacterial inner membrane proteins was by [31]. The proposed strategy for predicting the topology of this class of membrane proteins was based on an initial hydrophobicity analysis, followed by automatic generation of a set of possible topologies and finally a ranking of these by application of the positive-inside rule. The hydrophobicity analysis step is unremarkable in that although efforts were made to produce a reliable, 'clean' prediction of potential membrane-spanning segments, the hydrophobicity analysis was not significantly different from any of those described previously. The addition of topology evaluation, was however, a very novel step. The predicted transmembrane helices were divided into two sets: strongly predicted helices and weakly predicted helices. These predictions were used to construct a list of all the possible transmembrane topologies which included all the strongly predicted helices and any or none of the weakly predicted helices. The fundamental assumption in this work is that the membrane topology is a simple inside-outside meander, but given the assumption that most membrane structures are based on completely-spanning transmembrane segments, this is not unreasonable. The final list of alternative predicted topologies was then assessed by counting the number of positively charged residues which would be placed in inside-facing loops and comparing this number to the number in outside-facing loops. Any topology that places more positively charged residues on the outside than the inside was assumed to be incorrect, and the topology with the highest inside/outside ratio of positively charged residues was taken to be the final prediction.

Using this simple strategy, with no attempts at optimization, the topology of 23 out of 24 inner membrane proteins was predicted correctly. This level of success is very impressive. One point that should be made, however, is that in some of these cases, all the transmembrane helices were strongly predicted, and so the application of the positive inside rule only served to decide whether the N-terminus was inside or outside. In addition, the success rate of the initial prediction of transmembrane helix locations was somewhat optimal in the cases shown. This is not to say that the results were in any way invalid, only that the quality of the final prediction depends mostly on the success of the first stage and not the application of topogenic rules.

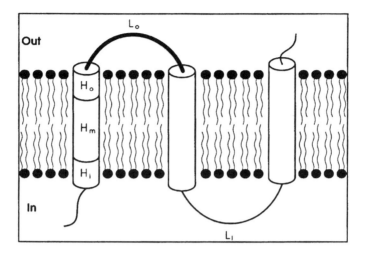

Figure 1: Structural states in a helical transmembrane protein. The α-helices are represented as cylinders crossing the lipid bilayer. Each helix is divided into three states relative to its orientation with respect to the cytoplasmic (inner) surface and the extracellular (outer) surface of the membrane — giving an inner cap (H_i) an outer cap (H_o) and a middle section (H_m). Similarly, the loops are distinguished as outer (L_o) and (L_i) inner. The cooperative identification of these states along the sequences helps distinguish both the location of the helices and their topology (out-in-out-... or in-out-in-...).

2.2   Cooperative prediction method

An attempt was made to integrate topogenic rules into the heart of the prediction process [14]. In this work a method is described that simultaneously takes into account the prediction of transmembrane secondary structure and the location of topogenic signals. For any given topology and scoring scheme, a mathematically optimal solution is found, which enables the likelihood of each suggested topology to be objectively assessed. The core idea here is the idea of expectation maximization, a simple statistical method which is concerned with the generation and fitting of models to data. Traditional prediction schemes attempt to determine the most reasonable underlying model based on an analysis of one or more sequences. In contrast, expectation maximization attempts to search for the model which best explains the given data. In other words, the task here is not to extract a model from the data, but to evaluate every possible model and determine which model is most likely to have produced the observed data. Given a function which calculates the total probability for the match of a given model with a given sequence, the resulting model from this methodology should correspond to the maximum of this function, hence the term expectation maximization.

Jones *et al.* classify residues into 5 structural states, as shown in figure 1. The 5 states are as follows: L_i (inside loop), L_o (outside loop), H_i (inside helix end), H_m (helix middle), and H_o (outside helix end). The number of residues taken to be in the helix end caps was arbitrarily taken as being 4, though other cap definitions could easily be used. Using this definition of membrane protein topology, a set of statistical tables (log likelihood ratios, or log likelihoods for short) compiled from well-characterized membrane protein data, and a novel dynamic programming algorithm to recognize membrane topology models by expectation maximization. The statistical tables show definite biases towards certain amino acid species on the inside, middle and outside of a cellular membrane. The most significant components of the propensities merely determine the lipophilic preferences of amino acids, or in other words that hydrophobic residues occur more frequently in the helical segments than the flanking regions. The signals that cannot be explained away by hydrophobicity alone are perhaps of more interest. The previously described preference for positively charged residues to be found in the inside loops is clearly seen, but it is also interesting to note that a similar effect is seen between the inside and outside helix caps, though this could be due to errors in assigning the boundaries between the membrane-spanning segments and their flanking regions. For multi-spanning proteins, the most significant preferences for inside/outside loop are Arg, Gly, His, Lys and Pro, whereas for single-spanning proteins, Ala, Arg, Asp, Gln, Lys, Pro, Thr, Trp and Val have the most significant propensities. For inside/outside helix caps, only Phe and Trp have highly significant topogenic propensities for multi-spanning helices whereas Cys, Gly, His, Leu, Lys, Phe, Pro, Ser, Thr, Tyr and Val show clear inside/outside preferences for single-spanning helix caps. The unusual abundance of tryptophan residues in outside locations of the photosynthetic reaction centre has been noted by Schiffer *et al.* (1992), and has also been seen in porin, but it would appear from these results that this is a general feature of transmembrane proteins as a whole.

To determine the most likely transmembrane models, a dynamic programming method was used, similar in principle to dynamic programming sequence alignment algorithms [20]. This algorithm was used to find the best set of variables (number, position, length and direction) for each considered model. This computation of membrane topology models by a process of expectation maximization is highly successful, with 64 out of 83 topologies being correctly predicted (34 out of 37 of the multi-spanning topologies were correct). Of the proteins with known structures, all 6 of the topologies have been correctly predicted, with success rates of 13/15 being achieved for the G-coupled receptors, 40/56 for proteins with experimentally well-determined topologies, and 5/6 for proteins with partial topological data. The locations of predicted helices were in close agreement with the experimental data. Most of the failures were due to overpredictions for large globular (eukaryotic) proteins with single membrane anchoring segments. Presumably in these cases, buried β-strands (or more rarely buried α-helices) are mistaken for membrane-spanning segments, which is a recurrent problem in all membrane protein structure prediction methods.

3   Modelling by "homology"

The use of a known protein structure to interpret the sequence of a related protein sequence of unknown structure is a common activity [2]. Its success relies heavily on having sufficient protein structures and a good method of sequence alignment. Transfer of this approach to the world of transmembrane proteins is therefore greatly limited by the lack of known structures of this class. Despite this, many models have been proposed for transmembrane structures based on what would be considered very dubious sequence similarities by the standards of globular protein sequence comparison. Such models, however, are often accepted because the constraints of crossing the membrane (with a polar main-chain) greatly restrict the possible forms of the structures.

Modelling interest has focused on the signal transduction proteins of the G-protein coupled receptor (GPCR) super-family. The widespread involvement of this super-family in physiological functions (and the importance of the control of these functions by drug action) has motivated considerable effort (e.g. [18, 4, 22, 13, 3]). All these studies, with one exception ([22] based their model on very weak specific sequence similarity), have followed the fold of the analogous light-driven proton pump bacteriorhodopsin [12]. This choice of modelling framework, however, is based only on the correspondence of seven observed and predicted helices and the binding of a similar chromophore in the opsin/rhodopsin sub-family of the GPCRs and otherwise ignores the completely different functions of the two proteins.

Having adopted a fold, the modelling problem is reduced to deciding the relative juxtaposition of the helices. This can be broken into an angular component in the plane of the membrane and a translation component normal to the membrane. If it is assumed that the predicted transmembrane helix is centred in the membrane then the latter part of the problem reduces to the prediction of the segment, and errors in this will directly result in errors in the model. Fortunately, the required length and the hydrophobic nature of these helices make their detection from sequence data a relatively simple matter compared to secondary structure prediction in globular proteins. The angular orientation of the helices, however, relies on detecting a more subtle signal within each helix and various methods have been devised.

3.1   Angular moments

The majority of methods rely on the detection of a periodic signal in the sequence with a frequency corresponding to the period of the α-helix. Graphically, such periodicity can be recognised when the sequence is plotted on a helical wheel [24]. Numerically, the preferred method is the Fourier transform which, generally, can identify the strength of fluctuations over a range of frequencies. The method was originally applied to the identification of the hydrophobic face of helices in globular proteins [8, 9] but can equally be applied to membrane helices [7, 23]. At a given frequency, a vector is derived (normal to the helix axis) pointing in the direction of the hydrophobic face. This hydrophobic moment vector typically points towards the core of the globular protein. (For general reviews, see [6, 10]). In globular proteins this orientation can be reinforced if multiple aligned sequences are available as the most conserved hydrophobic residues can be expected to lie more deeply in the core [26].

In transmembrane helix bundles, however, the hydrophobic moment would be expected to be in the reverse direction, pointing to the lipid solvent [13]. With a single sequence, little progress can be made beyond this assumption. However, with multiple aligned sequences the orientation can be refined through the analysis of conservation [16]. In the lipid environment there is no strong pressure on the type of hydrophobic residue. Hydrophobic positions interfacing with lipid will therefore appear in a multiple alignment as variable (equivalent to variable hydrophilic positions in water soluble proteins). By contrast, positions facing the interior, whether hydrophobic or not, will typically be relatively conserved.

These general principles have been treated in different ways by various groups and have often been refined by the use of more specific residue interaction preferences.

3.2   Packing preference methods

Residue preference parameters were derived by [3] from the structure of bacteriorhodopsin in which the environment of a residue was characterised by its angular orientation relative to the nearest packed helix. The sequence of each helix in the protein of unknown structure was displaced (or threaded) over the framework of bacteriorhodopsin and the preference parameters summed to calculate a measure of fit. Applying the method to the sequence of the β-2-adrenoreceptor, two of the seven helices had a clear unique minimum but for the others, multiple equivalent minima were generally observed. Because the preference parameters were specified only in terms of lipid or protein interaction, the optimal fit for each helix is independent, so avoiding the more difficult consideration of pairwise residue interactions.

At first sight the method appears simply to derive preference parameters for being directed towards lipid or the protein interior. However, comparison with the orientation of the helices predicted by a simple hydrophobic moment vector revealed considerable differences, indicating that additional information was being gained. The method suffers from a lack of sufficient data to derive good preference parameters and also possibly from the definition of the angular frame based on only one packing helix. In addition it also ignores information available from multiple sequences.

Blundell and co-workers also applied a preference parameter approach [21], developed on globular proteins, to membrane structures [5]. Where a multitude of residue environments were considered in globular proteins, only lipid accessibility was used for the transmembrane application. Using the structures of the photosynthetic reaction centre with all available sequences a table of amino acid substitution probabilities was calculated for buried residues and residues exposed to lipid. These were then combined in a single difference matrix and the pairwise sum (S_j) of these values over all residues at a position (j) in a multiple alignment indicated whether the position was buried or accessible. This somewhat convoluted approach has the advantage that it simultaneously considers amino acid composition and conservation, although it is not clear that the method has any advantage over the explicit treatment of these components.

Having calculated a lipid preference value for each position, a Fourier transform was calculated and the power spectrum summed for a region around the expected helical periodicity. The orientations calculated using the S values were compared with those using a simpler measure (V) based only on conservation [16] using the structure of bacteriorhodopsin (which was not used in parameter estimation) as a test model. The results were compared to the correct answer based on observed lipid accessibilities. While three of the orientations calculated using the S values were more accurate than those from the V values, three were worse (with errors of 30° and over) giving no overall improvement.

4   Fold prediction

All the above studies have assumed that the the fold of the sequence being modelled is known. This is clearly true when fitting the sequence of bacteriorhodopsin to its own structure, but to progress beyond test-data is difficult to justify when no clear sequence similarities can be found. This uncertainty of isomorphism in the main application area of modelling the GPCRs prompted prediction studies which make no fold assumptions.

Compared to the prediction of the tertiary structure of globular proteins, the prediction of the structure of membrane proteins is, in principle, a much easier problem. The constraint of aligned helix packing reduces the solution-space of the problem from three dimensions to two. Despite the relative simplicity of the two dimensional world and the central importance of the proteins involved, relatively little attention has been focused on prediction of membrane protein structure. This neglect may have resulted through of a lack of interest in the limited variety of anticipated forms, or (more probably) because the empirical based prediction methods currently used for globular protein require a large database from which to derive their rules.

4.1   Baldwin's method

Based on a helical wheel representation, [1] assembled a wide variety of conservation data for the aligned sequences of representatives across the entire GPCR super-family. Using a complex notation, this analysis concentrated on the identification of variability but also marked highly conserved (especially charged) residues and those known to interact with ligands. From the assembled data it was initially possible to rank the helices in order of exposure. Assuming packing between sequentially adjacent helices it was concluded that only two packing arrangements could accommodate this pattern of exposure. This included a fold corresponding to that found in bacteriorhodopsin and its mirror image — since simple helix exposure information cannot distinguish these possibilities.

To try and discriminate between enantiomers, arguments similar to those used in the interpretation of the electron density of bacteriorhodopsin [11] were applied. In particular, a pair of residues was considered that were known from biochemical experiments to interact in rhodopsin via the chromophore. Since the hand of the α-helix remains the same in both models, one conformation places the two residues at a suitable separation while in the other they are too distant. This selected the fold corresponding to bacteriorhodopsin as the preferred solution.

From consideration of further specific pairwise interactions (including a disulphide bridge) it was concluded that the rhodopsin structure may differ slightly from bacteriorhodopsin.

4.2 Taylor *et al.* method

The application to transmembrane protein structure modelling developed from methods originally used for the prediction and modelling of globular protein structure [27, 28]. The essential difference in reapplying these earlier methods was the substitution of variable hydrophilic positions in a multiple sequence alignment (as an indicator of exposure to solvent) with variable hydrophobic (*variphobic*) positions (as indicative of exposure to lipid). Otherwise, the methods remain the same.

Sequences were aligned using the multiple sequence alignment program MULTAL [25] using an amino acid relatedness matrix derived from a large number of transmembrane segments from proteins with more than one membrane spanning helix [15]. The prediction of transmembrane segments [14] (Section 2) allowed further constraints to be applied to the alignments. Two residues defined as being in a transmembrane helix were given a slight bias to preferentially align and any gaps in these regions were discouraged. These constraints made little difference to most of the alignments but eliminated a few weakly justified insertions at the ends of some helices.

A simple average hydrophobicity was calculated for each position in the multiple alignment but rather than use a hydrophobicity scale derived form globular proteins, a measure of the preference of amino acids to be found in the middle section of single membrane spanning helices was used [14] (Section 2). The conservation of residues at a position in a multiple alignment was defined as the pairwise sum of amino acid similarity but using a relatedness table derived from the helices of multiple spanning integral membrane proteins [15]. In addition, an option was allowed to give greater importance to the differences between closely similar sequences. These measures of hydrophobicity and conservation were combined to produce a score (v, referred to as *variphobicity*) which achieved a high value for unconserved hydrophobic positions. A variphobic moment was then calculated for each helix based on these values.

A model was constructed for bacteriorhodopsin based, not on the known structure, but on an idealised lattice of hexagonally packed helix axes, all with a uniform relative tilt corresponding to that predominantly found in the known structure. Each helix was centred on its axis with its variphobic moment directed away from a local centre-of-gravity defined by the lattice end-points of all neighbouring (packed) helices. This local definition may be important for larger problems where the assumption of approximate globularity cannot be made.

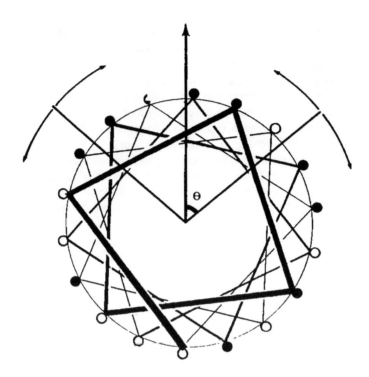

Figure 2:   Refinement of the variphobic arc — viewed down a helix axis the variable-hydrophobic (variphobic) positions (filled dots), which form a face of the helix, appear as an arc. The arc is bisected by the variphobic moment (radial arrow) and the angle θ defining this arc was varied to optimise the variphobic positions in the arc and the other positions outside. The optimal value of θ was used to evaluate the packing of the helix in predicted models.

The modelling method of [29] was used in combination with a combinatorial investigation of possible folds for both bacteriorhodopsin (as a test) and rhodopsin. This approach attempted to estimate not only the direction of the lipid exposed face (the *variphobic* moment vector), but also the extent of the face. As in the analysis of [1], this additional information was used to assess different folds.

Exposure to lipid is difficult to evaluate in absolute terms as the number and degree of similarity of the sequences in the alignment will set the scale and range of the variphobic values (v). However, as a first approximation, it is not unreasonable to assume that roughly half of all the residues in the protein will be exposed to lipid. From this, exposed and buried residues were defined as those with values of v above and below zero, respectively. Assuming that the exposed face of each helix forms a continuous arc on the helical wheel, its size can be calculated simply from the fraction of hydrophobic residues. This estimate of exposure was then be refined using the continuous range of values of v. (Fig. 2).

The framework, or lattice, over which the chain will be traced was a twisted bundle of close-packed cylinders, giving two layers of hexagonally spaced points. Given this set of points, those that lie within a prescribed distance of each other can be taken as possible connections (neighbours), then, beginning at any point, each neighbour can be visited in turn with the link taken to correspond to the path of the polypeptide chain. Applying this procedure recursively (with the condition that each point can be visited only once) leads to the exhaustive enumeration of all windings of the chain over the points. The number of neighbours each helix has dictates the expected size of its variphobic arc (from 0° for six neighbours to a maximum of 300° for one neighbour). This expectation can be matched to the size of arc calculated from the sequence and the squared difference accumulated over all helices provides a score of the degree to which the sequence fits the fold.

It was found that the angular size of the lipid exposed faces must be predicted quite accurately to give a good chance of selecting the native fold. With the inherent uncertainties in the prediction of helix end-points (and parameter choice) it was further found that, while the required accuracy could not be guaranteed, the correct fold was typically ranked within the top six folds (ignoring mirror images, which are not distinguished by the method). This result was obtained by imposing the packing of sequentially adjacent helices, however, when this constraint was relaxed, despite the enormous increase in possible folds, the rank of the correct fold generally remained high.

5   Conclusions

Despite being, in principle, a relatively tractable problem (compared to the prediction of globular protein structure), few methods have been developed for the prediction of membrane protein structure that are not based on the use of an 'homologous' structure. Furthermore, in many applications, this approach has been followed even though there was no significant sequence similarity between the template sequence and that being modelled. An exception is the approach of [1] to the G-protein coupled receptors which avoided any assumption of similarity to the bacterial rhodopsin family. This approach, however, is only partially automated and still relies on some biological insight on the part of the investigator to identify functionally equivalent sub-families. The methods developed by the authors, while inspired by the works of von Heijne and co-workers (topology) and Baldwin (folds), represents a step towards a more completely automatic route in the progression from sequence databank searching to the construction of a three dimensional model.

References

[1] J. M. Baldwin, The probable arrangement of the helices in G-protein coupled receptors, *EMBO J.*, 12, 1693–103, 1993.

[2] T. L. Blundell, D. Carney, S. Gardner, F. Hayes, B. Howlin, T. Hubbard, J. Overington, D. A. Singh, B. L. Sibanda, and M. Sutcliffe, Knowledge-based protein modelling and design, *Eur. J. Biochem.*, 172, 513–520, 1988.

[3] P. Cronet, C. Sander, and G. Vriend, Modelling of transmembrane 7 helix bundles, *Prot. Engng.*, 6, 59–64, 1993.

[4] D. Donnelly, M. S. Johnson, T. L. Blundell, and J. Saunders, An analysis of the periodicity of conserved residues in sequence alignments of G protein-coupled receptors, implications for the three dimensional structure, *FEBS Lett.*, 251, 109–116, 1989.

[5] D. Donnelly, J. P. Overington, S. V. Ruffle, J. H. A. Nugent, and T. L. Blundell, Modelling α-helical transmembrane domains, the calculation and use of substitution tables for lipid-facing residues, *Protein Sc.*, 2, 55–70, 1993.

[6] D. Eisenberg, Three-dimensional structure of membrane and surface proteins, *Ann. Rev. Biochem.*, 53, 595–623, 1984.

[7] D. Eisenberg, E. Schwarz, M. Komaromy, and R. Wall, Analysis of membrane and surface protein sequences with the hydrophobic moment plot, *J. Mol. Biol.*, 179, 125–142, 1984.

[8] D. Eisenberg, R. M. Weiss, and T. C. Terwilliger, The helical hydrophobic moment, a measure of the amphiphilicity of a helix, *Nature*, 299, 371–374, 1982.

[9] D. Eisenberg, R. M. Weiss, and T. C. Terwilliger, The hydrophobic moment detects periodicity in protein hydrophobicity, *Proc. Natl. Acad. Sci. U. S. A.*, 81, 140–144, 1984.

[10] D. Eisenberg, M. Wesson, and W. Wilcox, Hydrophobic moments as tools for analyzing protein sequences and structures. In G. D. Fasman (ed.), *Prediction of Protein Structure and the Principles of Protein Conformation*, chapter 16, page 635–646, Plenum Press, New York, 1989.

[11] D. M. Engleman, R. Henderson, A. D. McLachlan, and B. A. Wallace, Path of the polypeptide in bacteriorhodopsin, *Proc. Natl. Acad. Sci. U. S. A.*, 77, 2023–2027, 1980.

[12] R. Henderson, J. M. Baldwin, T. A. Ceska, F. Zemlin, E. Beckman, and K. H. Downing, Model for the structure of bacteriorhodopsin based on high-resolution electron cryo-microscopy, *J. Mol. Biol.*, 213, 899–929, 1990.

[13] M. F. Hilbert, S. Trumpp-Kallmeyer, A. Bruinvels, and J. Hoflack, Three-dimensional models of neurotransmitter G-binding protein-coupled receptors, *Mol. Pharm.*, 40, 8–15, 1991.

[14] D. T. Jones, W. R. Taylor, and J. M. Thornton, A model recognition approach to the prediction of all-helical membrane protein structure and topology, *Biochemistry*, 33, 3038–3049, 1994.

[15] D. T. Jones, W. R. Taylor, and J. M. Thornton, A mutation data matrix for transmembrane proteins, *FEBS Lett.*, pages 269–275, 1994.

[16] H. Komiya, T. O. Yeats, D. C. Rees, J. P. Allen, and G. Feher, Structure of the reaction centre from *Rhodobacter sphaeroides* R-26: symmetry relations and sequence comparisons between different species, *Proc. Natl. Acad. Sci. U. S. A.*, 85, 9012–9016, 1988.

[17] C. Landolt-Marticorena, K. A. Williams, C. M. Deber, and R. A. F. Reithmeier, The amino acid composition is different between the cytoplasmic and extracellular sides in membrane-proteins, *J. Mol. Biol.*, 229, 602–608, 1993.

[18] T. J. Mitchell, M. S. Tute, and G. A. Webb, A molecular modeling study of the interaction of noradrenaline with the beta-2-adrenegeric receptor, *J. Comp. Aided Mol. Des.*, 3, 211–223, 1989.

[19] H. Nakashima and K. Nishikawa, The amino acid composition is different between the cytoplasmic and extracellular sides in membrane-proteins, *FEBS Lett.*, 303, 141–146, 1992.

[20] S. B. Needleman and C. D. Wunsch, A general method applicable to the search for similarities in the amino acid sequence of two proteins, *J. Mol. Biol.*, 48, 443–453, 1970.

[21] J. Overington, D. Donnelly, M. S. Johnson, A. Šali, and T. L. Blundell, Environment-specific amino-acid substitution tables - tertiary templates and prediction of protein folds, *Protein Science*, 1, 216–226, 1992.

[22] L. Pardo, J. A. Ballesteros, R. Osman, and H. Weinstein, On the use of the transmembrane domain of bacteriorhodopsin as a template for modelling the 3-D structure of the G-protein coupled receptors, *Proc. Natl. Acad. Sci. U. S. A.*, 89, 4009–4012, 1992.

[23] D. C. Rees, L. Deantonio, and D. Eisenberg, The hydrophobic organisation of membrane proteins, *Science*, 245, 510–513, 1989.

[24] M. Schiffer and A. B. Edmunson, Use of helical wheels to represent the structures of proteins and to identify segments with helical potential, *Biophys. J.*, 7, 121–135, 1967.

[25] W. R. Taylor, Pattern matching methods in protein sequence comparison and structure prediction, *Prot. Engng.*, 2, 77–86, 1988.

[26] W. R. Taylor, Sequence analysis, spinning in hyperspace, *Nature*, 353, 388–389, 1991. (News and Views).

[27] W. R. Taylor, Towards protein tertiary fold prediction using distance and motif constraints, *Prot. Engng.*, 4, 853–870, 1991.

[28] W. R. Taylor, Protein fold refinement, building models from idealised folds using motif constraints and multiple sequence data, *Prot. Engng.*, 6, 593–604, 1993.

[29] W. R. Taylor, D. T. Jones, and N. M. Green, A method for α-helical integral membrane protein fold prediction, *Prot. Struct. Funct. Genet.*, 18, 281–294, 1994.

[30] N. Unwin, Nicotinic acetylcholine-receptor at 9-ångstrom resolution, *J. Mol. Biol.*, 229, 1101–1124, 1993.

[31] G. von Heijne, Membrane-protein structure prediction, hydrophobicity analysis and the positive-inside rule, *J. Mol. Biol.*, 225, 487–494, 1992.

[32] G. von Heijne and Y. Gavel, Topogenic signals in integral membrane proteins, *Eur. J. Biochem.*, 174, 671–678, 1988.

HIV GP120 Docking Interactions and Inhibitor Design Based on an Atomic Structure Derived by Molecular Modeling Using the DREIDING II Force Field

Jerome L. Gabriel* and William M. Mitchell†

* Department of Biochemistry, Temple University School of Medicine, Philadelphia, PA 19140, USA
† Department of Pathology, Vanderbilt University School of Medicine, Nashville, TN 37232, USA

Abstract

Despite substantial advances in knowledge pertaining to the structure and replicative cycle of the Human Immunodeficiency Virus (HIV), significant clinical gains derived from anti-HIV agents have been modest. The rational design of HIV inhibitors would optimally be guided by the availability of x-ray crystallographic structures of all HIV-encoded proteins. The recent development of potent HIV-protease inhibitors is one of the better examples of crystallographic structure driven drug design. Unfortunately, resistant mutants are quickly developed which will limit their usefulness as single agents for the inhibition of HIV replication. Another attractive site for anti-HIV drug development is the initial binding event of the virus to its cellular receptor, CD4, through the envelope gp120. Unfortunately, it is unlikely that crystallographic structures will be made available for the HIV envelope proteins due to their high degree of glycosylation. This consideration was the initial emphasis for our proposed atomic structure of gp120 derived by molecular dynamics and free energy minimization calculations using the generic DREIDING II force field. In the absence of direct crystallographic confirmation, the model is in agreement with available experimental data including site-directed mutagenesis and ligand binding studies. Docking of the proposed structure of gp120 to the x-ray derived structure of a CD4 fragment indicates that the primary mechanism of recognition lies in the placement of a solvent exposed F43 residue on CD4 into a solvent accessible aromatic binding site on gp120 composed of W427 and Y435. Mindful of the fact that molecular dynamics calculations cannot predict x-ray crystal quality structures, we have generated a working hypothesis that our model of the CD4 binding domain on gp120 is sufficiently accurate to enable the rational design of HIV inhibitors which specifically bind to gp120. We have calculated the interaction energies of a series of known inhibitors of HIV and have established a negative interaction

0-8493-4009-8/96$0.00+$.50

energy following computer simulated docking of each potential inhibitor with gp120. Refinement of ligand-protein interactions is provided by further molecular dynamics calculations. A quantitative relationship has been established between the computed interaction energy of a small number of HIV inhibitors and experimentally determined IC50 values from the literature, establishing a practical method with which small organic inhibitors of gp120/CD4 binding can be designed.

1   Introduction

The Human Immunodeficiency Virus (HIV) contains two heavily glycosylated proteins gp41 and gp120 as components of the viral envelope often referred to as viral coat proteins. One coat protein, gp41, contains a hydrophobic transmembrane sequence and is embedded into the lipid domain of the viral envelope. gp120 contains no transmembrane sequences and is associated with the extraviral domain of gp41 via non-covalent interactions. Together, the envelope proteins serve as the principle targets for functional immune response toward HIV (i.e., the generation of neutralizing and enhancing antibodies and cytotoxic lymphocytes). Both proteins play specific roles in the cell to cell membrane fusion process between the virus and its target cell. An essential step in this fusion process is a viral maturation step in which the polyprotein, gp160, is cleaved by a cellular protease to its gp120 and gp41 components. The recognition and subsequent noncovalent docking of gp120 to gp41 on the outer surface of the virus provides the infective form of the virus. The extracellular domain of the CD4 receptor of the target cell then binds to gp120 forming an activated ternary complex. Subsequent proteolytic cleavage of the V3 loop on gp120 has been suggested to be responsible at least in part for the cell tropism exhibited by the virus [1]. Following gp120/CD4 association it is generally believed that a conformational change occurs exposing a fusogenic peptide on the N-terminal of gp41 [2, 3]. Insertion of the hydrophobic gp41 fusion peptide into the membrane of the target cell is followed by cell fusion between the virus infected producer cell and uninfected target cells with resultant syncytium formation [4, 5]. Electron microscopy and isotopic labeling studies with the murine retroviruses clearly demonstrate that viral envelope on the producer cell fuses with the target cell plasma membrane resulting in the fusion of the plasma membranes of both infected and target cells with subsequent mixing of nuclei and cytoplasm from both cell types [6].

The coat proteins are initially synthesized and posttranslationally modified as a glycosylated protein, gp160, with gp120 occupying the N-terminal 511 residues of the IIIB isolate [7]. We will limit our comments here to our analysis of the structure of gp120. Our initial study used a truncated model of gp120 [8]. We have more recently modeled the entire protein with no significant alterations in functional sites on the molecule. The linear relationship of disulfide bonds and glycosylation sites on gp160 is shown in figure 1.

The amino terminal leader sequence is illustrated by a cross-hatched segment (L) with cleavage one amino acid distal to the only free sulfhydryl in the gp120 molecule. The disulfide bonding patterns are constant in all isolates and are indicated above the linear bar. Within the bar are stippled areas labeled V1 to V5 which indicate the hypervariable regions of gp120. The transmembrane anchor region is indicated by the TM legend. N-linked oligosaccharides include either a complex carbohydrate type (open circle) or a high mannose type (closed circle). Unknown glycosyl structures are indicated by a ?. Protein domains which elicit neutralizing antibody responses toward HIV infectivity are indicated as black boxes below the linear sequence and include the CD4 binding domain (horizontal stripes), aa 423-437, and the hypervariable V3 region, aa 296-311, defined by Modrow *et al.* [9]. Regions which induce

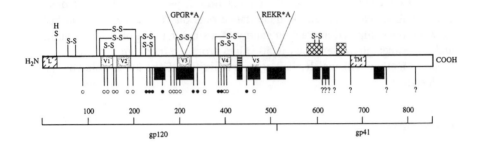

Figure 1: Linear relationship of disulfide bonds, glycosylation sites, and functional domains of gp160 based on the IIIB isolate and using the Los Alamos numbering system [48]. Details are provided in the text.

antibody-dependent enhancement are identified above the linear sequence box by double cross-hatched bars. The sequences for cellular based proteolysis within the V3 loop and the gp120/g41 cleavage site are expanded above the sequence box with hydrolytic sites identified by an asterisk.

2 Rationale

The elucidation of the molecular mechanism directing the binding of gp120 to the extracellular domain of the CD4 receptor requires atomic level structural information. It is unlikely that the x-ray crystal structure of gp120 will be forthcoming in the near future since half the mass of the native protein is N-glycosylated [10], making it not amenable to crystallization. In the absence of direct experimental structural information, we have been able to use molecular modeling techniques to generate a tertiary structure of this highly glycosylated protein which is amenable to a variety of experimental methods of validation.

Tertiary structure prediction of an unknown target protein using *homology molecular modeling* requires knowledge of the x-ray structure of a closely related protein. The underlying assumption behind homology modeling is the observation that proteins having similar amino acid sequences should have similar three-dimensional structures. Since no known homologs of HIV gp120 have been crystallized, we have chosen to evaluate *de novo* molecular modeling using molecular dynamics calculations as our approach to generating a testable model of the tertiary structure of gp120. We are mindful of the fact that molecular dynamics calculations will not generate x-ray crystal quality structures but a model of the general tertiary structural features of the protein which can be compared with the available experimental evidence for general structure verification and which can be used to guide future experiments including the design of HIV inhibitors.

Tertiary structure prediction using *de novo* modeling is based on the widely accepted premise that the information necessary to completely describe the folding of a protein and thus its tertiary structure resides in its primary structure, i.e. — the lowest free energy state determined by the linear array of amino acids which is often referred to as the "thermodynamic hypothesis" of Anfinsen [11]. Denaturation-renaturation experiments in support of this hypothesis [11] invalidate arguments for a pathway of progressive folding and the development of metastable states [12] as the polypeptide is synthesized. Of significant concern, however,

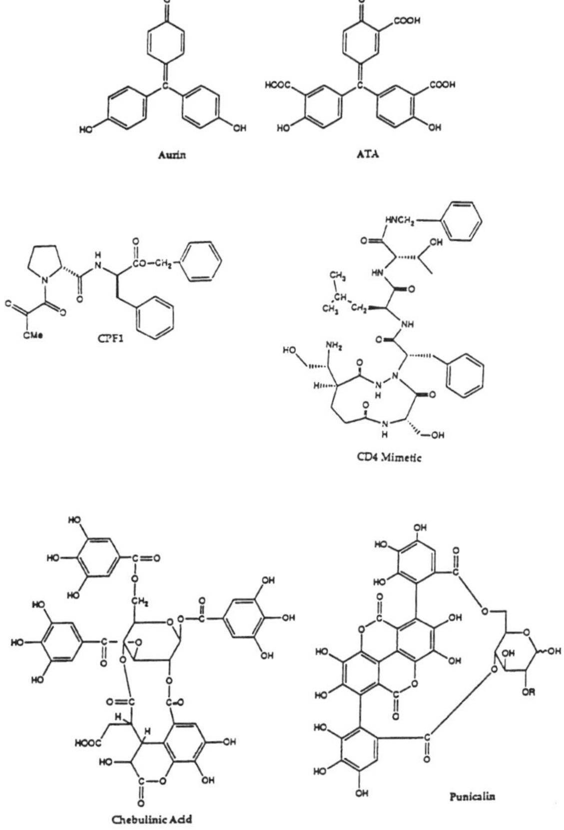

Figure 2: Structures of known inhibitors of gp120-CD4 binding.

to the protein folding process to a lowest free energy state is the consideration of Levinthal's paradox [13]. Levinthal [13] argued in support of his metastable state hypothesis that although protein folding can occur within seconds or less, finding a native protein conformation based solely by taking a given amino acid sequence and biologically searching for all possible conformations would consume an enormous amount of time which was inconsistent with known protein folding times. It has been shown, however, that Levinthal's paradox can be overcome, with calculated folding times greatly reduced, if certain interactions between amino acids are considered [14]. Using a simple mathematical model, Zwanzig and coworkers [14] demonstrated that biased searches against locally unfavorable configurations result in folding times which are biologically relevant.

In our procedure of *de novo* modeling, by including the appropriate secondary structural elements predicted from sequence specific algorithms [15, 16] in our initial model, we are imposing restrictions on the conformational search to limit the degrees of freedom for the molecular dynamics calculations, thus countering Levinthal's paradox. Our inclusion of secondary structural elements in the initial model is supported by the suggestion of Jaenicke that secondary structure is formed early in the folding process providing a framework for the

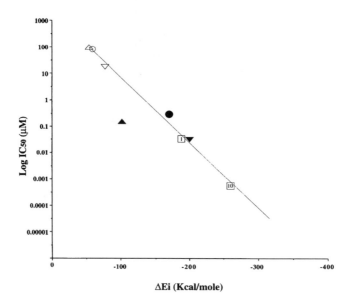

Figure 3: Plot of the log of experimentally determined IC_{50} values as a function of the computed ΔEi for various known binding inhibitors for gp120 with CD4 receptors. ΔEi is the differential internal energy of the protein ligand complex versus the sum of the free reactants. ATA ($\triangle$), CPF ($\bigcirc$), CD4 mimetic ($\triangledown$), punicallin (●), chebullinic acid (black triangle pointing up), SCD4 (black triangle pointing down). Predicted IC_{50} for analog 1 (1) and analog 10 (10) based on computed ΔEi.

rest of the protein [17, 18]. By including the location of native disulfide bonds where present in the initial model [8], one can further limit the degrees of freedom for the molecular dynamics calculations. A recent report on the oxidative folding of bovine trypsin inhibitor demonstrated that the pathway for the folding of this protein proceeded through the formation of oxidative intermediates found in the native protein [19]. Thus in the *de novo* modeling of proteins, one can construct the native disulfide pairings in the initial model without considering non-native intermediates and their metastable conformations.

3   Methods used

All molecular modeling was performed on a Silicon Graphics Personal Iris 4D/35 workstation using Biograf software (Molecular Simulations, Inc., Waltham, MA). The calculations involved energy minimizations, or molecular mechanics, coupled with molecular dynamics simulations in order to generate minimal energy structures for the HIV envelope protein, gp120. The following sections will include a generalized discussion of the force field used in the calculations of potential energy values and molecular dynamics. For a more detailed discussion see Mayo *et al.* [20].

3.1 Initial conditions

Protein secondary structure analysis was determined using both the Genetic Computer Group sequence analysis package [21] which utilizes both the Chou-Fasman [15] and Garnier [16] algorithms or the PHD profile method available from EMBL [22]. The secondary structure used in constructing the initial model was taken as the union of the results from all algorithms, i.e., only where the methods agreed. Using the peptide builder within the main Biograf program, the initial gp120 structure was constructed by adding amino acid residues with the desired secondary structure to the growing peptide chain. Secondary structural elements were defined according to their (Φ, Ψ) angles, e.g. $(-57°, -47°)$ for a residue in an α-helix and $(-119°, 113°)$ for a residue in a β-sheet. β-turns were defined by residues two $(-50°, -40°)$ and three $(-75°, -20°)$ of the four residue β-turn. In the absence of any predicted secondary structure for a given position in the primary sequence, an amino acid was added to the protein chain in the extended conformation $(180°, 180°)$. The predicted secondary structure was used to define the initial starting point for molecular dynamics in order to limit the degrees of freedom during the calculations; no constraints were placed on the system to maintain this initial secondary structure. To further limit the degrees of freedom during the molecular dynamics calculations, intrachain disulfide bonds were constructed by rotating the peptide chain until appropriate Cys residues were in close proximity for disulfide bond formation. This initial model was then minimized to convergence.

An iterative procedure of molecular dynamics calculations followed by energy minimization was then used until a stable low energy, tertiary structure was obtained. Thus, the calculations were discontinued if two or more sequential structures had the same mainchain or backbone structure and approximately the same low potential energy. Although the structure derived in this manner is at a minimum in the potential energy curve, it is uncertain whether a local minimum or the global minimum has been reached. The validity of the structure so obtained, however, lies in how well the model agrees with the structural information available for the protein in question. This structural information is not used to define the model but only to test its validity.

3.2 Force field

Potential energy (E) was described using the generic DREIDING force field[20] in which each atom is treated explicitly and atomic parameters are based solely on the element and its hybridization. The potential energy is calculated as a sum of bonded and non-bonded interactions, as indicated by equation 1. All calculations were carried out using default limits of the program.

$$E = E_B + E_\vartheta + E_\Phi + E_i + E_{elect} + E_{VDW} + E_{HB} \tag{1}$$

Thus, the bonded interactions consisted of terms for harmonic bond stretching (E_B), theta expansion bond angle bending (E_ϑ) dihedral angle torsion (E_Φ), and inversion (improper torsion) (E_i). Nonbonded interactions included electrostatic or coulombic terms (E_{elect}) of the form $Q_i Q_j / \varepsilon R_{ij}$ where R_{ij} is the distance between two atoms, ε is the dielectric constant, and Q_i, Q_j are point charges representing the atoms. Predetermined point charges for each amino acid residue are contained within the default limits of the program. For nonmacromolecular structures such as organic ligands, the calculation of point charges was based either on the method described by Gasteiger & Marsili [23] or by charge equilibration [24]. Also included in the nonbonded portion of the potential energy were van der Waals (E_{VDW}) terms, described by a Lennard-Jones 12-6 potential and hydrogen bonding terms (E_{HB}), described by a Lennard-Jones 12-10 potential [20]. Nonbonded interactions were calculated for atomic pairs within a 9 Å cutoff distance. Not included in the nonbonded energy calculations were interactions between atoms bonded to one another or atoms involved in angle interactions. Energy minimization by the method of conjugate gradients [25] was used to minimize the potential energy of the molecule and thus is capable of relieving strain generated by sidechain-sidechain interactions.

3.3 Molecular dynamics

During molecular dynamics, both the forces on the atoms and the movement of the atoms in response to these forces are computed, according to Newton's equations of motion, as described by equation 2.

$$\mathbf{F}_i = m_i \frac{d^2 \mathbf{r}_i}{dt^2} = -\nabla_i [E(\mathbf{r}_1, \ldots, \mathbf{r}_n)], \quad i = 1, n \tag{2}$$

where $\mathbf{F}_i$ is the force on atom i due to all other atoms, m_i is the mass of atom i, r_i is the position vector of atom i, and t is time. Dynamics calculations were performed using the Verlet algorithm [26] in Biograf version 2.2 and the summed Verlet algorithm [27] in version 3.0.

In the present study, molecular dynamics (quenched dynamics) calculations are allowed to proceed for 0.1 psec, at 0.002 psec intervals, for a total of 50 steps, followed by limited energy minimization to relieve strain. This constitutes an equilibration cycle. After each equilibration cycle a temperature T is calculated in terms of the average kinetic energy given by equation 3 [28],

$$\frac{3}{2} nkT = \left\langle \sum_i \frac{1}{2} m_i v_{i^2} \right\rangle, \quad i = 1, n \tag{3}$$

where the average is over an equilibration cycle. The calculated temperature is then compared to the selected initial temperature T_0 and if it is outside of a prescribed range, velocities are scaled according to equation 4 [28].

$$v_{new}/v_{old} = (T_0/T)^{1/2} \tag{4}$$

Dynamics calculations as described above are allowed to proceed for at least 25 psec, after which time the lowest energy structure is minimized until convergence is obtained. This procedure of molecular dynamics calculations followed by energy minimization is repeated until a minimal energy structure is obtained. All dynamics calculations were carried out at a value of $T_0 = 450°K$.

4 Features of gp120 structure

In order to limit computer CPU time requirements, the sequence of a truncated fragment of gp120, spanning residues 101 to 456, was initially modeled. A nonglycosylated minimal energy structure was obtained after 195 psec of molecular dynamics calculations. The resulting structure, shown in color plate 13A (page xxvii), is globular with approximate dimensions 60 Å x 30 Å x 20 Å. Eight of the nine disulfide bonds present in gp120 (Fig. 1) are present in the truncated model. Each of the protein domains which elicit neutralizing antibody response (see Fig. 1), including the CD4 binding domain, residues 423-437, and the V3 loop, residues 296-311, lie on the surface of the protein (Color plate 14A). The solvent accessibility of these protein domains as depicted by the model confirms their experimental antigenicity. The truncated gp120 used in our study contains 22 N-linked oligosaccharides of two types, 11 high mannose core and 11 complex oligosaccharides. (For structures see Fig. 1 of Gabriel and Mitchell, [8]). Earlier hydrophobicity plot analysis [29] suggested that only one-third of the N-glycosylation sites were maximally accessible, although all 22 sites have been found to be glycosylated in the virus. All glycosylation sites in the model are on the surface of the protein, maximally accessible for N-linked glycosylation.

The appropriate N-glycosyl units were added to the minimal energy gp120 structure previously obtained as described by Leonard *et al.* [30]. The resulting model was further subjected to an additional 100 psec of molecular dynamics calculations until a minimal energy glycosylated structure was obtained after a total time of 295 psec. As shown in Color Plate 14B (page xxvii), the oligosaccharide residues are not evenly distributed on the surface of gp120 but occur in clusters that block access to large areas of the polypeptide surface. All known antigenic sites that have been shown to induce neutralizing antibody responses occur on the surface, solvent accessible regions, not covered by carbohydrates. The highly conserved sequence GPGR-A, which occurs at the midpoint of the V3 loop, is essential for HIV infectivity although it is not directly involved in viral binding to the CD4 receptor. We have demonstrated by molecular modeling that proteolytic cleavage of the R-A bond results in a protein conformational change with a predicted tighter gp120/CD4 association [31]. Our fully glycosylated model of gp120 predicts that this conserved GPGR sequence is exposed and accessible to the appropriate proteolytic enzyme responsible for hydrolyzing the R-A bond (Color plate 14C, page xxvii).

4.1   The gp120/CD4 interaction

Although the extra cellular domain of the CD4 receptor contains 375 amino acid residues, an N-terminal 113 amino acid fragment contains epitopes for anti-CD4 monoclonal antibodies which block binding to gp120 within this fragment [32]. The gp120 binding site on CD4 has been further localized by site-directed mutagenesis to a region between residues 29-85. This region on CD4 contains the highly mutationally sensitive F43 residue, the solvent accessibility of which is a prominent feature in the crystal structure of an N-terminal truncated fragment of CD4 [33, 34]. A similar mutagenic analysis of gp120 has localized the CD4 binding domain on this protein to the region between residues 423-437, containing the highly conserved W427 and Y435 residues, essential elements in CD4 binding and viral infectivity.

It has been suggested in the literature that the driving force for the binding between CD4 and gp120 relies on the interaction between residue F43 on CD4 and its reciprocal binding site on gp120 containing residues W427 and Y435. Support for this is exemplified by frequent reports in the literature concerning the inhibition of HIV activity by small, aromatic containing, organic ligands [35, 36, 37, 38]. The docking of gp120 with the crystal structure of CD4 was accomplished by manually orienting the CD4 crystal structure into a position with respect to our gp120 model such that the solvent accessible F43 residue could interact with the aromatic residues W427 and Y435 on gp120. After minimizing the energy of the entire complex, protein-protein interactions were refined by continuing molecular dynamics calculations on the complex, followed again by energy minimization. Favorable docking between gp120 and CD4 was demonstrated by calculating an interaction energy, i.e., the decrease in potential energy of the complex as compared to the sum of the potential energy of the individual proteins in the complex. The interaction energy for the fully glycosylated complex was -200 Kcal/mole which decreased to -75 Kcal/mole when the non-glycosylated gp120 model was docked with CD4, independently confirming the importance of glycosylation to binding [39, 40, 41] and infectivity [42, 43, 44, 45].

The refined binding interactions between the two proteins is shown in color plate 13D (page xxvii). One readily observes a binding pocket on the surface of gp120 consisting of the highly conserved aromatic residues W427 and Y435 into which snugly fits the solvent exposed F43 residue on CD4. The driving force for the binding interaction appears to be $\pi - \pi*$ interactions between these aromatic residues and is consistent with the usual ring orientation observed in protein crystals [46]. Lining one side of this binding pocket is the high mannose oligosaccharide N-linked to N230. Other aromatic residues localized within the binding pocket include gp120-Y191 and CD4-W62. Alanine-scanning mutagenesis of CD4 resulting in a W62 to A62 mutation abolishes the binding of gp120 to CD4 [47]. While Y435 is present in all sequenced HIV-1 isolates, W427 is similarly conserved with one exception, isolate Eli, where no aromatic residue is present at this position [48]. Y191 which is in close proximity to W427 in our model could provide the potential hydrophobic environment required for CD4 binding for the rare viable mutations of W427. Notably, Y191 although occurring in the hypervariable V2 region of gp120 is highly conserved [48].

4.2   Ligand design

Throughout the literature, several classes of organic molecules containing aromatic rings have been examined for their ability to inhibit HIV infectivity on the premise that these compounds may mimic the solvent accessible F43 residue on CD4 and bind to gp120 in the neighborhood of W427/Y435 (Fig. 2).

One of the earlier components examined for inhibition of HIV infectivity is aurin tricarboxylic acid (ATA) which binds to CD4 [38]. Based on inhibition of syncytium formation we estimate an IC-50 value of 100 μM for gp120/CD4 inhibition while its decarboxylated counterpart aurin exhibits no bioactivity [38]. A class of compounds with affinity for gp120 termed CPF's, n-carbomethoxy carbonyl-propyl-phenylalanyl benzyl esters, is approximately as active as ATA, IC$_{50}$ = 90μM, in preventing gp120 to binding to CD4 [35]. More recently, other gp120 binding analogs have been identified which are more potent inhibitors of gp120 binding to CD4. A CD4 β turn mimetic, designed to mimic the β turn at position Q40-F43 observed in the crystal structure of CD4 has been synthesized by investigators at the University of Illinois; binding assays for the inhibition of CD4 binding to gp120 demonstrated an IC$_{50}$ value of 18 μM [36]. The screening of a series of natural products termed tannins, as inhibitors of HIV replication, demonstrated that this class of aromatic ring containing compounds could inhibit the replication of HIV [49]. Two such tannins, chebulinic acid and punicalin, have been shown to inhibit the binding of CD4 to gp120 with an approximate IC$_{50}$ value of 0.15 to 0.3 μM [37].

In the rational design of novel inhibitors of HIV, one must use all available information currently in the literature. Although the crystal structure of an N-terminal fragment of the CD4 receptor has been derived [33, 34], it is unlikely that the x-ray derived structure of gp120 will be forthcoming in the near future. The model of the HIV envelope protein gp120 presented here, although not experimentally derived, agrees with all known structure features of gp120 and represents our "best estimate" for the structure of this protein. Is the model of gp120 defined well enough to direct the rational design of new HIV inhibitors? To answer this question, we have constructed models of each of the known HIV inhibitor analogs shown in Figure 3 and docked them into the CD4 binding pocket observed in our model of gp120, which is comprised of residues 101-255 and 369-456 (Color plate 15A, page xxviii).

Initially, each analog was docked into the binding pocket by orienting one of the aromatic rings contained within each compound into the position occupied by CD4 residue F43 in the model of the complex. After energy minimization, we again used molecular dynamics calculations (25 psec) to refine the intermolecular interactions of the gp120-ligand complex and calculated an interaction energy for each inhibitor as previously described for the gp120/CD4 complex. Thus, a more negative interaction energy represents tighter ligand binding to gp120.

Since it has been demonstrated that aurin tricarboxylic acid (ATA) inhibits HIV by preferentially binding to CD4[38], ATA was docked into both the CD4 binding site on gp120 and the complimentary gp120 binding site on CD4. Interaction energy calculations supported the experimental results yielding a more negative value for ATA bound to CD4 <u>versus</u> ATA binding to gp120, i.e. -51 Kcal/mole and -28 Kcal/mole respectively.

Similar energy calculations were performed after docking each potential HIV inhibitor (shown in Fig. 2) into the proposed CD4 binding site on gp120 (Color plate 15A, page xxviii). Although each inhibitor analog was initially placed in approximately the same orientation within the binding site, two potential subsites, an upper and a lower site, were evident upon completion of the molecular dynamics calculations. As shown in Figure 4B, minimum energy gp120-ligand complexes involving the CPF's or the two tannins, punicalin and chebulinic acid, suggested that these inhibitor analogs preferentially bind to the lower portion of the CD4 binding site. On the other hand, similar calculations involving the CD4 mimetics reveal that this class of gp120 inhibitors appear to bind preferentially to the upper portion of the CD4 binding site. It was interesting to note that both the CD4 mimetic and the CPF analogs could be simultaneously accommodated into the full CD4 binding site with minimal overlap. This finding suggests the possibility of designing a new class of novel gp120/CD4 inhibitors representing single molecules containing functional groups from both the CD4 mimetic and CPF analog classes. Using molecular modeling techniques, we have begun to construct a new class of bifunctional inhibitors which apparently bind to the total CD4 binding site (Color plate 15, page xxviii) with interaction energies ranging from -167 Kcal/mole (analog 1) to -270 Kcal/mole (analog 10).

The latter is significantly more negative than the value of -200 Kcal/mole obtained for CD4. Although our calculations suggest that this class of computer modeled inhibitors may be more potent inhibitors of gp120/CD4 binding interaction than soluble CD4, proof of this awaits analog synthesis and biological testing. The *de novo* predicted CD4 binding site on gp120 presented here provides a rational mechanism for the observed binding affinities of known analogs to the envelope glycoprotein. As shown in figure 3, a linear correlation has been obtained between log IC_{50} values for inhibition of CD4/gp120 binding obtained from the literature [35, 36, 37] and interaction energies calculated on the basis of the currently proposed model of gp120.

5   Conclusions

At the present time, we have constructed a working model of the HIV envelope glycoprotein gp120 which agrees with the available experimental evidence in the literature to date. Our docked model of the gp120-CD4 receptor complex is in accordance with the docking orientation for these proteins suggested in the literature. A proposed binding pocket has been localized on our model of gp120 which accommodates CD4 residues 29-85 containing the mutationally sensitive and solvent accessible F43 residue. The affinity (IC_{50} values) of known inhibitors of the gp120/CD4 binding interaction correlates with interaction energy values calculated on the basis of the presented model. In looking toward the future, we anticipate that the current model will enable us to design more effective HIV inhibitors.

Acknowledgements

This work was supported in part by NIH grants AI 33815 and AI 31371.

References

[1] C. Ebenbichler, P. Westervelt, A. Carrillo, T. Henkel, D. Johnson and L. Ratner, Structure-function relationships of the HIV-1 envelope V3 loop tropism determinant: evidence for two distinct conformations, *AIDS*, 7, 639–646, 1993.

[2] J. P. Moore, B. A. Jameson, R. A. Weiss and Q. J. Sattenau, The HIV-cell fusion reaction, in *Viral Fusion Mechanisms*, Bentz, J., Eds., CRC Press, Boca Raton, FL, 234–289, 1993.

[3] H. Ellens and C. Larsen, CD4-induced change in gp120/41 conformation and its potential relationship to fusion, in *Viral Fusion Mechanisms*, Bentz, J., Eds., CRC Press, Boca Raton, FL, 291–312, 1993.

[4] M. L. Bosch, P. L. Earl, K. Fargnoli, S. Picciafaoco, F. Giombini, F. Wong-Staal and G. Franchini, Identification of the fusion peptide of primate immunodeficiency viruses, *Science*, 244, 694–697, 1989.

[5] E. O. Freed, D. J. Myers and R. Risser, Characterization of the fusion domain of the human immunodeficiency virus type 1 envelope glycoprotein gp41, *Proc. Natl. Acad. Sci.*, 87, 4650–4654, 1990.

[6] J. Korinek, H. L. Moses, W. M. Mitchell and D. N. Orth, Mechanism of syncytium formation between XC sarcoma cells and murine endocrine carcinoma cells, *J. Natl. Cancer Inst.*, 49, 1269–1275, 1972.

[7] F. M. Veronese, A. L. DeVico, T. D. Copeland, S. Oroszlan, R. C. Gallo, and M. G. Sarngadharan, Characterization of gp41 as the transmembrane protein coded by the HTLV-III/LAV envelope gene, *Science*, 229, 1402–1405, 1985.

[8] J. L. Gabriel and W. M. Mitchell, Proposed atomic structure of a truncated human immunodeficiency virus glycoprotein (HIV) gp120 derived by molecular modeling: target CD4 recognition and docking mechanism, *Proc. Natl. Acad. Sci.*, 90, 4186–4192, 1992.

[9] S. Modrow, B. H. Hahn, G. W. Shaw, R. C. Gallo, F. Wong-Staal, and H. Wolf, Computer-assisted analysis of envelope protein sequences of seven human immunodeficiency virus isolates: prediction of antigenic epitopes in conserved and variable regions, *J. Virol.*, 61, 570–578, 1987.

[10] M. A. Muesing, D. H. Smith, C. D. Cabradilla, C. V. Benton, L. A. Lasky and D. J. Dapon, Nucleic acids structure and expression of the human AIDS/lymphadenopathy retroviruses, *Nature* (London), 313, 450–458, 1985.

[11] C. B. Anfinsen, Principles that govern the folding of protein chains, *Science*, 181, 223–230, 1973.

[12] C. Levinthal, Are there pathways for protein folding? *J. Chim. Phys.*, 65, 44–45, 1968.

[13] C. Levinthal, How to fold graciously, in *Mössbauer Spectroscopy in Biological Systems*, Proceedings of a Meeting held at Allerton House, Monticello, IL, Debrunner, P., Tsibris, J. C. M. and Münch, E., Eds., University of Illinois Press, Urbana, Illinois, 22–24, 1969.

[14] R. Zwanzig, A. Szabo and B. Bagchi, Levinthal's paradox, *Proc. Natl. Acad. Sci.*, 89, 20–22, 1992.

[15] Chou, P. Y. and Fasman, G. D., Prediction of protein conformation, *Biochemistry*, 13, 221–244, 1974.

[16] J. Garnier, D. J. Oguthorpe and B. Robson, Analysis of the accuracy and implications of simple methods for predicting the secondary structure of globular proteins, *J. Mol. Biol.*, 120, 97–120, 1979.

[17] R. Jaenicke, Folding and association of proteins, Prog. Biophys, *Mol. Biol.*, 49, 117–327, 1987.

[18] R. Jaenicke, Protein folding: local structures, domains, subunits and assemblies, *Biochemistry*, 30, 3147–3160, 1991.

[19] J. S. Weissman and P. S. Kim, Reexamination of the folding of BPTI: predominance of native intermediates, *Science*, 253, 1386–1393, 1991.

[20] S. L. Mayo, B. D. Olafson and W. A. Goddard, III, Dreiding: a generic force field for molecular simulations, *J. Phys. Chem.*, 94, 8897-8909, 1990.

[21] J. Devereux, P. Haeberli and O. Smithies, A comprehensive set of sequence analysis programs for the VAX, *Nucleic Acids Res.*, 12, 387–395, 1984.

[22] B. Rost, R. Schneider and C. Sander, Progress in protein structure prediction, *TIBS*, April, 120–123, 1993.

[23] J. Gasteiger and M. Marsili , Iterative partial equilization of orbital electronegativity — a rapid access to atomic charges, *Tetrahedron*, 36, 3219–3228, 1980.

[24] A. K. Rappe and W. A. Goddard, III, A charge equilibration method for calculating electrostatic charges, *Biograf Reference Manual*, pp. 25, Molecular Simulations, Inc., 1994, chap. 3.

[25] R. Fletcher and C. M. Reeves , Function minimization by conjugate gradients, *Comput. J.*, 149–154, 1964.

[26] L. Verlet, Computer "experiments" on classical fluids. I. Thermodynamical properties of Lennard-Jones molecules, *Physical Rev.*, 159, 98–103, 1967.

[27] W. C. Swope, H. C. Andersen, P. H. Berens and K. R. Wilson, A computer simulation method for the calculation of equilibrium constants for the formation of physical clusters of molecules: application to small water clusters, *J. Chem. Phys.*, 76, 637–649, 1982.

[28] C. L. Brooks III, M. Karplus and B. M. Pettitt, Dynamical simulation methods, in *Proteins: A Theoretical Perspective of Dynamics, Structure and Thermodynamics*, pp. 33–58, John Wiley and Sons, 1988, chap. 4.

[29] W. E. Robinson Jr., D. C. Montefiori and W. M. Mitchell, Evidence that mannosyl residues are involved in human immunodeficiency virus type 1 (HIV-1) pathogenesis, *AIDS Res. Hum. Retroviruses*, 3, 265–282, 1987.

[30] C. K. Leonard, M. W. Spellman, L. Riddle, R. J. Harris, J. N. Thomas and T. J. Gregory, Assignment of intrachain disulfide bonds and characterization of potential glycosylation sites of the type 1 recombinant human immunodeficiency virus envelope glycoprotein (gp120) expressed in Chinese hamster ovary cells, *J. Biol. Chem.*, 265, 10373–10382, 1990.

[31] W. M. Mitchell and J. L. Gabriel, Cleavage of the GR*AFV sequence of gp120 results in a predicted conformational change leading to tighter CD4 binding, *Ninth International Conference on AIDS*, Berlin, Germany, WS-A01-6, 1993.

[32] B. H. Chao, D. S. Costopoulos, T. Curiel, J. M. Bertonis, P. Chisholm, C. Williams, R. T. Schooley, J. J. Rosa, R. A. Fisher and J. M. Maraganore, 113-amino-acid fragment of CD4 produced in Esherichia coli blocks human immunodeficiency virus-induced cell fusion, *J. Biol. Chem.*, 264, 5812–5817, 1989.

[33] J. Wang, Y. Yan, T. P. J. Garrett, J. Liu, D. W. Rodgers, R. L. Garlick, G. E. Tarr, Y. Husain, E. L. Reinherz and S. C. Harrison, Atomic structure of a fragment of human CD4 containing two immunoglobulin-like domains, *Nature* (London), 348, 411–418, 1990.

[34] S. -E. Ryu, P. D. Kwong, A. Trunah, T. G. Porter, J. Arthos, M. Rosenberg, X. Dai,

N. -h. Xuong, R. Axel, R. W. Sweet and W. A. Hendrickson, Crystal structure of an HIV-binding recombinant fragment of human CD4, *Nature* (London), 348, 419-426, 1990.

[35] R. W. Finberg, D. C. Diamond, D. B. Mitchell, Y. Rosenstein, G. Soman, T. C. Norman, S. L. Schreiber and S. J. Burakoff, Prevention of HIV-1 infection and preservation of CD4 function by the binding of CPF's to gp120, *Science*, 249, 287-291, 1990.

[36] S. Chen, R. A. Chrusciel, H. Nakanishi, A. Raktabutr, M. E. Johnson, A. Sato, D. Weiner, J. Hotie, H. V. Saragovi, M. L. Greene and M. Kahn, Design and synthesis of a CD4 β-turn mimetic that inhibits human immunodeficiency virus envelope glycoprotein gp120 binding and infection of human lymphocytes, *Proc. Natl. Acad. Sci.*, 89, 5872–5876, 1992.

[37] J. L. Weaver, P. S. Pine, G. Dutschman, Y. -C. Cheng, K. H. Lee and A. Aszalos, , Prevention of binding of rgp120 by anti-HIV tannins, *Biochem. Pharmacol.*, 43, 2479–2480, 1992.

[38] D. Schols, M. Baba, R. Panwels, J. Desmyter and E. DeClercq, Specific interaction of aurintricarboxylic acid with the human immunodeficiency virus/CD4 cell receptor, *Proc. Natl. Acad. Sci.*, 86, 3322–3326, 1989.

[39] E. Fenouillet, B. Clerget-Raslain, J. C. Gluckman, D. Guetard, L. Montagnier and E. Bahraoui, Role of N-linked glycans in the interaction between the envelope glycoprotein of human immunodeficiency virus and its CD4 cellular receptor, *J. Exp. Med.*, 169, 807–822, 1989.

[40] E. Fenouillet, J. C. Gluckman and E. Bahraoui , Role of N-linked glycans of envelope glycoproteins in infectivity of human immunodeficiency virus type 1, *J. Virol.*, 64, 2841-2848, 1990.

[41] T. J. Matthews, K. J. Weinhold, H. K. Lyerly, A. J. Langlois, H. Wigzel and D. Bolognesi, Interaction between the human T-cell lymphotropic virus type IIIB envelope glycoprotein gp120 and the surface antigen CD4: role of carbohydrate in binding and cell fusion, *Proc. Natl. Acad. Sci.*, 84, 5424–5428, 1987.

[42] R. A. Gruters, J. J. Neefjes, M. Tersmette, R. E. Y. deGoede, A. Tulp, H. G. Huisman, F. Miedema and H. L. Ploegh, Interference with HIV-induced syncytium formation and viral infectivity by inhibitors of trimming glucosidase, *Nature*, 330, 74–77, 1987.

[43] D. C. Montefiori, W. E. Robinson Jr. and W. M. Mitchell, Role of protein N-glycosylation in pathogenesis of human immunodeficiency virus type 1, *Proc. Natl. Acad. Sci.*, 85, 9248–9252, 1988.

[44] A. Karpas, G. W. J. Fllet, R. A. Dwek, S. Petursson, S. K. Namgoong, N. G. Ramsden, G. S. Jacob and T. W. Rademacher, Aminosugar derivatives as potential anti-human immunodeficiency virus agents, *Proc. Natl. Acad. Sci.*, 85, 9229–9233, 1988.

[45] R. Pal, G. M. Hoke and M. G. Sarngadharan , Role of oligosaccharides in the processing and maturation of envelope glycoproteins of human immunodeficiency virus type 1, *Proc. Natl. Acad. Sci.*, 86, 3384–3388, 1989.

[46] S. K. Burley and G. A. Petsko, Aromatic-aromatic interactions: a mechanism of protein structure stabilization, *Science*, 229, 23–28, 1985.

[47] A. Ashkenazi, L. G. Presta, S. A. Marsters, T. R. Camerato, K. A. Rosenthal, B. M. Fendly and D. J. Capon, Mapping the CD4 binding site for human immunodeficiency virus by alanine-scanning mutagenesis, *Proc. Natl. Acad. Sci.*, 87, 7150–7154, 1990.

[48] G. Myers, B. Korber, S. Wain-Hobson, K-T. Jeang, L. E. Henderson and G. N. Pavlakis II, Amino acid alignments, in *Human Retroviruses and AIDS*, II-A34–IIA-63, Los Alamos National Laboratory, Los Alamos, NM, 1994.

[49] M. Nishizawa, T. Yamagishi, G. E. Dutsehman, W. B. Parker, A. J. Bodner, R. E.

Kilkuskie, Y. C. Cheng and K. H. Lee, Anti-AIDS agents, 1. Isolation and characterization of four new tetragalloylquinic acids as a new class of HIV reverse transcriptase inhibitors from tannic acid, *J. Natl. Prod.*, 52, 762–768, 1989.

A Model of the 3D Structure of Obelin — the Photoprotein from *Obelia longissima*

Tatyana Sandalova

Institute of Biophysics, Siberian Branch of RAS, Krasnoyarsk, 660036, Russia
Present address: Department of Molecular Biology, Swedish University of Agricultural
Sciences, BioMedical Center, Box 590, S-75124 Uppsala, Sweden

Abstract

A model of the 3D structure of obelin — a photoprotein from sea organism *Obelia longissima* is suggested. Based on a 3D profile search of the compatibility of the sequence of photoproteins with the structure of calmodulin, troponin C, parvalbumin, and sarcoplasmic calcium binding protein (SCBP), the latter was chosen as template for modeling of the 3D structure of photoproteins. After substitution of the amino acid sequence of SCBP to that of obelin according to the alignment of their primary and secondary structures, the model was subjected to some rounds of energy minimization and the model obtained was analyzed. The structure contains a cavity which is lined by residues that have been shown to be important for the bioluminescence of photoproteins. To prove the suggested 3D structure of photoproteins and the suggested binding site for the photoactive compound some residues are proposed for mutational experiments.

1 Introduction

Among the proteins involved in bioluminescent reactions in various organisms, photoproteins found in some coelenterates differ by a special property: they emit light only in the presence of Ca^{2+} [1]. Four different photoproteins: aequorin, clytin, mitrocomin, and obelin, have been purified and characterized [2, 3, 4, 5, 6]. Aequorin found in the jellyfish *Aequoria victoria* is the most studied among the photoproteins: two different isoenzymes were obtained [2, 3] and many mutant aequorins have been characterized [7, 8, 9, 10, 11], but the mechanism of the bioluminescence as well as 3D structure of photoproteins remain obscure.

Photoproteins are composed from coelenterazine (an imidazopyrazine compound) which together with molecular oxygen is covalently bound to apoprotein [1]. In the presence of calcium ions coelenterazine is oxidized to coelenteramide and one molecule of carbon dioxide and one photon are released. Coelenteramide is bound to apoprotein non-covalently, and the phenolate anion of coelenteramide is believed to be an excited light emitter [12].

The amino acid sequence of the photoproteins from four different organisms have been published [2, 3, 4, 5, 6]. They share high level of sequence identity with each others and much less sequence identity with other members of the Ca^{2+}-binding protein family (Table 1). It is known that proteins with more than 30% sequence identity usually have a similar

Table 1: Results of the compatibility search of sequences of different photoproteins with the 3D structure of some calcium-binding proteins with EF-hand type binding site.
In the right part of the Table, Z score of sequences are shown, in the left half of the Table, below the diagonal, the percent of identical residues with respect to longer protein are displayed. Four Ca^{2+} — binding proteins with known 3D structure and four photoproteins are compared: 2SCP — sarcoplasmic Ca^{2+}-binding protein from *N. diversicolor*, 1CLL — calmodulin, 5TNC — troponin C, 5CPV — parvalbumin, AEQ — aequorin, OBEL — obelin, CLYT — clytin, MITR — mitrocomin.

| Profiled | % of identity and Z-score | | | | | | | |
| protein | Calcium-binding | | | proteins | | Photoproteins | | |
	2SCP	1CLL	5TNC	5CPV	AEQ	OBEL	CLYT	MITR
2SCP	28.1	8.4	5.2	<3	3.1	8.1	9.2	6.7
1CLL	19%	34.6	27.2	15.1	4.6	7.9	6.2	5.6
5TNC	19%	53%	38.6	16.3	4.8	6.4	6.7	6.6
5CPV	16%	26%	28%	25.0	<3	<3	4.2	3.8
AEQ	17%	19%	18%	18%				
OBEL	18%	19%	20%	16%	65%			
CLYT	20%	19%	20%	20%	63%	77%		
MITR	18%	16%	15%	18%	70%	63%	60%	

overall fold. The spatial similarity is more obscure if the amount of identity is 15-20% as we have in photoprotein in comparison to parvalbumin, troponin C, calmodulin, or SCBP the most similar among other Ca^{2+}-binding proteins. Nevertheless, photoproteins are likely to have a 3D structure similar to these Ca^{2+}-binding proteins. Crystals of aequorin have been obtained and preliminary results have been published [13] but no structure has been reported yet, therefore, the modeling of the 3D structure of a photoprotein is described here. Knowledge of the photoprotein structure can be a guide in mutational experiments and in understanding the mechanism of the reaction and process of bioluminescence.

2 Methods

Secondary structure predictions were obtained from EMBL (Heidelberg) via an electronic mail service. It was performed by the neural network [14] using multiple sequence alignment. The sequence of obelin was aligned with aequorin, mitrocomin, clytin, calmodulin, troponin C, and sarcoplasmic calcium-binding protein from *Nereis diversicolor* by the program CLUSTAL V [15]. The alignment was sent to EMBL to be used as input for the neural network system.

A study of the compatibility of any photoprotein chain with known 3D structures was performed by the 3D profile methods [16]. The profiles were computed from four different Ca^{2+}-binding proteins with well-refined 3D structure from Brookhaven Protein Data Bank [17]: calmodulin (1CLL) [18], troponin C (5TNC) [19], parvalbumin (5CPV) [20], sarcoplasmic Ca^{2+}-binding protein from *N. diversicolor* (2SCP) [21].

In order to check whether the sequences of photoproteins are consistent with the fold of other Ca^{2+}-binding proteins the profiles made from these proteins were scanned against a test dataset of 945 protein sequences from SwissProt. The dataset contains 134 Ca^{2+}-binding proteins: besides 4 sequences of the photoproteins and proteins which were profiled, the dataset includes 41 sequences of calmodulins and calmodulin-like proteins, 21 sequences of troponins C, 31 sequences of myosin light chains, 31 sequences of parvalbumins, and 8 sequences of sarcoplasmic Ca^{2+}-binding proteins. The rest, 811 proteins, either have another fold or their 3D structure is not known so far. The quality of the sequence - structure fit is given by the Z-score — numbers of standard deviations above the mean score for the sequence of similar length [16].

The construction of the 3D model of obelin from the 2SCP coordinates was performed using the program O [22]. The amino acids of 2SCP were replaced by obelin according to the alignment by option MUTATE of O. The initial conformations of loop regions which are absent in 2SCP were chosen in the fragment dataset of O. After changing the primary structure, all hydrogen atoms were introduced at their positions using the XPLOR [23] and the model was subjected to some rounds of energy minimization by XPLOR. In the first steps of the minimization, the Ca atoms and residues were restrained to their position in 2SCP and all charges of side chains were switched off. After minimization, some residues were found in unfavored regions in a Ramachandran plot. The conformation of these residues were changed manually and one additional round of energy minimization was made. During this round no constraints were used and all charges were taken into the calculation.

The stereochemistry and quality of the model was analysed using the programs XPLOR [23], PROCHECK [24], DSSP [25]. The surface accessible area was calculated by DSSP [25]. The volume of the model and cavity search was performed by VOIDOO [26].

3 Results

3.1 Sequence alignment

About 200 protein sequences are known which contain the EF-hand motif - a rather famous fold consisting of 29 amino acid residues arranged in an helix-loop-helix conformation [27]. Most of these proteins contain 2-8 copies of EF-hand domains. The majority of Ca^{2+}- binding sites contribute seven oxygen ligands to the metal ion. All these ligand atoms are from the 12-residue loop between the two helices. Each of these 12 residues is important for Ca^{2+}-binding, but five of them (first, third, 5th, 6th, and 12th) are rather conserved and directly involved in calcium binding [28].

All these proteins consisting of similar domains are homologous, but some of them have diverged very far. The search against SwissProt showed that photoproteins have the highest percentage of identical residues with parvalbumin from carp, but parvalbumin is only half the length of the photoprotein. Other Ca^{2+}-binding proteins, such as calmodulins, troponin C, or SCBP have a similar number of identical residues to photoproteins. Sarcoplasmic Ca^{2+}-binding protein from sandworm N. *diversicolor* has the largest length of alignment while still having similar number of identical residues.

The aligned sequences of all photoproteins together with calmodulin (1CLL) and sarcoplasmic Ca^{2+}-binding protein from *N.diversicolor* (2SCP) are shown in Figure 1. One can see that three active Ca^{2+}-binding sites of photoproteins are aligned well with Ca^{2+}-binding sites of both 1CLL and 2SCP. The second non-functional Ca^{2+}-binding site of photoproteins differs from both 1CLL, which has normal working Ca^{2+}-binding site, and from 2SCP, which second site is non-functional like in photoproteins.

3.2 The prediction of secondary structure

The prediction of secondary structure of obelin, performed from multiple sequence alignment by neural networks at EMBL, showed a good agreement between predicted secondary struc-

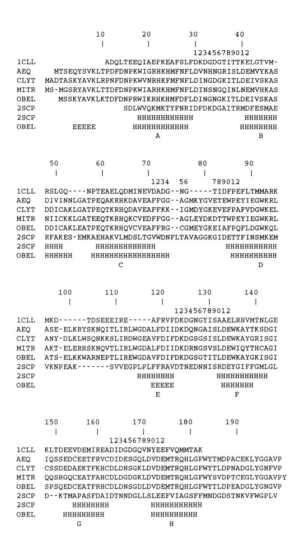

```
                    10        20        30        40
                     |         |         |         |
                                         123456789012
        1CLL              ADQLTEEQIAEFKEAFSLFDKDGDGTITTKELGTVM-
        AEQ        MTSEQYSVKLTPDFDNPKWIGRHKHMFNFLDVNHNGRISLDEMVYKAS
        CLYT       MADTASKYAVKLRPNFDNPKWVNRHKFMFNFLDINGDGKITLDEIVSKAS
        MITR       MS-MGSRYAVKLTTDFDNPKWIARHKHMFNFLDINSNGQINLNEMVHKAS
        OBEL       MSSKYAVKLKTDFDNPRWIKRHKHMFDFLDINGNGKITLDEIVSKAS
        2SCP              SDLWVQKMKTYFNRIDFDKDGAITRMDFESMAE
        2SCP              HHHHHHHHHHH             HHHHHHH
        OBEL       EEEEE        HHHHHHHHHHH        HHHHHHH
                                   A                    B

                    50        60        70        80        90
                     |         |         |         |         |
                                        1234  56    789012
        1CLL       RSLGQ----NPTEAELQDMINEVDADG--NG-----TIDFPEFLTMMARK
        AEQ        DIVINNLGATPEQAKRHKDAVEAFFGG--AGMKYGVETEWPEYIEGWKRL
        CLYT       DDICAKLGATPEQTKRHQDAVEAFFKK--IGMDYGKEVEFPAFVDGWKEL
        MITR       NIICKKLGATEEQTKRHQKCVEDFFGG--AGLEYDKDTTWPEYIEGWKRL
        OBEL       DDICAKLEATPEQTKRHQVCVEAFFRG--CGMEYGKEIAFPQFLDGWKQL
        2SCP       RFAKES-EMKAEHAKVLMDSLTGVWDNFLTAVAGGKGIDETTFINSMKEM
        2SCP       HHHH   HHHHHHHHHHH                 HHHHHHHHHH
        OBEL       HHHHHH    HHHHHHHHHHHHHHHHHH        HHHHHHHHHH
                       C                                  D

                    100       110       120       130       140
                     |         |         |         |         |
                                        123456789012
        1CLL       MKD------TDSEEEIRE-----AFRVFDKDGNGYISAAELRHVMTNLGE
        AEQ        ASE-ELKRYSKNQITLIRLWGDALFDIIDKDQNGAISLDEWKAYTKSDGI
        CLYT       ANY-DLKLWSQNKKSLIRDWGEAVFDIFDKDGSGSISLDEWKAYGRISGI
        MITR       AKT-ELERHSKNQVTLIRLWGDALFDIIDKDRNGSVSLDEWIQYTHCAGI
        OBEL       ATS-ELKKWARNEPTLIREWGDAVFDIFDKDGSGTITLDEWKAYGKISGI
        2SCP       VKNPEAK-------SVVEGPLPLFFRAVDTNEDNNISRDEYGIFFGMLGL
        2SCP                       HHHHHHHH         HHHHHHHHHH
        OBEL                       EEEEE            HHHHHHH
                                     E                  F

                    150       160       170       180       190
                     |         |         |         |         |
                                        123456789012
        1CLL       KLTDEEVDEMIREADIDGDGQVNYEEFVQMMTAK
        AEQ        IQSSEDCEETFRVCDIDESGQLDVDEMTRQHLGFWYTMDPACEKLYGGAVP
        CLYT       CSSDEDAEKTFKHCDLDNSGKLDVDEMTRQHLGFWYTLDPNADGLYGNFVP
        MITR       QQSRGQCEATFAHCDLDGDGKLDVDEMTRQHLGFWYSVDPTCEGLYGGAVPY
        OBEL       SPSQEDCEATFRHCDLDNSGDLDVDEMTRQHLGFWYTLDPEADGLYGNGVP
        2SCP       D--KTMAPASFDAIDTNNDGLLSLEEFVIAGSFFMNDGDSTNKVFWGPLV
        2SCP       HHHHHHHH         HHHHHHHHHHH
        OBEL       HHHHHHHHH        HHHHHHHHHH
                       G                  H
```

Figure 1: Alignment of the sequences of calmodulin (1CLL), four different photoproteins: aequorin (AEQ), clytin (CLYT),mitrocomin (MITR), obelin (OBEL), sarcoplasmic calcium binding protein (2SCP), made by CLUSTAL V [15]. The predicted secondary structure of obelin and the secondary structure of 2SCP, deduced from its 3D structure are shown below sequences. Calcium binding loops are identified by conventional numbering of residues participating in calcium binding.

tures of obelin and the secondary structures of 1CLL and 2SCP deduced from their known three- dimensional structures. There is only one (but important) difference - a β-strand was predicted instead of helix E for obelin. However, the secondary structure of this region seems to be wrongly predicted since there is a very strong homology between photoproteins and other Ca^{2+}-binding proteins which have a classical EF-hand domain at least at the end of a helix. The result of this prediction shown in Fig.1 confirms that photoproteins are folded as

Table 2: Top-scoring list of sequences after the compatibility search with profiles computed from parvalbumin (5CPV) [21], troponin C (5TNC) [22], calmodulin (1CLL) [20], and sarcoplasmic calcium binding protein (2SCP) [17] against test dataset of 945 protein sequences containing 130 different Ca^{2+}-binding proteins.

NonCa — first sequence in the top-scoring list which has not EF-hand domain. TNC — a troponin C, CALM — a calmodulin, AEQ — aequorin, CLYT — clytin, MITR — mitrocomin, OBEL — obelin.

	PROFILED					PROTEIN					
5CPV			5TNC			1CLL			2SCP		
N	protein	Z	N	protein	Z	N	protein	Z	N	protein	Z
1.	5CPV	25.	1.	5TNC	39.	1.	1CLL	40.	1.	2SCP	28.
2.	tNC	15.	2.	tNC	38.	2.	CALM	39.	2.	CALM	10.
..	..	..	..	..	..	..	..	..	3.	CLYT	9.
95.	CLYT	4.	91.	CLYT	7.	96.	OBEL	8.	4.	OBEL	8.
96.	MITR	4.	92.	MITR	7.	97.	CLYT	6.	..	..	..
97.	NonCa	3.	93.	OBEL	6.	98.	MITR	6.	9.	MITR	7.
..	..	..	..	..	..	99.	2SCP	6.	..	..	..
..	..	..	98.	AEQ	5.	100.	AEQ	5.	74.	AEQ	3.
..	..	..	99.	NonCa	4.	101.	SCBP	5.	..	...	..
..	..	..	..	..	..	102.	NonsA	4.	78.	NonsA	2.

other Ca^{2+}-binding proteins.

3.3   Choice of template

It is not clear which protein is best to use as a template to model the 3D structure of photoproteins: the sequence identities of all compared proteins are rather low and approximately the same. Therefore, the number of identical residues is not a good parameter for the choice of template in this case.

To find the best template the profile method [16] was used to evaluate the compatibility of the Ca^{2+}-binding protein 3D structure and the amino acid sequence of photoproteins. The profiles were built for the 3D structures of calmodulin (1CLL), troponin C (5TNC), parvalbumin (5CPV), and SCBP (2SCP). The results of the search performed against the dataset of 945 protein sequences are shown in the Table 1, where the obtained Z-scores are presented and in the Table 2, where the top-scored sequences for every profile are shown.

One can see that the profile method is able to detect sequences of Ca^{2+}-binding proteins even when there is very poor sequence identity. The profiles calculated from calmodulins and troponin C detect almost all sequences in our dataset, which are supposed to be Ca^{2+}-binding proteins. Profiles from 1CLL do not detect 6 sequences of SCBP out of 8, and 2 sequences of calcitonins. Despite the difference of the 3D structure of parvalbumins and calmodulins, troponin C, myosin light regulatory chains, the profile made from 5CPV detects all sequences of these proteins. The Z score of photoproteins and of SCBP were rather small in this case. Photoproteins had lower score than all other Ca^{2+}-binding proteins except SCBP, when profiles were calculated from 1CLL, 5CPV, 5TNC. Another distribution of Ca^{2+}-binding proteins in top-scoring list is obtained when 2SCP was used to calculate the profile. The photoproteins Z scores are higher than those obtained with other profiles (Table 2), and photoproteins are situated in the upper part of the top-scoring list before the majority of Ca^{2+}-binding proteins: third, fourth, 8th, and 74th for clytin, obelin, mitrocomin, and aequorin, respectively.

It is interesting that aequorin, which has the same sequence identity with calmodulin and troponin C as other photoproteins, has the lowest Z score among photoproteins if one compares the profiles of those proteins with aequorin sequence (Tables 1 and 2). According to the Z score aequorin has the most different 3D structure from the Ca^{2+}-binding proteins.

It is believed that proteins with a score of more than 6 share the fold of the profiled protein [16]. One can see that Z score of obelin, as well as of other photoproteins except aequorin are high enough to assume that their fold is similar to 2SCP, 1CLL, or 5TNC. The Z scores of photoproteins were the highest when 2SCP was used to calculate the profile. Thus, according to the profiles, 2SCP is the best template for modeling the photoproteins.

Information available about essential residues of photoproteins confirms this choice of template [7, 8, 9, 10, 11]. Apart from mutations of the Ca^{2+}-binding loops, five residues have been found in aequorin for which point mutations decreased the bioluminescence level by a factor of 100: His22, His64, His175, Trp179, and Pro195 (numeration of residues of all photoproteins is according to the obelin sequence as in Fig. 1.). If calmodulin or troponin C are used to model the 3D structure of photoproteins, the distance between His22 and His175 would be about 45A. Even in the bent form of calmodulin [29] (2BBM PDB code) these residues are far away from each other. When 2SCP was used as a template all residues were found near each other (see below). Besides, 2SCP is the only Ca^{2+}-binding protein with four putative Ca^{2+}-binding domains but with non-functional second domain like all known photoproteins. Therefore, the final model of the obelin 3D structure was built from 2SCP.

3.4 Model of obelin structure

Substitution of the amino acid sequence of 2SCP to that of obelin and a following energy minimization resulted in minor shift in the main-chain position of the protein: The root mean square deviation between 2SCP and the obelin model is 0.38A for 169 Ca atoms. The model obtained is a compact globule of volume $18740A^3$, which corresponds to a sphere of radius 16.5A. The accessible surface area is $10190A^2$. There are 128 hydrogen bonds (calculated by DSSP) and no buried charged residues inside the globule except three glutamates: E41, E134, and E170. All these glutamic acids are 12th residues in Ca^{2+}-binding loops; the side chain of these glutamates provide two oxygen ligands for calcium ions, and they are buried in the most EF-hand domains.

The overall 3D structure of the obelin model is shown in figure 2. The globule has a clear hydrophobic core but there is a cavity inside between His175, His 64, and His22. The cavity might be the coelenterazine binding site, because the volume of the cavity is about $800A^3$ which is enough to harbor the coelenterazine. Residues lining the cavity are mostly from helical regions, therefore even if loop conformations differ from the predicted structure it does not strongly affect the cavity. The region is very hydrophobic: 4 tryptophanes, 4 phenylalanines, 4 isoleucines, 2 valines, leucine, methionine, and alanine participate in the cavity formation. All residues of photoproteins for which mutation have been shown to be crucial for the bioluminescence either are included in Ca^{2+}-binding loops or participate in formation of this cavity.

It has been shown that the emitter of the bioluminescence is a phenolate anion [12]. There are some residues which might form a salt bridge with the phenolate of coelenterazine. The distance between His175 which has been proposed as oxygen-binding site and His64, which mutation changes the bioluminescence spectrum, is about 12-14A just expected for residues located near the oxygen-binding site and the phenolate binding residue. Alternatively, if coelenterazine is bound in a different way, Arg112 can be the phenolate-binding residue.

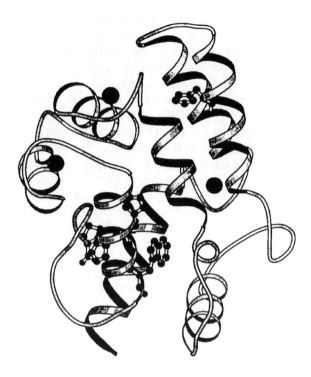

Figure 2: Schematic representation of the 3D model of obelin drawn by MOLSCRIPT [30]. Residues essential for the bioluminescence are shown in ball-and-sticks.

The existence and importance of disulfide bond in photoproteins has been discussed [31]. According to this model and to the alignment of known photoprotein sequences there are no cysteins which can form a disulfide bridge. It was suggested that Cys151 and Cys158 form a disulfide bond, however, and they are located in a helix (which means that their position is rather rigid) at a distance of more than 5A between their sulfides which therefore makes the formation of a disulfide impossible. Besides, Cys151 is not conserved: there is Ala at this position in clytin.

If we assume that the active site of photoproteins is located in this cavity then mutation of residues Met25, Leu29, Phe88, Arg112, Tyr190 might result in an essential decrease in the level of bioluminescence due to lower affinity for coelenterazine. All these residues are conserved among photoproteins. Besides the above mentioned, mutation of hydrophobic residues near to His175 (Phe71, Ile118, Phe119, Phe(Ile)122, Ile(Val)130, Cys158, Met171, Phe178)might result in lowering of the bioluminescence if the mutation decreases the size of the side chain (substitution by Ala) and might result in a shift of the bioluminescence wavelength for the aromatic residues, if they form a stacking interaction with coelenterazine.

Acknowledgements

I wish to thank Dr. Ylva Lindqvist for numerous helpful discussions. The work was supported by a stipend from the Swedish University of Agricultural Science which is gratefully acknowledged.

References

[1] M. J. Sormier, D. C. Prasher, M. Longiaru and R. O. McCann, *Photochem. Photobiol.*, 4, p. 509-512, 1989.

[2] S. Inouye, M. Noguchi, Y. Sakaki, Y. Takagi, T. Miyata, S. Iwanaga and F. I. Tsuji, *Proc. Natl. Acad. Sci. USA*, 82, p. 3154-3158, 1985.

[3] D. C. Prasher, R. O. McCann, M. Longiaru, and M. J. Cormier, *Biochemistry*, 26, p. 1326-1332, 1987.

[4] S. Inouye and F. I. Tsuji, *FEBS Letters*, 315, p. 343-346, 1993.

[5] T. F. Fagan, Y. Ohmiya, J. R. Blinks, S. Inouye and F. I. Tsuji, *FEBS Letters*, 333, p. 301-305, 1994.

[6] B. A. Illarionov and V. Illarionova, V. S. Bondar and E. S. Vysotski, *Gene*, in press.

[7] Y. Ohmiya and F. I. Tsuji, *FEBS Letters*, 320, p. 267-270, 1993.

[8] F. I. Tsuji, S. Inouye, T. Goto and Y. Sakaki, *Proc. Natl. Acad. Sci. USA*, 83, p. 8107-8111, 1986.

[9] Y. Ohmiya, M. Ohashi and F. I. Tsuji, *FEBS Letters*, 301, p. 197-201, 1992.

[10] J. M. Kendall, G. Sala-Newby, V. Ghalaut, R. L. Dormer and A. K. Campbell, *Biochem. Biophys. Res. Commun.*, 187, p. 1091-1097, 1992.

[11] K. Kurose, S. Inouye, Y. Sakaki and F. I. Tsuji, *Proc. Natl. Acad. Sci. USA*, 86, p. 80-84, 1989.

[12] T. Hirano, I. Mizoguchi and M. Yamaguchi, *J. Chem. Soc.*, 2, p. 165-168, 1994.

[13] L. I. Hannick, D. C. Prasher and L. W. Schultz, *Proteins*, 15, p. 103-107, 1993.

[14] S. Rost and C. Sander, *J. Mol. Biol.*, 232, p. 584-589, 1993.

[15] D. G. Higgins, A. J. Bleasby and R. Fuchs, *Comp. App. in Biosci.*, 8, p. 189-191, 1992.

[16] J. Bowie, R. Luthi and D. Eisenberg, *Science*, 253, p. 164-170, 1991.

[17] F. C. Bernstein, T. F. Koetzle, G. Williams, D. J. Meyer, M. D. Brice, J. R. Rodgers, O. Kennard, T. Shimanouchi and M. Tasumi, *J. Mol. Biol.*, 112, p. 535-542, 1977.

[18] R. Shattopadhyaya, W. E. Meador, A. R. Means and F. A. Quiocho, *J. Mol. Biol.*, 228, p. 1177-1192, 1992.

[19] O. Herzberg and M. N. G. James, *J. Mol. Biol.*, 203, p. 761-779, 1988.

[20] A. L. Swain, R. H. Kretsinger and E. L. Amma, *J. Biol. Chem.* 264, p. 16620-16628, 1989.

[21] S. Vijay-Kumar and W. J. Cook, *J. Mol. Biol.*, 229, p. 461-471, 1993.

[22] T. A. Jones, Y. Zou and S. W. Cowan, *Acta Crystallogr.*, A47, p. 110-119, 1991.

[23] A. T. Bruenger, A. Krukowski and J. Erickson, *Acta Crystallogr.*, A46, p. 585-593, 1989.

[24] R. A. Laskovski, D. S. Moss and J. M. Thornton, *J. Mol. Biol.*, 231, p. 1049-1067, 1993.

[25] W. Kabsch and C. Sander, *Biopolymers*, 22, p. 2577-2637, 1984.

[26] G. T. Kleywegt and A. Jones, *Acta Crystallogr.*, D50, p. 178-185, 1994.

[27] R. H. Kretsinger and C. E. Nickolds, *J. Biol. Chem.*, 248, p. 3313-3326, 1973.

[28] N. C. J. Strynadka and M. N. G. James, *Annu. Rev. Biochem.*, 58, p. 951-998, 1989.

[29] M. Ikura, G. M. Clore, A. M. Gronenborn, G. Zhu and C. B. Klee, *Science*, 256, p. 632-640, 1992.

[30] P. Kraulis, *J. Appl. Crystallogr.*, 24, p. 946-950, 1991.

[31] Y. Ohmiya, S. Kurono, M. Ohashi, T. F. Fagan and F. I. Tsuji, *FEBS Letters*, 332, p. 226-228, 1993.

Index